INJECTION TECHNIQUES
IN MUSCULOSKELETAL MEDICINE
A PRACTICAL MANUAL FOR CLINICIANS IN PRIMARY AND SECONDARY CARE

Log on to:

www.injectiontechniquesonline.com

- your virtual trainer on the top most common injection techniques by body region
- >50 video clips
- animations & self-testing

INJECTION TECHNIQUES
IN MUSCULOSKELETAL MEDICINE

A PRACTICAL MANUAL FOR CLINICIANS IN PRIMARY AND SECONDARY CARE

FIFTH EDITION

Stephanie Saunders, FCSP, FSOM

Founder and Director, Orthopaedic Medicine Seminars, London, England

Steve Longworth, MB, ChB, MSc (Sport and Ex Med), FRCGP, FRACGP, DM-SMed DPCR, FSOM

General Practitioner, CY O'Connor Village Medical Centre, Piara Waters, Perth, Western Australia

Foreword by Jonathan Botting, FRCGP

ELSEVIER

EDINBURGH LONDON NEW YORK OXFORD PHILADELPHIA ST LOUIS SYDNEY TORONTO 2019

ELSEVIER

First edition 1997
Second edition 2002
Third edition 2006
    Reprinted 2007, 2008, 2009
Fourth edition 2012
Fifth edition 2019

ISBN 978-0-7020-6957-4

Notices

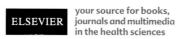

ELSEVIER your source for books, journals and multimedia in the health sciences
www.elsevierhealth.com

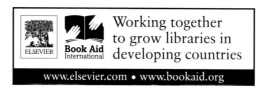

Working together to grow libraries in developing countries

www.elsevier.com • www.bookaid.org

The publisher's policy is to use paper manufactured from sustainable forests

Printed in China
Last digit is the print number: 9   8   7   6   5

For Elsevier
Content Strategists: Poppy Garraway Smith and Serena Castelnovo
Content Development Specialist: Katie Golsby
Project Manager: Joanna Souch
Designer: Miles Hitchen
Illustration Manager: Nichole Beard
Illustrator: Graphic World

Contents

Dedication

To Alan – with my thanks for his quiet patience during the writing of this edition (despite having no idea what it was about), and to my family for their amused tolerance.

SS

To Stephanie, who taught me such a lot, and to my patients, who taught me even more.

SL

Acknowledgements

Thanks to the supportive team at Elsevier and to Ryan Probyn for baring his body for the photos.

Foreword

Stephanie Saunders helped me transform the care I give my patients; her teaching continues to influence my everyday practice as a GP. We met on her Orthopaedic Medicine course; I was a GP outnumbered by physiotherapists. Outnumbered and out of my depth. Through her expert teaching I have progressed from pupil to practitioner to teacher.

What she and Steve Longworth (a GP and musculo-skeletal expert) bring to this book is their clarity and depth of thought combined with a forensically detailed approach to diagnosis and treatment. This is delivered in very easy to follow steps, laid out with great clarity which makes the book both an effortless and intuitive source of reference.

Stephanie's Orthopaedic Medicine course exposed my own inadequate level of musculoskeletal knowledge gained in training as a doctor. My experience as a GP and GP trainer has uncovered similar gaps in knowledge in many of the doctors I meet.

This book should be considered a core reference in every GP practice, and every physiotherapy, rheumatology and orthopaedic department. It should also be considered an essential read for every trainee in those specialties.

The opening chapters succinctly and clearly provide detailed references for evidence based joint injection practice. Next the reader is introduced to a logical, chapter structure based on anatomical location, each encompassing how to diagnose specific conditions and how to treat them.

For physiotherapists extending their practice to incorporate injection therapy this book is invaluable. For rheumatology and orthopaedic departments this book provides an excellent guide to assessing and injecting patients without the need for imaging. For GPs and for doctors in training the book does all of the above, and in addition it introduces them to a range of conditions not covered in most generic medical training.

Almost 30 years in GP practice has taught me how often colleagues and trainees fit their patients and their symptoms to conditions that they are familiar with. This book will not only give clinicians the skill to diagnose and treat more with confidence but also to know when not to treat.

In writing this foreword I have come to realise that in our on-line world where every fact is available at the touch of a button I have but three reference books that never gather dust in my clinic. One is a photographic atlas of anatomy (now sadly out of print), the second is the British National Formulary (on-line but better in print) and the third is my copy of *Injection Techniques in Musculoskeletal Medicine*. It is the last of these that deserves the title of vade mecum.

Jonathan Botting, FRCGP
London
2018

Preface

I have always found the process of diagnosis fascinating. It is somewhat like doing a complicated crossword puzzle, where one is given faint clues and hints. These may or may not assist in helping one to process waves of superfluous information in order to arrive, hopefully, at a final answer – the all-important diagnosis.

For me, this is always the most challenging and rewarding part of clinical practice. Choice of treatment tends to be dictated by the diagnosis and the clinician's skills, so is slightly less challenging but, for successful injections, correct diagnosis is the key, together with an intimate knowledge of anatomy. The actual process of giving the injection is simple.

For this reason, we have added a section on diagnosis in this edition, which is based on many years of experience in treating musculoskeletal conditions. This experience not only taught us much about human behaviour, but also enabled us to teach a method of diagnostic reasoning to clinicians attending our injection therapy courses. We hope it will also aid you.

For new readers, the purpose of this text is to provide a clear practical manual on the basic principles of injection therapy, which can be easily used in primary care and outpatient settings. It is not intended to be an academic text with detailed discussion of alternatives to injection therapy, of which there are many, so further reading is recommended.

In this edition, we have added more diagnostic guides, simplified some of the instructions, re-shot the examination process, included boxed Practical Points and updated references, which were current when we went to print in 2018.

This is the fifth edition of our textbook, and we are grateful for the success of previous editions. My final thank you is, as before, to the many wonderful patients I was fortunate enough to encounter, to the questioning students who kept me on my toes and, of course, to my co-author Steve Longworth, whose enthusiasm for the subject has never waned – despite his emigration to Australia!

Stephanie Saunders, FCSP, FSOM
Richmond, England
2018

About the Authors

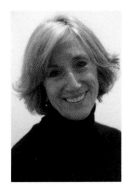

Stephanie Saunders, FCSP, FSOM, trained at St Thomas' Hospital, London, and joined the Orthopaedic Medicine team there, headed by Dr James Cyriax. He became her mentor and, in 1977, invited her to lead a teaching group on a lecture tour in Atlanta, Georgia. This led to many years of teaching courses in orthopaedic medicine in the United Kingdom, United States, Canada, Australia, South Africa and several European countries, in between running a busy private practice in London.

She was the founding Vice-Chairman of the Society of Orthopaedic Medicine (SOM) and, as Director of Teacher Training, instructed many clinicians in how to teach these courses. She was also founding chair and journal editor for the Association of Chartered Physiotherapists in Orthopaedic Medicine. In 1995, she designed and led the first injection therapy course for chartered physiotherapists in the United Kingdom and has continued to promote this skill in connection with the Chartered Society of Physiotherapy (CSP) and the Department of Health. Fellowship of the CSP was awarded for her work in achieving injection rights for allied health professionals in the UK.

As well as being the keynote speaker at several international meetings worldwide, she has published many papers and clinical guidelines. Her textbook, originally entitled *Injection Techniques in Orthopaedic Medicine*, now entitled *Injection Techniques in Musculoskeletal Medicine*, was first published in 1997 and is now in its fifth edition. On her recent retirement, she is even busier with family, friends and travelling with her new husband.

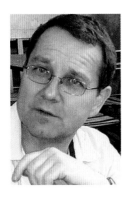

Dr. Stephen Longworth, MSc (Sport and Exercise Medicine), FRCGP, FRACGP, DM-SMed, DPCR, FSOM – graduated from the University of Manchester in the United Kingdom in 1981 and was a full-time general practitioner (GP) in Leicester for 30 years before moving to Western Australia, where he has worked as a GP since 2015.

For 15 years, he also worked as a Specialist Doctor in the Orthopaedic Spine Clinic at Leicester General Hospital for one session per week, having previously worked there in the Shoulder Clinic. He was the first General Practitioner with Special Interest in Musculoskeletal Medicine in Leicester and, for several years, was a musculoskeletal mentor to a number of other GP practices in Leicester.

He has a Master's degree in Sport and Exercise Medicine and diplomas in Musculoskeletal Medicine and Primary Care Rheumatology. He is a past president of the Primary Care Rheumatology Society and was a tutor and examiner for the Diploma in Primary Care Rheumatology at the University of Bath. He was a GP Trainer, appraiser and undergraduate tutor and has served on more committees and boards than he cares to remember. He was a Visiting Professor in the Department of Clinical Skills at St. George's University Medical School, Grenada, West Indies, in the Caribbean.

SECTION 1

INJECTION THERAPY – THE EVIDENCE

CHAPTER 1: THE EVIDENCE BASE FOR INJECTION THERAPY

OVERVIEW

Injection therapy is the treatment of musculoskeletal disorders by the targeted injection of drugs into joints and soft tissues. Corticosteroid (CS) and local anaesthetic (LA) injection therapy has been in use for almost 70 years and has stood the test of time.[1] There is a wealth of anecdotal evidence for its efficacy, but few, if any, definitive studies[1-5] and few studies comparing injection therapy with other treatments; the comparative studies that do exist mainly concern the shoulder and elbow, and their conclusions are contradictory.[6-20] Consequently, there are few facts and a mass of opinions – many of them dogmatic and contradictory – about almost every aspect of injection therapy.[21-24] Published guidelines for joint and soft tissue injections are based more on personal experience and anecdote than on evidence.[1-4] This state of affairs is surprising because injection therapy is the most common therapeutic intervention in rheumatological practice.[25]

Interpretation of injection therapy studies is compounded by a disconcerting lack of expert agreement about definitions, diagnosis and outcome measures in musculoskeletal medicine,[1,26-31] coupled with wide variations in methodology and quality between trials. Because of this, most authoritative reviews tend to be conservative in their estimates of the presence and size of treatment effects in injection therapy.[3,5,32-43]

Nonetheless, injection therapy is recommended for musculoskeletal (mainly knee and shoulder) disorders in national and international guidelines[3,44-48] and is used extensively for other musculoskeletal conditions.[49,50] Given its relative safety,[1,3,5,51-53] ease of application in trained hands and cost-effectiveness,[3] plus the frequent lack of convincing systematic evidence for the effectiveness of alternatives,[38] injection therapy is a very useful treatment modality.[54] This is supported by the collective experience of most clinicians in primary care and the locomotor specialties.[55]

Remarkably, there are hardly any double-blind randomized controlled trials of intraarticular versus systemic CS injection therapy for the treatment of any inflammatory arthropathies.

The superior clinical efficacy of joint injection therapy has been reported in two trials comparing intraarticular injections with the systemic injection of the same total dosage of triamcinolone in the treatment of rheumatoid arthritis. In the first randomized study, patients with polyarticular disease who were treated with intraarticular injections of triamcinolone demonstrated significantly better pain control and range of motion than those who were treated with the same total dosage of minipulse systemic steroids. Patient evaluation of disease activity, tender joint count, blood pressure, side effects, physician contacts and hospital visits were significantly better for those treated with intraarticular steroids.[56]

The second study compared the efficacy and safety of intraarticular CS injection with the systemic injection of the same dose of triamcinolone for the treatment of monoarthritis of the knee in rheumatoid arthritis patients. The intraarticular approach showed better results in terms of local inflammatory variables and improvement evaluation by the patient and physician.[57]

However, in both studies, the systemic treatment was given with triamcinolone acetonide, whereas the joints were injected with the far less soluble and longer acting triamcinolone hexacetonide. It could be argued that what these studies demonstrate is the superiority of the hexacetonide formulation of triamcinolone, rather than the route of administration.

The definitive randomized trial to demonstrate the superiority of the intraarticular route of CS administration in those with inflammatory joint disease is still awaited. Nonetheless, authoritative international guidelines have recommended that intraarticular CS injections should be considered for the relief of local symptoms in patients with inflammatory arthritis.[58]

As with other treatment modalities, the challenge for all clinicians delivering injection therapy is to implement evidence-based practice by applying the best research-based treatments, tempered by clinical experience and patients' values.[59] Where good research evidence is lacking, clinicians should become involved in research that will provide that evidence.

Problems with injection therapy may arise when the following occurs.

- An inappropriate drug is chosen.
- Too large a dose or volume is given.
- The drug is put into the wrong tissue.
- Poor technique allows the spread of drugs to adjacent tissue.
- Injections are given too frequently.
- Insufficient attention is directed to the cause of the lesion.
- No regard is given to aftercare and rehabilitation.

The art of good injection therapy is to select the appropriate patient and place the minimal effective amount of an appropriate drug into the exact site of the affected tissue at an appropriate time. This means that the clinician using injection therapy must possess a high level of diagnostic and technical skill.

DELIVERY OF INJECTION THERAPY

Doctors in rheumatology, orthopaedics, musculoskeletal medicine, sports medicine, pain management and interventional radiology are the main medical specialists who deliver injection therapy. Most general practitioners (GPs) in the United Kingdom carry out some joint and soft tissue injections, but limit themselves to knees, shoulders and elbows.[60] A small, highly active group receives referrals from colleagues.[60,61] Most of the injections in the community are performed by just 5 to 15% of GPs.[61,62] The main perceived barriers to performing these injections are inadequate training, the inability to maintain injection skills and discomfort or lack of confidence with the performance of the technique.[60-62] Training improves GPs' injection activity and their level of confidence.[63]

In 1995, chartered physiotherapists in the United Kingdom were granted the right to use injection therapy, whereupon we developed the first training programme in this field and were lead contributors to the first published injection therapy guidelines.[64] Guidelines for GPs have since been developed by the Primary Care Rheumatology Society and can be seen at www.pcrsociety.org/resources/other/joint-injections-guidelines.

Injections administered by physiotherapists have been shown to be part of a very effective way of managing orthopaedic[65] and rheumatology[66] outpatients and patients in the community with musculoskeletal lesions.[67] Extended-scope practitioners in physiotherapy have been shown to be as effective as orthopaedic surgeons and to generate lower initial direct hospital costs.[68]

Podiatrists also deliver injection therapy for lower limb disorders, and nurses have also been trained in musculoskeletal injection therapy.[69,70]

CURRENT CONTROVERSIES IN INJECTION THERAPY

Almost every aspect of injection therapy is nonstandardized. Notwithstanding controversies about diagnosis, there is no universal agreement about the following questions.

- What are we treating? What is the pathological or biochemical abnormality responsible for the pain?
- Are we always treating inflammation or is the CS and/or LA doing something else, such as modifying the action of nociceptors?
- Are there subgroups of potential injection responders within broad diagnostic categories, such as shoulder pain or back pain and, if so, how can we identify them?
- Which options – which specific CS and LA, dosage, volume, injection technique, venue, aftercare, co-intervention and/or rehabilitation – should we advocate?
- When is the optimal time to inject during any disorder?
- Should injections be repeated? If so, at what intervals, and how often?
- Who should be followed up? At what intervals, and for how long?
- How much benefit is attributable to the placebo, the acupuncture or the fluid volume effect rather than any specific pharmacological effect?
- What is the role of other injectable drugs in addition to CS and LA? (see Chapter 3)
- Is injected saline an analgesic? This may influence the interpretation of trials in which saline was used as an (assumed) inactive control.[71,72]
- How useful is imaging control? (see Chapter 4)
- Is a targeted injection more effective than a nonspecific systemic one?[73-75]
- How much do patients' expectations and preferences affect the outcome?[76]
- How much mythology is there about injection therapy, and how can we correct it?

THE RESEARCH AGENDA IN INJECTION THERAPY

Given the large number of questions listed above, we might reflect on why, after 7 decades, there is such a dearth of first-rate evidence for a therapeutic approach that is so well established and widely used (a problem common to many areas of practice in the locomotor specialties[77]). Certainly, the research agenda should seek to address the points raised, but why are published studies in the recent medical literature concerning injection therapy with CS and LA so relatively sparse? It may be that to some, the benefits are so well established and self-evident that further research is unnecessary (we would vigorously disagree).

Certainly, newer agents (see Chapter 3) may attract more interest because of their novelty value and (often unfulfilled) theoretical potential.[78] Perhaps research into novel treatments is generously funded by manufacturers, with the potential for partial reporting of results, whereas research into inexpensive and familiar treatments attracts little or no support from industry and academia. There are undoubtedly other reasons.

Recommendations for future research abound in the papers cited in this text, which are far too numerous to mention here. A particular issue is that double-blind randomized controlled studies comparing CS injection therapy with a placebo or another treatment all test a single injection (or initial cluster of injections) at the outset with the comparator. However, in real life, most clinicians empirically use repeated injections, but the strategy of repeating the injection as required has never been explicitly tested for efficacy, safety and cost-effectiveness in a prospective trial.

One suggestion we fully endorse is that those systematically reviewing and meta-analysing the musculoskeletal literature should provide model research protocols, methodologies and frameworks. These could be taken off the shelf and used by anyone sufficiently enthused to participate in injection therapy research.

In the previous edition of this text, we noted that 2010 was the 350th anniversary of that bastion of scientific enquiry, the Royal Society. Anyone who aspires to best evidence-based practice should bear in mind the society's motto: *nulius in verba* (take nobody's word for it).

We would like to take this opportunity to mention Buxton's Law. "It is always too early for rigorous evaluation, until, unfortunately, it is suddenly too late."[79]

APPROACH TO PATIENTS WITH MUSCULOSKELETAL DISORDERS

OPTIONS AND SHARED DECISION MAKING

Anyone who has spent any time researching the evidence base for the treatment of nonsystemic musculoskeletal disorders will have been dismayed by the startling paucity and poor quality of evidence for interventions, be they physical, pharmacological or surgical.[78] What little evidence there is to be found is often contradictory (see Key References in Sections 3, 4 and 5). Given our professional obligation to evidence-based practice, how should we approach our patients?

A common misunderstanding of evidence-based medicine (EBM) is that it makes us slaves to the published research,[80] implying that if the evidence does not support our treatment modalities, we should simply shrug our shoulders, smile apologetically and send the patient away, possibly into the hands of those who are not so rigorous about applying the evidence.

The current definition of EBM is the conscientious, explicit and judicious use of current best evidence in making decisions about the care of individual patients. The practice of EBM means integrating individual clinical expertise with the best available external clinical evidence from systematic research. By individual clinical expertise, we mean the proficiency and judgment that individual clinicians acquire through clinical experience and clinical practice. Increased expertise is reflected in many ways, but especially in more effective and efficient diagnosis and in the more thoughtful identification and compassionate use of individual patients' predicaments, rights and preferences in making clinical decisions about their care. By best available external clinical evidence, we mean clinically relevant research.[81] To put it briefly, EBM integrates clinical experience and patients' values with the best available research information.

When taking into account our own expertise and experience, we have to be honest with ourselves – we are all prone to confirmation bias – and honest with our patients. It is important to find out the patient's perspective on his or her problem and discover how bothersome the problem is and their preferences.[82]

According to the UK National Institute for Health and Care Excellence, shared decision making starts with a conversation between the person receiving care and the person delivering care (nice.org.uk).

When discussing treatment options, the following should be addressed.

- Be frank about the current state of knowledge.
- Explain, where appropriate, that we are uncertain about the best treatment.
- When there are options; explain the pros and cons.
- Support the discussion with good-quality written information (e.g., as found on websites such Patient.co.uk or NHS Choices at www.nhs.uk) or specific patient decision aids.

For many musculoskeletal conditions, options include the following.

1. Wait and see
2. Painkillers (oral, topical)
3. Devices (e.g., clasps, orthotics)
4. Physical therapy
5. Injection therapy
6. Surgery
7. Combinations and sequences of treatments that may be individually negotiated with the patient

The patient retains the right to choose not to choose and to defer to the clinician; in this case, in the absence of a clear-cut best choice, it may be judicious to start with the most conservative therapy and arrange a review.

Patients who are allowed to express their preferences and are involved in choosing therapy may have better outcomes than those who are not.[12] There are potential obstacles to this collaborative approach, but they are not insurmountable.[83] Mind sets and social context affect every medical encounter and we should be "mindful of mind sets."[84,85]

As an example, consider the treatment of tennis elbow. The evidence for treatment in primary care is summarized in Fig. 1.1. The different-coloured lines represent different treatments in a number of comparative studies. In the

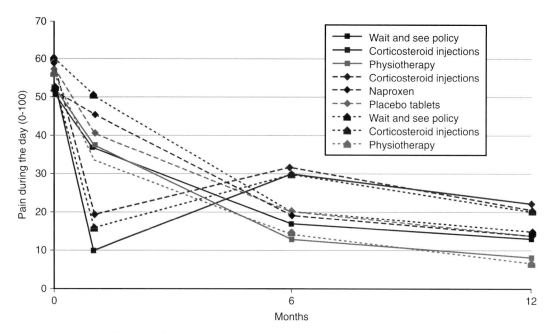

Fig. 1.1 Treatment of tennis elbow. From Smidt N, van der Windt DA. Tennis elbow in primary care. *BMJ*. 2006;333:927-928.

short term, injection therapy clearly gives the best results, but in the longer run is less effective than the alternatives, although after injection the pain is still significantly better than at the outset.

- Does the patient value a short-term result over a longer term one?
- Can she or he commit to a rehabilitation programme?
- Is such a programme available in a reasonable time frame?
- What happens if the injection is repeated at the point that the lines on the graph cross over? (The evidence base is silent on this issue.)

There are many other considerations. The skilful blending of clinical wisdom with the patient's values, especially when the research evidence is lacking or contradictory, offers a route to the best available outcome.

REFERENCES

1. Ines LPBS, da Silva JAP. Soft tissue injections. *Best Pract Res Clin Rheumatol.* 2005;19(3):503–527.
2. Peterson C, Holder J. Evidence-based radiology (part 2): is there sufficient research to support the use of therapeutic injections into the peripheral joints? *Skeletal Radiol.* 2010;39(1):11–18.
3. National Institute for Health and Care Excellence. Osteoarthritis: care and management clinical guideline. https://www.nice.org.uk/Guidance/CG177.
4. Speed CA. Injection therapies for soft-tissue lesions. *Best Pract Res Clin Rheumatol.* 2007;21(2):333–347.

5. Cole BJ, Schumacher HR Jr. Injectable corticosteroids in modern practice. *J Am Acad Orthop Surg.* 2005;13(1):37–46.
6. Skedros JG, Hunt KJ, Pitts TC. Variations in corticosteroid/anaesthetic injections for painful shoulder conditions: comparisons among orthopaedic surgeons, rheumatologists, and physical medicine and primary-care physicians. *BMC Musculoskelet Disord.* 2007;8:63.
7. Gaujoux-Viala C, Dougados M, Gossec L. Efficacy and safety of steroid injections for shoulder and elbow tendonitis: a meta-analysis of randomised controlled trials. *Ann Rheum Dis.* 2009;68(12):1843–1849.
8. Crashaw DP, Helliwell PS, Hensor EMA, et al. Exercise therapy after corticosteroid injection for moderate to severe shoulder pain: large pragmatic randomised trial. *BMJ.* 2010;340:c3037.
9. Karthikeyan S, Kwong HT, Upadhyay PK, et al. A double-blind randomized controlled study comparing subacromial injection of tenoxicam or methylprednisolone in patients with subacromial impingement. *J Bone Joint Surg Br.* 2010;92(1):77–82.
10. Ryans I, Montgomery A, Galway R, et al. A randomized controlled trial of intra-articular triamcinolone and/or physiotherapy in shoulder capsulitis. *Rheumatology.* 2005;44(4):529–535.
11. Hay EM, Thomas E, Paterson SM, et al. A pragmatic randomised controlled trial of local corticosteroid injection and physiotherapy for the treatment of new episodes of unilateral shoulder pain in primary care. *Ann Rheum Dis.* 2003;62:394–399.
12. van der Windt DAWM, Bouter LM. Physiotherapy or corticosteroid injection for shoulder pain? *Ann Rheum Dis.* 2003;62:385–387.
13. Carette S, Moffet H, Tardif J, et al. Intraarticular corticosteroids, supervised physiotherapy, or a combination of the two in the treatment of adhesive capsulitis of the shoulder: a placebo-controlled trial. *Arthritis Rheum.* 2003;48:829–838.
14. Winters JC, Jorritsma W, Groenier KH, et al. Treatment of shoulder complaints in general practice: long-term results of a randomised, single blind study comparing physiotherapy, manipulation, and corticosteroid injection. *BMJ.* 1999;318:1395–1396.
15. van der Windt DAWM, Koes BW, Deville W, et al. Effectiveness of corticosteroid injections versus physiotherapy for treatment of painful stiff shoulder in primary care: randomised trial. *BMJ.* 1998;317:1292–1296.
16. Winters JC, Sobel JS, Groenier KH, et al. Comparison of physiotherapy manipulation and corticosteroid injection for treating shoulder complaints in general practice: randomised single blind study. *BMJ.* 1997;314:1320–1325.
17. Tonks JH, Pai SK, Murali SR. Steroid injection therapy is the best conservative treatment for lateral epicondylitis: a prospective randomised controlled trial. *Int J Clin Pract.* 2007;61(2):240–246.
18. Bisset L, Beller E, Jull G, et al. Mobilisation with movement and exercise, corticosteroid injection, or wait and see for tennis elbow: randomized trial. *BMJ.* 2006;333:939.
19. Hay EM, Paterson SM, Lewis M, et al. Pragmatic randomised controlled trial of local corticosteroid injection and naproxen for treatment of lateral epicondylitis of elbow in primary care. *BMJ.* 1999;319:964–968.

20. Verhaar JAN, Walenkamp GHIM, van Mameren H, et al. Local corticosteroid injection versus Cyriax type physiotherapy for tennis elbow. *J Bone Joint Surg Br*. 1995;77:128–132.
21. Charalambous CP, Tryfonidis M, Sadiq S, et al. Septic arthritis following intra-articular steroid injection of the knee – a survey of current practice regarding antiseptic technique used during intra-articular steroid injection of the knee. *Clin Rheumatol*. 2003;22:386–390.
22. Haslock I, Macfarlane D, Speed C. Intra-articular and soft tissue injections: a survey of current practice. *Br J Rheumatol*. 1995;34:449–452.
23. Cluff R, Mehio AK, Cohen SP, et al. The technical aspects of epidural steroid injections: a national survey. *Anesth Analg*. 2002;95:403–408.
24. Masi AT, Driessnack RP, Yunus MB, et al. Techniques for "blind" glucocorticosteroid injections into glenohumeral joints [letter]. *J Rheumatol*. 2007;34(5):1201–1202.
25. Bamji AM, Dieppe PA, Haslock DI, et al. What do rheumatologists do? A pilot audit study. *Br J Rheumatol*. 1990;29:295–298.
26. Kassimos G, Panayi G, van der Windt DAWM. Differences in the management of shoulder pain between primary and secondary care in Europe: time for a consensus. *Ann Rheum Dis*. 2004;63:111–112.
27. Hoving JL, Buchbinder R, Green S, et al. How reliably do rheumatologists measure shoulder movement? *Ann Rheum Dis*. 2002;7:612–616.
28. Nørregaard J, Krogsgaard MR, Lorenzen T, et al. Diagnosing patients with long-standing shoulder joint pain. *Ann Rheum Dis*. 2002;61:646–649.
29. Carette S. Adhesive Capsulitis – research advances frozen in time? *J Rheumatol*. 2000;27:1329–1331.
30. Marx RG, Bombardier C, Wright JG. What do we know about the reliability and validity of physical examination tests used to examine the upper extremity? *J Hand Surg Am*. 1999;24A:185–193.
31. Bamji AN, Erhardt CC, Price TR, et al. The painful shoulder: can consultants agree? *Br J Rheumatol*. 1996;35:1172–1174.
32. Gaujoux-Viala C, Dougados M, Gossec L. Efficacy and safety of steroid injections for shoulder and elbow tendonitis: a meta-analysis of randomised controlled trials. *Ann Rheum Dis*. 2009;68:1843–1849.
33. Dorrestijn O, Stevens M, Winters JC, et al. Conservative or surgical treatment for subacromial impingement syndrome: a systematic review. *J Shoulder Elbow Surg*. 2009;18(4):652–660.
34. Buchbinder R, Green S, Youd JM. Corticosteroid injections for shoulder pain. *Cochrane Database Syst Rev*. 2003;(1):CD004016.
35. Shah N, Lewis M. Shoulder adhesive capsulitis: systematic review of randomised trials using multiple corticosteroid injections. *Br J Gen Pract*. 2007;57:662–667.
36. Koester MC, Dunn WR, Kuhn JE, et al. The efficacy of subacromial corticosteroid injection in the treatment of rotator cuff disease: a systematic review. *J Am Acad Orthop Surg*. 2007;15(1):3–11.
37. Faber E, Kuiper JI, Burdorf A, et al. Treatment of impingement syndrome: a systematic review of the effects on functional limitations and return to work. *J Occup Rehabil*. 2006;16(1):7–25.
38. Assendelft W, Green S, Buchbinder R. Tennis elbow. *BMJ*. 2003;327:329.

39. Hepper CT, Halvorson JJ, Duncan ST. The efficacy and duration of intraarticular corticosteroid injection for knee osteoarthritis: a systematic review of Level I Studies. *J Am Acad Orthop Surg*. 2009;17(10):638–646.

40. Bellamy N, Campbell J, Welch V, et al. Intraarticular corticosteroid for treatment of osteoarthritis of the knee. *Cochrane Database Syst Rev*. 2006;(2):Art. No.: CD005328, doi:10.1002/14651858.CD005328.pub2. [Edited - no change to conclusions - published in Issue 2, 2009].

41. Godwin M Dawes. Intraarticular steroid injections for painful knees: systematic review with meta-analysis. *Can Fam Physician*. 2004;50:241–248.

42. Arroll B, Goodyear-Smith F. Corticosteroid injections for osteoarthritis of the knee: meta-analysis. *BMJ*. 2004;328:869–870.

43. Gossec L, Dougados M. Intraarticular treatments in osteoarthritis: from the symptomatic to the structure modifying. *Ann Rheum Dis*. 2004;63:478–482.

44. Geraets JJ, de Jongh AC, Boeke AJ, et al. Summary of the practice guideline for shoulder complaints from the Dutch College of General Practitioners. *Ned Tijdschr Geneeskd*. 2009;153:A164.

45. New Zealand Guidelines Group. Diagnosis and management of soft tissue shoulder injuries and related disorders. *Best Practice Evidence Based Guideline* 2004.

46. American College of Rheumatology subcommittee on osteoarthritis guidelines. Recommendations for the medical management of osteoarthritis of the hip and knee. *Arthritis Rheum*. 2000;43:1905–1915.

47. Jordan KM, Arden NK, Doherty M, et al. EULAR Recommendations 2003: an evidence-based approach to the management of knee osteoarthritis: report of a Task Force of the Standing Committee for International Clinical Studies Including Therapeutic Trials (ESCISIT). *Ann Rheum Dis*. 2003;62:1145–1155.

48. American Academy of Orthopaedic Surgeons. *Management of Carpal Tunnel Syndrome Evidence-Based Clinical Practice Guideline*. www.aaos.org/ctsguideline. Published February 29, 2016.

49. Creamer P. Intra-articular corticosteroid injections in osteoarthritis: do they work, and if so, how? *Ann Rheum Dis*. 1997;56:634–636.

50. Fanciullo GJ, Hanscom B, Seville J, et al. An observational study of the frequency and pattern of use of epidural steroid injection in 25,479 patients with spinal and radicular pain. *Reg Anesth Pain Med*. 2001;26(1):5–11.

51. Nichols AW. Complications associated with the use of corticosteroids in the treatment of athletic injuries. *Clin J Sport Med*. 2005;15(5):E370.

52. Kumar N, Newman R. Complications of intra- and peri-articular steroid injections. *Br J Gen Pract*. 1999;49:465–466.

53. Seror P, Pluvinage P, Lecoq d'Andre F, et al. Frequency of sepsis after local corticosteroid injection (an inquiry on 1160000 injections in rheumatological private practice in France). *Rheumatology* (Oxford). 1999;38:1272–1274.

54. Holden J, Wooff E. Is our evidence-based practice effective? Review of 435 steroid injections given by a general practitioner over eight years. *Clin Gov*. 2005;10(4):276–280.

55. Croft P. Admissible evidence. *Ann Rheum Dis*. 1998;57:387–389.

56. Furtado RN, Oliveira LM, Natour J. Polyarticular corticosteroid injection versus systemic administration in treatment of rheumatoid arthritis patients: a randomized controlled study. *J Rheumatol.* 2005;32(9):1691–1698.

57. Konai MS, Vilar Furtado RN, Dos Santos MF, et al. Monoarticular corticosteroid injection versus systemic administration in the treatment of rheumatoid arthritis patients: a randomized double-blind controlled study. *Clin Exp Rheumatol.* 2009;27(2):214–221.

58. Combe B, Landewe R, Daien CI, et al. 2016 update of the EULAR recommendations for the management of early arthritis. *Ann Rheum Dis.* 2017;76:948–959.

59. Haynes RB, Devereaux PJ, Guyatt GH. Physicians' and patients' choices in evidence-based practice. *BMJ.* 2002;324:1350.

60. Liddell WG, Carmichael CR, McHugh NJ. Joint and soft tissue injections: a survey of general practitioners. *Rheumatology* (Oxford). 2005;44(8):1043–1046.

61. Gormley GJ, Corrigan M, Steele WK, et al. Joint and soft tissue injections in the community: questionnaire survey of general practitioners' experiences and attitudes. *Ann Rheum Dis.* 2003;62:61–64.

62. Jolly M, Curran JJ. Underuse of intra-articular and periarticular corticosteroid injections by primary care physicians: discomfort with the technique. *J Clin Rheumatol.* 2003;9(3):187–192.

63. Gormley GJ, Steele WK, Stevenson M, et al. A randomised study of two training programmes for general practitioners in the techniques of shoulder injection. *Ann Rheum Dis.* 2003;62:1006–1009.

64. Chartered Society of Physiotherapy. *A Clinical Guideline for the Use of Injection Therapy by Physiotherapists.* London: ACPRC; 1999.

65. Weale A, Bannister GC. Who should see orthopaedic outpatients – physiotherapists or surgeons? *Ann R Coll Surg Engl.* 1995;77(suppl):71–73.

66. Dyce C, Biddle P, Hall K, et al. Evaluation of extended role of physio and occupational therapists in rheumatology practice. *Br J Rheumatol.* 1996;35(suppl 1):130.

67. Hattam P, Smeatham A. Evaluation of an orthopaedic screening service in primary care. *Clin Perform Qual Health Care.* 1999;7(3): 121–124.

68. Daker-White G, Carr AJ, Harvey I, et al. A randomised controlled trial – shifting boundaries of doctors and physiotherapists in orthopaedic outpatient departments. *J Epidemiol Community Health.* 1999;53:643–650.

69. Edwards J, Hannah B, Brailsford-Atkinson K, et al. Intra-articular and soft tissue injections: assessment of the service provided by nurses [letter]. *Ann Rheum Dis.* 2002;61:656–657.

70. Edwards J, Hassell A. Intraarticular and soft tissue injections by nurses: preparation for expanded practice. *Nurs Stand.* 2000;14(33): 43–46.

71. Yelland MJ, Glasziou PP, Bogduk N, et al. Prolotherapy injections, saline injections, and exercises for chronic low-back pain: a randomized trial. *Spine.* 2004;29(1):9–16.

72. Rosseland LA, Helgesen KG, Breivik H, et al. Moderate-to-severe pain after knee arthroscopy is relieved by intraarticular saline: a randomized controlled trial. *Anesth Analg.* 2004;98:1546–1551.
73. Koes BW. Corticosteroid injection for rotator cuff disease. *BMJ.* 2009;338:a2599.
74. Ekeberg OM, Bautz-Holter E, Tveita EK, et al. Subacromial ultrasound guided or systemic steroid injection for rotator cuff disease: randomised double-blind study. *BMJ.* 2009;338:a3112.
75. Ghahreman A, Ferch R, Bogduk N. The efficacy of transforaminal injection of steroids for the treatment of lumbar radicular pain. *Pain Med.* 2010;11(8):1149–1168.
76. van der Windt DAWM, Bouter LM. Physiotherapy or corticosteroid injection for shoulder pain? *Ann Rheum Dis.* 2003;62:385–387.
77. Lohmander LS, Roos EM. The evidence base for orthopaedics and sports medicine: scandalously poor in parts. *Br J Sports Med.* 2016;50(9):564–565.
78. Gerwin N, Hops C, Lucke A. Intraarticular drug delivery in osteoarthritis. *Adv Drug Deliv Rev.* 2006;58(2):226–242.
79. Buxton MJ. Problems in the economic appraisal of new health technology: the evaluation of heart transplants in the UK. In: Drummond MF, ed. *Economic Appraisal Of Health Technology in the European Community.* New York: Oxford University Press; 1987:103–118.
80. Greenhalgh T, Howick J, Maskrey N. Evidence based medicine; a movement in crisis? *BMJ.* 2014;348:g3725.
81. Sackett DL, Rosenberg WMC, Muir Gray JA, et al. Evidence-based medicine: what it is and what it isn't. *BMJ.* 1996;312:71–72.
82. Hoffmann TC, Legare F, Simmons MB, et al. Shared decision making: what do clinicians need to know and why should they bother? *Med J Aust.* 2014;201(1):35–39.
83. Joseph-Williams N, Lloyd A, Edwards A, et al. Implementing shared decision making in the NHS: lessons from the MAGIC programme. *BMJ.* 2017;357:1744.
84 Crum AJ, Leibowitz KA, Verghese A. Making mindset matter. *BMJ.* 2017;356:j674.
85 Mallows A, Debenham J, Walker T, et al. Association of psychological variables and outcomes in tendinopathy: a systematic review. *Br J Sports Med.* 2017;51:743–748.

CHAPTER 2: CORTICOSTEROIDS AND LOCAL ANAESTHETICS

CORTICOSTEROIDS

Corticosteroids were first administered systemically in 1948 by Philip Hench in the United States[1] and were hailed as the new universal panacea, but it soon became apparent that there were major side effects greatly limiting their systemic use.[2,3] In 1951, Hollander, in the United States, reported the first use of local hydrocortisone injections for arthritic joints.[4]

The commonly used injectable corticosteroids are synthetic analogues of the adrenal glucocorticoid hormone cortisol (hydrocortisone), which is secreted by the middle layer (zona fasciculata) of the adrenal cortex. Cortisol has many important actions, including antiinflammatory activity. Corticosteroids influence the cells involved in the immune and inflammatory responses primarily by modulating the transcription of a large number of genes. They act directly on nuclear steroid receptors to control the rate of synthesis of mRNA.[5] However, they also reduce the production of a wide range of proinflammatory mediators, including cytokines and other important enzymes.[2,3,6-8]

RATIONALE FOR USING CORTICO-STEROIDS

We know surprisingly little about the precise pharmacological effects of corticosteroids when they are injected directly into joints and soft tissues.[9-11] There are few injection-therapy studies comparing different doses of the same corticosteroid for the same condition, but those that have been performed suggest that lower doses may be as effective as higher ones.[12,13]

Local corticosteroid injections are thought to work by a number of mechanisms.

Suppressing inflammation

They suppress inflammation in inflammatory systemic diseases such as rheumatoid or psoriatic arthritis and gout.[3,6,14-17] Synovial cell infiltration and proinflammatory cytokine expression are reduced in a multifaceted manner by intraarticular corticosteroid injection.[6] The role of inflammation in tendinopathy is controversial and in recent years, mainstream opinion has asserted that the condition is purely degenerative. However, this view is being challenged because it has been found that increased numbers of specific inflammatory cells are present in pathological tendons, consistent with a chronic inflammatory process.[18-23]

Suppressing inflammatory flares

They appear to suppress inflammatory flares in degenerative joint disease.[5,16,24,25] However, the pathophysiology of osteoarthritis is poorly understood,[26] and there are no reliable clinical features that predict which osteoarthritic joints will respond to injection. Often, the only way to find out is with an empirical trial of injection therapy.[16,24]

Breaking up the inflammatory damage-repair-damage cycle

This is postulated to set up a continuous, low-grade, inflammatory response, inhibiting tissue repair and sound scar formation while forming adverse adhesions.[27,28] However, there is little direct evidence to support this.[10]

Protecting cartilage

There may be a direct chondroprotective effect on cartilage metabolism or other effects not related to the antiinflammatory activity of the steroids, such as promotion of articular surfactant production.[5,8,29-37]

Direct analgesic effect:

Inflammation is a complex cascade of molecular and cellular events.[38,39] The precise role of inflammation in tendinitis is the subject of considerable debate, and many authors prefer the terms *tendinosis* or *tendinopathy* to describe the pathological changes.[38,39] Tendon pain may not be caused by inflammation (tendinitis) or structural disruption of the tendon fibres (tendinosis), but might instead be caused by the stimulation of nociceptors by chemicals such as glutamate, substance P and chondroitin sulphate released from the damaged tendon.[40,41] Corticosteroids (and possibly local anaesthetics) may inhibit the release of noxious chemicals and/or the long-term behaviour of local nociceptors. In vitro, corticosteroids have also been shown to inhibit the transmission of pain along unmyelinated C fibres by a direct membrane action.[42]

Other effects

Intraarticular corticosteroid given over 3 months protects against periarticular bone loss in inflamed finger joints in rheumatoid arthritis.[43]

Note: The authors strongly advise that all clinicians thoroughly study the most up to date manufacturers' data sheets for the drugs that they propose to use for injection therapy and stay abreast of any subsequent modifications.

COMMONLY USED CORTICO-STEROIDS

The following are commonly used corticosteroids. The dosages and concentrations are shown in parentheses.

- **Triamcinolone acetonide**
  Adcortyl   (10 mg/ml, dilute)
  Kenalog   (40 mg/ml, concentrated)

Throughout this text, Kenalog is our reference drug, but we appreciate that other clinicians, for various reasons (e.g., being licensed to mix with local anaesthetics), prefer to use different corticosteroids. Dosage conversions may be made using the antiinflammatory equivalence (Box 1.1).

> **Box 1.1 Equivalent antiinflammatory doses of corticosteroids**
>
> Triamcinolone acetonide – 40 mg is equivalent to the following:
>
> - Triamcinolone hexacetonide, 20 mg
> - Methylprednisolone, 40 mg
> - Hydrocortisone, 200 mg
> - Betamethasone, 7.5 mg
> - Dexamethasone, 7.5 mg
> - Prednisolone, 50 mg

Kenalog can be used in very small quantities, so it is ideal for small joints and tendon entheses, in which distension may increase pain. Adcortyl, however, is useful when a larger volume is required, as in larger joints and bursae. The duration of action of the drug is approximately 2 to 3 weeks.[44,45]

● Triamcinolone hexacetonide
    Lederspan   (20 mg/ml, concentrated)

The least soluble and longest lasting injectable corticosteroid, Lederspan was unavailable in the United Kingdom from 2001 to 2013. It is licensed to be mixed with 1% or 2% lidocaine or other similar local anaesthetics. Pharmacokinetic studies have shown that the biological effect of triamcinolone acetonide is equivalent to that of triamcinolone hexacetonide if used at double the dosage, but even when triamcinolone acetonide is given at higher doses, triamcinolone hexacetonide has proven to be more effective, with a greater duration of action in head-to-head studies.[46-48] It is available in the United States as Aristospa

● Methylprednisolone acetate
    Depo-Medrone   (40 mg/ml, concentrated)

This drug may cause more postinjection pain than triamcinalone acetonide.[49] It is also available premixed with local anaesthetic as Depo-Medrone (40 mg/ml) with lidocaine (10 mg/ml) in 1- and 2 ml vials, which we do not use because it is a fixed-dose combination and therefore difficult to adjust.

● Betamethasone
    Celestone   (United States; betamethasone sodium phosphate,
    Soluspan   3 mg, and betamethasone acetate, 3 mg = 6 mg/ml,
                     concentrated)

The dose of Celestone Chronodose in Australia is slightly different. Celestone is licensed to be mixed (in the syringe, not the ampoule) with 1% or 2% lidocaine.

● Hydrocortisone
    Hydrocortistab   (25 mg/ml, very dilute)

This is very soluble and has the shortest duration of action of the corticosteroids mentioned here, perhaps as little as 6 days.[11] It may be particularly useful for superficial injections in thin, dark-skinned patients, in whom depigmentation or local fat atrophy may be more noticeable.

LOCAL ANAESTHETICS

These membrane-stabilizing drugs act by causing a reversible block to conduction along nerve fibres. The smaller nerve fibres are more sensitive, so that a differential block may occur where the small fibres carrying pain and autonomic impulses are blocked, sparing coarse touch and movement. Uptake into the systemic circulation is important for terminating their action and also for producing toxicity. Following most regional anaesthetic procedures, maximum arterial plasma concentrations of local anaesthetic develop within about 10 to 25 minutes, so careful surveillance for toxic effects is recommended for the first 30 minutes after injection if significant volumes are used.[50]

RATIONALE FOR USING LOCAL ANAESTHETICS

Analgesic

Although the effect is temporary, this may make the overall procedure less unpleasant for the patient, break the pain cycle (by reducing nociceptive input to the gate in the dorsal horn of the spinal cord) and increase the confidence of the patient in the clinician, the diagnosis and the treatment. In one study, pain inhibition was better with bupivacaine than lidocaine during the first 6 hours, presumably because of its longer half-life; in later evaluations, no differences in outcomes were observed.[51] In another study, bupivacaine was superior to lidocaine at 2 weeks, but not at 3 and 12 months.[52] Some practitioners inject a mixture of short- and long-acting local anaesthetic to obtain both the immediate diagnostic effect and more prolonged pain relief.

Diagnostic

The pain relief following an injection confirms the diagnosis and the correct placement of the solution.[10] Sometimes, even the most experienced practitioner will be unsure exactly which tissue is at fault; in this situation, a small amount of local anaesthetic may be injected into the most likely tissue and the patient re-examined after a few minutes. If the pain is relieved, then the source of the problem has been identified, and further treatment can be accurately directed.

Dilution

The internal surface area of joints and bursae is surprisingly large because of the highly convoluted synovial lining, with its many villae, so an increased volume of the injected solution helps spread the steroid around this surface.[10]

Distension

There is a beneficial volume effect in joints and bursae, which may be the physical stretching of the capsule or bursa with physical disruption of adhesions.[53-56] There is silver level evidence that arthrographic distension with saline and steroid provides short-term benefits in pain, range of movement and function in adhesive capsulitis of the shoulder.[57] Distension is not required at entheses, so the smallest practicable volume should be used; distension in tendons by the bolus injection of a relatively large volume of solution may physically disrupt the fibres, compress the relatively poor arterial supply and also give rise to distension pain.

COMMONLY USED LOCAL ANAESTHETICS

Local anaesthetics vary widely in their potency, duration of action and toxicity.[50] The most commonly used anaesthetics for joint and soft tissue injection are as follows.

● Lidocaine hydrochloride

This was previously lignocaine hydrochloride in the United Kingdom. It is the most widely used local anaesthetic, acts more rapidly and is more stable than others. The effects occur within seconds and the duration of block is about 30 minutes; this is the local anaesthetic recommended in this text.

● Marcaine (bupivacaine)

It has a slow onset of action (≈30 minutes for full effect), but the duration of block is up to 8 hours. It is the principal drug used for spinal anaesthesia in the United Kingdom.[50] We do not use it for routine outpatient injections because the delayed onset of action precludes the immediate diagnostic effect available with lidocaine and, if there is an adverse effect, this will take a long time to dissipate. There is no evidence of any long-term benefit from using bupivacaine instead of lidocaine.[52] Compared with placebo, the effect of intraarticular bupivacaine wears off in less than 24 hours.[58]

● Prilocaine

This has low toxicity, similar to that of lidocaine, but is not as commonly used. Procaine is now also seldom used. It is as potent as lidocaine but with a shorter duration of action.

Lidocaine (under the brand name Xylocaine) and Marcaine are also manufactured with added adrenaline, which causes vasoconstriction when used for skin anaesthesia, and so prolongs the local anaesthetic effect. These preparations are not recommended for procedures involving the appendages because of the risk of ischaemic necrosis.[9] Xylocaine with adrenaline added is clearly marked in red. We recommend that clinicians who administer injection therapy avoid these combination products altogether.

Recommended maximum doses are given in Table 1.1. In practice, however, we suggest that much lower maximum doses be used (see Chapter 6).

Table 1.1 Commonly used local anaesthetics with maximum doses

Drug	Strength	Maximum dose and volume	Suggested maximum
Lidocaine	0.5%, 5 mg/ml	200 mg, 40 ml	100 mg, 20 ml
	1.0%, 10 mg/ml	200 mg, 20 ml	100 mg, 10 ml
	2.0%, 20 mg/ml	200 mg, 10 ml	100 mg, 5 ml
Bupivacaine	0.25%, 2.5 mg/ml	150 mg, 60 ml	75 mg, 30 ml
	0.5%, 5 mg/ml	150 mg, 30 ml	75 mg,15 ml

Modified from British Medical Association and Royal Pharmaceutical Society. *British National Formulary No. 72*. London: British Medical Association and Royal Pharmaceutical Society; 2017:1181.

POTENTIAL SIDE EFFECTS

Side effects from injection therapy with corticosteroids and/or local anaesthetics are uncommon and, when they do occur, are usually mild and transient.[59-61] Nonetheless, it is incumbent on the clinician practicing injection therapy to be aware of the presentation and management of all the potential minor and more serious side effects associated with this treatment (Table 1.2).[62]

	Systemic side effects	Local side effects
Table 1.2 Potential side effects of locally injected corticosteroids	Facial flushing Impaired diabetic control Menstrual irregularity Hypothalamic-pituitary axis suppression Fall in erythrocyte sedimentation rate, C-reactive protein level Anaphylaxis (very rare)	Postinjection flare of pain Skin depigmentation Fat atrophy Bleeding, bruising Steroid chalk, calcification Steroid arthropathy Tendon rupture, atrophy Joint, soft tissue infection

Practice point: The wrong drug

Injection of the wrong drug is a potentially serious and totally avoidable problem, with severe consequences for all concerned.[63] Strict attention to the preparation protocol should prevent this (see Section 2). We always draw up our own injections and do not delegate this task.

Practice point: Pregnancy and breastfeeding

Consider carefully before giving corticosteroid injections to pregnant or breastfeeding women. This therapy has been recommended for carpal tunnel syndrome and De Quervain tendovaginitis in these patients,[64,65] but these conditions usually resolve following delivery. If used, a detailed discussion of the pros and cons of injection therapy should be carefully documented.

Practice point: Injecting a patient with a psychotic illness

Because systemic corticosteroids may precipitate or aggravate a psychotic episode in a patient with a psychotic illness, consider discussing this with the patient's psychiatrist before giving an injection.[66]

LOCAL SIDE EFFECTS

Local side effects may occur when an injection is misdirected or too large a dose in too large a volume is injected too often. Subcutaneous placement of the steroid and the injection of a drug bolus at entheses must both be avoided. Serious local side effects are rare.[59,67] Local side effects include the following.

Postinjection flare of pain

The quoted figures are from about 2 to 10%,[61,68] but this is well in excess of our own experience. When it does happen, it is usually after a soft tissue injection and rarely follows a joint injection.[61] When a corticosteroid is mixed with a local anaesthetic, the solution should be inspected carefully for flocculation or precipitation before injecting because this may be related to postinjection flare of pain.[11] It may also be caused by the rapid intracellular ingestion of the microcrystalline steroid ester and must always be distinguished from sepsis.[69] There may be more frequent postinjection flares with methylprednisolone, but this may have more to do with the preservative in the drug than with the corticosteroid itself.[70] An early increase in joint stiffness following intraarticular corticosteroids is consistent with a transient synovitis.[71]

Multidose bottles of lidocaine contain parabens as a preservative. Many steroids will precipitate when added to it, and this precipitate may be responsible for some cases of postinjection flare of pain and steroid chalk (see later). Parabens may also be responsible for some allergic reactions to local injections. The use of multidose bottles increases the risk of cross infection and must be avoided.[72] Single-dose vials of lidocaine do not contain parabens.

Subcutaneous atrophy and/or skin depigmentation[68,73]

In one meta-analysis of shoulder and elbow injections, skin modification had a frequency of 4%.[69] Skin changes may be more likely to occur when superficial lesions are injected, especially in dark-skinned patients. The injected drugs should not be allowed to reflux back through the needle tract; pressure applied around the needle with cotton wool when withdrawing may help. In thin dark-skinned patients especially, it may be preferable to use hydrocortisone for superficial lesions. These patients must always be advised of the possibility of this side effect, and this should be recorded. Local atrophy appears within 1 to 4 months after injection and characteristically proceeds to resolution 6 to 24 months later, but may take longer.[74] Fat atrophy following corticosteroid injection may rarely have significant functional consequences.[75,76]

Bleeding or bruising

This may occur at the injection site. Apply firm pressure to the injection site immediately following needle withdrawal. Joint and soft tissue injections and aspirations in selected patients taking stable doses of warfarin sodium are associated with a low risk of haemorrhage.[77-81] There is no need to stop this medication before injection therapy. There is little information to guide the clinician when considering injection therapy in patients taking an antiplatelet drug such as aspirin, dipyridamole or clopidogrel, an oral nonsteroidal antiinflammatory drug (NSAID) or a novel oral anticoagulant, nonvitamin K antagonist oral anticoagulant (NOAC). Unsurprisingly, there is a wide variation in practice when faced with this issue.[82]

Practice point: Patients on warfarin

In patents taking warfarin, make sure that the international normalized ratio (INR) is in the therapeutic range for the condition being treated and that the patient is not currently experiencing any unexplained bleeding or bruising.[83] The possibility of bleeding, bruising or haemarthrosis should be discussed and documented.

> **Practice point: Patients on antiplatelet drugs, oral NSAIDS and NOACs**
>
> Each case will need to be considered on its own merits. Make sure that the patient is not currently experiencing any unexplained bleeding or bruising. The possibility of bleeding, bruising and/or haemarthrosis should be discussed and documented. In our experience, there is no need to stop this medication before injection therapy, which is in keeping with advice from the manufacturers of the NOACs dabigatran and rivaroxaban. This states that "patients undergoing minor procedures may not require interruption of anticoagulation." NOACs have a shorter half-life than warfarin and consideration should be given to avoiding interventional procedures during peak drug activity. For example, for rivaroxaban this peak activity would be 2 to 4 hours after the last dose.

Steroid chalk or paste

This may be found on the surface of previously injected tendons and joints during surgery. Suspension flocculation, resulting from the mixture of steroid with a local anaesthetic containing preservative, may be responsible. The clinical significance of these deposits is uncertain.[84]

Soft tissue calcification

Periarticular calcification may be associated with large numbers of repeated injections into the small joints of the hand.[85] Corticosteroid injections into osteoarthritic interphalangeal joints of the hand may possibly result in calcification or joint fusion because of pericapsular leakage of steroids as a result of raised intraarticular pressure.[86] No deleterious effects have been ascribed to this calcification. Calcifications have been reported after intradiscal injection in the coccygeal region for coccydynia.[87]

Steroid arthropathy

This is a well-known and much feared complication of local injection treatment, but it is also largely a myth.[88] In many cases, injected steroid can be chondroprotective rather than destructive.[29-37] There is good evidence linking prolonged high-dose *oral* steroid usage with osteonecrosis,[60] but almost all the reports linking injected steroids with accelerated nonseptic joint destruction are anecdotal and mainly relate to joints receiving huge numbers of injections.[88] A reasonable guide is to give injections into the major joints in the lower limbs at no less than 3- to 4-month intervals, although this advice is based on consensus rather than evidence.[9,89,90] Reports of Charcot-like accelerated joint destruction after steroid injection in human hip osteoarthritis may reflect the disease itself rather than the treatment.[86,90] Currently, no evidence supports the promotion of disease progression by steroid injections; repeat injections into the osteoarthritic knee joint every 3 months seem to be safe over 2 years.[91]

One study has determined the relationship between frequent intraarticular steroid injection and subsequent joint replacement surgery in patients with rheumatoid arthritis who had received four or more injections in an asymmetric pattern in a single year. A subset of 13 patients with an average of 7.4 years of follow-up was established as the cohort of a 5-year prospective study. This highly selected cohort received 1622 injections; joint replacement surgery was not significantly more common in the heavily injected joints. The authors concluded that frequent intraarticular steroid injection does not greatly increase the risk inherent in continued disease activity for these patients and may offer some chondroprotection.[92]

Tendon rupture and atrophy

The literature does not provide precise estimates for complication rates following the therapeutic use of injected or systemic steroids in the treatment of athletic injuries, but tendon and fascial ruptures are reported complications of injection.[60] Tendon[93-95] and fascial rupture[96,97] or atrophy[98] is probably minimized by withdrawing the needle a little if an unusual amount of resistance is encountered[93] and by using a peppering technique at entheses with the smallest effective dose and volume of steroid.[99] The whole issue of steroid-associated tendon rupture is controversial,[94,97,100] disputed[101] and anecdotal,[60,93,102] and in humans is not well supported in the literature,[95] although it is widely accepted that repeated injection of steroids into load-bearing tendons carries the risk of rupture.[103] The risk of this unusual complication might be reduced by minimizing the dose and frequency of corticosteroid injections and extending the interval between injections to a minimum of 3 months.[104]

The current climate of opinion is antithetical towards steroid injection into and around the Achilles tendon. If this is being contemplated, it is advisable to image the tendon first to confirm it is a peritendinitis with no degenerative change (with or without tears) in the body of the tendon. Low-dose peritendinous steroid injections appear to be safe,[105] but it might be safer to infiltrate with local anaesthetic alone. The patient should rest from provocative activity for 6 to 8 weeks.[94] In rabbits, injections of steroid, both within the tendon substance and into the retrocalcaneal bursa adversely affect the biomechanical properties of Achilles tendons. Additionally, rabbit tendons that received bilateral injections demonstrated significantly worse biomechanical properties compared with unilaterally injected tendons. Bilateral injections should be avoided because they may have a systemic effect in conjunction with the local effect, further weakening the tendon.[106] Surgery for chronic Achilles tendinopathy has a complication rate of around 10% and should not be assumed to be a trouble-free treatment option.[107]

Delayed soft tissue healing

This may be associated with local steroid injection. In a study of rabbit ligaments, the tensile strength of the injected specimens returned to a value equal to that of the noninjected controls; however, the peak load of the injected specimens remained inferior, with a lag in histological maturation.[108] This has implications for the timing of return to activity following injection therapy.

Sepsis

Joint sepsis is the most feared complication of steroid injection treatment[109]; it may be lethal[110] but is a rarity.[59,111] In various studies local infection occurred in only 1 in 17,000 to 1 in 162,000 patients when joint and soft tissue injections were performed as an office procedure.[86,112,113] In one study, local sepsis following injection of a prepackaged corticosteroid in a sterile syringe was 1 in 162,000 injections compared with 1 in 21,000 injections using a nonprepackaged syringe.[112] Soft tissue infections and osteomyelitis can also occur after local soft tissue injection.[114,115]

Prompt recognition of infection is essential to prevent joint and soft tissue destruction, although diagnosis may be delayed if symptoms are mistaken for a postinjection flare or exacerbation of the underlying arthropathy.[116] Following an injection, swelling at the site, increased pain, fever, systemic upset (e.g., sweating, headaches) and severe pain on all attempted active and passive movements should raise clinical suspicion of infection. In the case of a patient who developed septic arthritis following a shoulder joint injection by her general practitioner (GP), the expert opinion was that infection is a rare hazard of the procedure for which the GP should not be blamed, but that failure to recognize and appropriately manage this side effect is difficult to defend.[62]

Fragments of skin may be carried into a joint on the tip of a needle and may be a source of infection.[117] Joint infections may also possibly occur by haematogenous spread, rather than by direct inoculation of organisms into the joint. Steroid injection may create a local focus of reduced immunity in a joint, thus rendering it more vulnerable to bloodborne spread. Rarely, injection of contaminated drugs or hormonal activation of a quiescent infection may be to blame.[111,116]

Practice point: Suspected septic arthritis following injection

All cases of suspected infection following injection must be promptly admitted to hospital for diagnosis and treatment.[111] Blood tests (e.g., erythrocyte sedimentation rate [ESR], C-reactive protein [CRP], plasma viscosity, white blood cell differential count, blood cultures) should be carried out along with diagnostic aspiration of the affected joint or any other localized swelling. The needle used for attempted aspiration may be sent for culture if no aspirate is obtained.[114] X-ray changes may be absent in the early stages of joint infection, and more sophisticated imaging techniques such as MRI and isotope bone scans may be helpful.

Practice point: Avoid injecting an already infected joint

To avoid injecting an already infected joint, have a high index of suspicion in rheumatoid patients,[118] older osteoarthritic patients with an acute monoarthritic flare (especially hip) and patients with coexistent infection elsewhere, such as the chest, urinary tract and skin, especially the legs. Visualize and dipstick the urine, and check the erythrocyte sedimentation rate.[119]

In the largest series of bacterial isolates reported from UK patients with septic arthritis, the most common organisms were *Staphylococcus aureus* and *Streptococci* spp. Others were *Escherichia coli, Haemophilus influenzae, Salmonella* and *Pseudomonas* spp. and *Mycobacterium tuberculosis*.[120] *M. tuberculosis* may be particularly difficult to diagnose and may require the study of synovial biopsy samples.[116] Infection was most common in children and older adults. Underlying risk factors were reported in 20% of cases, with the most frequent being a prosthetic joint (11%). Others included haematological malignancy, joint disease or connective tissue disorder, diabetes, oral steroid therapy, chemotherapy, presence of an intravenous line, intravenous drug abuse and postarthroscopy.[120] Steroid injection may also delay the presentation of sepsis by 6 to 12 days.[121]

In one study, the incidence of septic arthritis increased over a 12-year period as more invasive procedures (arthroscopies and arthrocenteses) were performed on the study population, although the frequency of sepsis per procedure remained static, with sepsis after arthroscopy being almost four times as frequent.[122] Joint infection has been reported as occurring between 4 days and 3 weeks after injection.[114] Exotic infections may occur in immunocompromised patients following joint injection.[123]

Aggressive therapy, including powerful immunosuppressive and cytotoxic drugs, is increasingly being used for the treatment of rheumatoid arthritis (RA) and confers increased susceptibility to infections. Antitumour necrosis factor (TNF) therapy use in RA is associated with a doubling of the risk of septic arthritis.[87] Septic arthritis is one infectious complication known to be overrepresented in RA; in one small series of patients with septic arthritis, six of nine had received an intraarticular injection into the infected joint within 3 months before the onset of the sepsis. Only one of these occurred immediately after joint injection. The annual frequency of septic arthritis was approximately 0.2%; during the 4-year period studied, the frequency was 0.5%. A frequency of 1/2,000 injections was found when late septic arthritis was included. The high frequency of delayed septic arthritis in rheumatoid patients after intraarticular steroid administration should alert clinicians to this complication.[124]

Concern has been raised that prior steroid injection of the knee and hip may increase the risk of a subsequent joint infection following joint replacement,[125,126] although this has been disputed.[127] One review has concluded that the risk of sepsis with a hip or knee implant does not seem to be increased by prior joint injections as long as the injection and surgery are separated by at least 2 months.[83] A systematic review has suggested that the included studies were underpowered and at risk of selection bias and recommended further research to settle the question.[128] Some surgeons deprecate the routine use of intraarticular steroids following knee surgery because of a perceived increased risk of infection,[121] whereas others advocate this for postprocedural pain relief.[129-132]

> **Practice point: Measures to prevent future injection related joint infections**
>
> If infection occurs following an injection, vigorous attempts must be made to isolate the causative organism. If this is *Staphylococcus aureus*, the clinician should have nasal swabs taken and, if positive, should receive appropriate antibiotic treatment and not give any more injections until further swabs confirm clearance. A review of the aseptic technique used should also be undertaken.[114]

Intraarticular corticosteroids may be effective following septic arthritis when pain and synovitis persist despite intravenous antibiotic treatment and when lavage and repeat synovial fluid and blood cultures are sterile.[133] Multidose bottles and vials should be avoided because they may become contaminated and act as a source of infection.[73] Drugs for injection must be stored in accordance with the manufacturer's instructions.

Rare local side effects

These include nerve damage (severe pain and electric shocks if you needle a nerve), transient paresis of an extremity (from an inadvertent motor nerve block) and needle fracture.[62,63]

SYSTEMIC SIDE EFFECTS

Systemic complications are rare.[11] They include the following.

Facial flushing

This is probably the most common systemic side effect,[89] occurring in from 5%[134] of patients to fewer than 1%.[84] It may come on within 24 to 48 hours after the injection and may last 1 to 2 days.

Deterioration of diabetic glycaemic control

Diabetic patients must be warned about this possible temporary side effect.[135] A common observation is that blood sugar levels undergo a modest rise for up to a week, rarely longer. When larger doses of corticosteroid than recommended here for single-site injection are given – or multiple sites are injected at one time or over a few days – this may lead to a more prolonged elevation of blood sugar levels (up to 3 weeks). This may require a short-term increase in diabetic drug dosage, so the patient should be informed about the steroid drug and dosage given. Recent injection therapy with a corticosteroid may affect the timing and interpretation of diagnostic and monitoring tests for diabetes.

Systolic blood pressure

This may be temporarily elevated by large doses of intraarticular corticosteroids.[136,137]

Uterine bleeding

Premenopausal and postmenopausal uterine bleeding may occur.[138] The exact mechanism is unknown but intraarticular corticosteroid treatment causes a temporary, but considerable, suppression of sex steroid hormone secretion in women,[139] with a transient decrease in oestradiol levels with no alteration in levels of follicle-stimulating hormone (FSH) and luteinizing hormone (LH).[83] In a postmenopausal woman, postinjection uterine bleeding creates a difficult dilemma. Is the bleeding related to the injection, or should the woman be investigated to exclude other, potentially serious causes? If this complication occurs, it must always be taken seriously. Other side effects with a low incidence in women include lactation disturbances and hirsutism.[140]

Suppression of the hypothalamic-pituitary axis

This occurs following intraarticular and intramuscular injection of corticosteroids,[141,142] but at the doses and frequencies described in this text, this usually appears to be of no significant clinical consequence.[71] We do not routinely issue a steroid card to patients after an injection.[50]

Rarely, systemic absorption of corticosteroid may evoke a secondary hypercortisolism similar to Cushing syndrome. Patients who develop a cushingoid state about 2 weeks after injection therapy (and their clinicians) often do not associate this with the corticosteroid injection, with the potential for the patient to undergo unnecessary investigation and treatment for a presumed primary endocrine disorder (Box 1.2). Screening the urine for corticosteroid drug metabolites helps with diagnosis. There may also be a transient eosinopenia on the differential blood white cell count.[143,144]

> **Box 1.2 Suppression of the hypothalamic-pituitary axis by corticosteroid injection therapy**
>
> Probably underrecognized
> May occur with single intraarticular injection of triamcinolone acetonide (TCA), 40 mg
> Possibly more likely with multiple injections of 40 mg TCA at one sitting or two or more injections within a minimum of 5 weeks
> Onset of clinical syndrome 10–14 days after injection
>
> **Clinical features**
> Moon face
> Buffalo hump
> Acne-like eruptions
> Flushing
> Palpitations
> Tremors
> Dyspnoea
> Weight gain, 5–8 kg
> Disturbed menstruation
>
> **Outcome**
> Spontaneous resolution at 3 months (one injection) and 6 months (two injections)
>
> Modified from Jansen T, van Roon E. Four cases of a secondary Cushingoid state following local triamcinolone acetonide injection. *Netherlands J Med.* 2002;60(3):151-153.

Children may be particularly susceptible and display features of Cushing syndrome following intraarticular corticosteroid injection.[145] Patients infected with HIV who are treated with ritonavir are at much greater risk for Cushing syndrome after epidural injection.[83]

Clinical improvement of distant joints in a polyarthritis is an early clinical feature suggestive of significant systemic absorption of locally administered corticosteroid. In one study, triamcinolone hexacetonide plasma levels reached their median serum peak 8 hours after injection into the rheumatoid knee.[146] This may account for the common observation of symptomatic improvement in joints other than the one injected. Higher serum levels of the injectate have been found in patients in whom the dose was divided into two joints rather than administering it into a single joint; a putative potentiation effect of divided doses has been attributed to a greater absorptive surface area in the divided doses.[84] However, in one study comparing the treatment of rheumatoid arthritis with equivalent doses of intraarticular and intramuscular minipulse therapy with triamcinolone, less significant adrenocorticotropic hormone level reduction was observed for those in the intraarticular group.[147]

Significant falls in the erythrocyte sedimentation rate and C-reactive protein level

There is a mean decrease of about 50% in these parameters. Intraarticular corticosteroid injections can cause this in patients with inflammatory arthritis, and this effect can last for up to 6 months. This needs to be taken into account when using these blood tests to assess the response of patients to disease-modifying drugs.[148]

> **Practice point: Injection therapy and vaccinations**
>
> Intraarticular corticosteroids do not cause systemic immunosuppression. Therefore, administration of live vaccines in not contraindicated.[149]

Anaphylaxis

Severe anaphylactic reactions to local anaesthetic injections are rare, but can be fatal.[150] Anaphylactic reactions to corticosteroid injections are extremely rare and are probably a reaction to the stabilizers with which the drug is mixed, rather than the drug itself.[71,131]

Nicolau syndrome

This is a livedo-like dermatitis secondary to acute arterial thrombosis that occurs immediately after the intravascular injection of an insoluble drug substance. It may rarely occur following an injection of a corticosteroid in a crystalline suspension in or about a joint. The pathophysiology of this syndrome probably involves acute vascular spasm related to the penetration of microcrystals into a blood vessel. Typically, the injection is followed immediately by excruciating pain at the injection site, sometimes with syncope. Cyanotic patches and a livedoid skin pattern develop. Rapid resolution of the pain and slower clearing of the skin changes occur in most patients. Incomplete variants without skin abnormalities may occur.[151]

Tachon syndrome

Local injections of corticosteroids can, in very rare cases, be complicated by intense lumbar and/or thoracic pain a few minutes after the injection, with rapid regression of the pain. Inadvertent intravenous injection could explain the pathophysiology of this disorder.[152]

Other rare systemic side effects

Rare side effects from a local corticosteroid injection include pancreatitis (patient presents with abdominal pain, and the serum amylase level is increased), nausea, dysphoria (emotional upset), acute psychosis, myopathy and posterior subcapsular cataracts.[62,66,153] Transient dysphonia may occur, but we consider that the incidence of 12% reported in one review[87] appears to be excessive unless this is a seriously underrecognised complication. Complex regional pain syndrome has been reported after trigger thumb injection.[154] In patients with sickle cell disease, a crisis may be precipitated by the intraarticular injection of corticosteroids; the mechanism is not clear, but it has been suggested that this treatment be used with caution in these patients.[155] Severe acneiform rashes have rarely been seen in adolescents with juvenile idiopathic arthritis following intraarticular injections of triamcinolone hexacetonide.[156] Tibial stress fractures and multifocal osteonecrosis have been reported with *systemic* but not locally injected corticosteroids used for athletic injuries.[60]

Despite all these considerations, injection therapy for joints and soft tissues is a relatively safe form of treatment. Adverse events can be minimized by ensuring that well-trained practitioners follow appropriate procedures.[68]

In a large prospective study of 1147 injections, complications of injection therapy were recorded in just under 12% of patients (7% of injections), but almost all these were transient. Only four patients (with tennis elbow) had subcutaneous atrophy, but the steroid dose was four times the one we recommend. The most common side effect was postinjection pain, but methylprednisolone was used, which we believe causes more pain than triamcinolone. Postinjection pain occurred in 12% of periarticular injections, but only 2% of intraarticular injections were painful. Other side effects were bleeding, fainting and dizziness.

It is safe to mix corticosteroids with local anaesthetics before injection. High-performance liquid chromatographic analysis to assess the stability of combinations of triamcinolone and hydrocortisone when mixed with combinations of lidocaine and bupivacaine has shown that the combinations are stable when mixed together, supporting the continued use of these products in combination.[157] Lederspan and Celestone are licensed to be mixed with 1% and 2% lidocaine and Depo-Medrone is available as a premixed, fixed-dose solution with lidocaine.

Compared with the safety profile of oral NSAIDs, the justification for using the minimum effective dose of injectable drugs in the correct place with appropriate preparation and aftercare becomes evident (Table 1.3).[158]

Table 1.3 Numbers needed to harm for patients prescribed an oral nonsteroidal antiinflammatory drug[a]

Number	Harm caused
1 in 5	Endoscopic ulcer
1 in 70	Symptomatic ulcer
1 in 150	Bleeding ulcer
1 in 1200	Death from bleeding ulcer

[a]For longer than 2 months.
From Tramer MR, Moore RA, Reynolds JM, McQuay HJ. Quantitative estimation of rare adverse events which follow a biological progression: a new model applied to chronic NSAID use. *Pain.* 2000;85:169-182.

COSTS

The injectable corticosteroids and local anaesthetics that we use are remarkably inexpensive (UK prices 2017).[50]

- 1 ml ampoule of Adcortyl (10 mg of triamcinolone acetonide): £0.91
- 1 ml vial of Kenalog (40 mg): £1.89
- 10 ml of 1% lidocaine: £0.40

Compare this with the cost of some commonly prescribed oral NSAIDs:

- Generic diclofenac, one month, 50 mg, three times daily: £4.57
- Generic ibuprofen, one month, 400 mg, three times daily: £3.26
- Generic naproxen, one month, 500 mg, three times daily: £3.99

Compare this also with the cost of hyaluronan injections:

- Ostenil (3 ×2 ml prefilled syringes of sodium hyaluronate): £101.88
- Synvisc (3 ×2 ml prefilled syringes of Hylan G-F 20): £205.00 (treatment usually consists of a course of three injections)

Compare also with this:

- Xiapex (collagenase), per vial: £650.00

Injection therapy may offer significant cost savings when compared with other treatment strategies for common musculoskeletal disorders.[159]

REFERENCES

1. Kirwan JR, Balint G, Szebenyi B. Anniversary: 50 years of glucocorticoid treatment in rheumatoid arthritis. *Rheumatology* (Oxford). 1999;38:100–102.
2. Goulding NJ. Corticosteroids – a case of mistaken identity? *Br J Rheumatol*. 1998;37:477–480.
3. Coombes GM, Bax DE. The use and abuse of steroids in rheumatology. *Rep Rheum Dis*. 1996;(Ser 3):1.
4. Hollander JL, Brown EM Jr, Jessar RA, et al. Hydrocortisone and cortisone injected into arthritic joints; comparative effects of a use of hydrocortisone as a local anti-arthritic agent. *JAMA*. 1951;147(17):1629–1635.
5. Creamer P. Intra-articular corticosteroid injections in osteoarthritis: do they work, and if so, how? *Ann Rheum Dis*. 1997;56:634–636.
6. af Klint E, Grundtman C, Engström M, et al. Intraarticular glucocorticoid treatment reduces inflammation in synovial cell infiltrations more efficiently than in synovial blood vessels. *Arthritis Rheum*. 2005;52(12):3880–3889.
7. Goulding NJ. Anti-inflammatory corticosteroids. *Rep Rheum Dis*. 1999;(Ser 3):1.
8. Cutolo M. The roles of steroid hormones in arthritis. *Br J Rheumatol*. 1998;37:597–599.
9. Speed CA. Injection therapies for soft-tissue lesions. *Best Pract Res Clin Rheumatol*. 2007;21(2):333–347.
10. Ines LPBS, da Silva JAP. Soft tissue injections. *Best Pract Res Clin Rheumatol*. 2005;19(3):503–527.
11. Cole BJ, Schumacher RH Jr. Injectable corticosteroids in modern practice. *J Am Acad Orthop Surg*. 2005;139(1):37–46.
12. Price R, Sinclair H, Heinrich I, et al. Local injection treatment of tennis elbow – hydrocortisone, triamcinolone and lignocaine compared. *Br J Rheumatol*. 1991;30(1):39–44.
13. Yoon SH, Lee HY, Lee HJ, et al. Optimal dose of intra-articular corticosteroids for adhesive capsulitis: a randomized, triple-blind, placebo-controlled trial. *Am J Sports Med*. 2013;41(5):1133–1139.
14. Anon. Gout in primary care. *Drugs Ther Bull*. 2004;42(5):37–40.
15. Gossec L, Dougados M. Intra-articular treatments in osteoarthritis: from the symptomatic to the structure modifying. *Ann Rheum Dis*. 2004;63:478–482.
16. Kirwan JR, Rankin E. Intraarticular therapy in osteoarthritis. *Baillieres Clin Rheumatol*. 1997;11(4):769–794.
17. Franz JK, Burmester GR. Antirheumatic treatment: the needle and the damage done. *Ann Rheum Dis*. 2005;64:798–800.
18. Rees JD, Stride M, Scott A. Tendons – time to revisit inflammation. *Br J Sports Med*. 2014;48:1553–1557.
19. Dean BJF, Gettings P, Dakin SJ, et al. Are inflammatory cells increased in painful human tendinopathy? A systematic review. *Br J Sports Med*. 2016;50:216–220.
20. Rees JD. The role of inflammatory cells in tendinopathy: is the picture getting any clearer? *Br J Sports Med*. 2016;50:201–202.

21. Millar NL, Dean BJ, Dakin SG. Inflammation and the continuum model: time to acknowledge the molecular era of tendinopathy. *Br J Sports Med*. 2016;50:1486.

22. Struglics A, Okroj M, Swärd P, et al. The complement system is activated in synovial fluid from subjects with knee injury and from patients with osteoarthritis. *Arthritis Res Ther*. 2016;18(1):223.

23. Haugeberg G, Morton S, Emery P, et al. Effect of intra-articular corticosteroid injections and inflammation on periarticular and generalised bone loss in early rheumatoid arthritis. *Ann Rheum Dis*. 2011;70:184–187.

24. Jones A, Doherty M. Intra-articular corticosteroid injections are effective in osteoarthritis but there are no clinical predictors of response. *Ann Rheum Dis*. 1996;55:829–832.

25. Zulian F, Martini G, Gobber D, et al. Comparison of intra-articular triamcinolone hexacetonide and triamcinolone acetonide in oligoarticular juvenile idiopathic arthritis. *Rheumatology*. 2003;42:1254–1259.

26. Brandt KD, Radin EL, Dieppe PA, et al. Yet more evidence that osteoarthritis is not a cartilage disease. *Ann Rheum Dis*. 2006;65:1261–1264.

27. Dorman T, Ravin T. *Diagnosis and Injection Techniques in Orthopaedic Medicine*. Baltimore, Maryland: Williams and Wilkins; 1991:33–34.

28. Daley CT, Stanish WD. Soft tissue injuries: overuse syndromes. In: Bull RC, ed. *Handbook of Sports Injuries*. New York: McGraw Hill; 1998:185.

29. Weitoft T, Larsson A, Ronnblom L. Serum levels of sex steroid hormones and matrix metalloproteinases after intra-articular glucocorticoid treatment in female patients with rheumatoid arthritis. *Ann Rheum Dis*. 2008;67:422–424.

30. Verbruggen G. Chondroprotective drugs in degenerative joint diseases. *Rheumatology* (Oxford). 2006;45(2):129–138.

31. Weitoft T, Larsson A, Saxne T, et al. Changes of cartilage and bone markers after intra-articular glucocorticoid treatment with and without postinjection rest in patients with rheumatoid arthritis. *Ann Rheum Dis*. 2005;64:1750–1753.

32. Larsson E, Erlandsson Harris H, Larsson A, et al. Corticosteroid treatment of experimental arthritis retards cartilage destruction as determined by histology and serum. *Rheumatology* (Oxford). 2004;43(4):428–434.

33. Raynauld JP. Clinical trials: impact of intra-articular steroid injections on the progression of knee osteoarthritis. *Osteoarthritis Cartilage*. 1999;7:348–349.

34. Hills BA, Ethell MT, Hodgson DR. Release of lubricating synovial surfactant by intra-articular steroid. *Br J Rheumatol*. 1998;37(6):649–652.

35. Pelletier JP, Mineau F, Raynauld JP, et al. Intraarticular injections with methylprednisolone acetate reduce osteoarthritic lesions in parallel with chondrocyte stromelysin synthesis in experimental osteoarthritis. *Arthritis Rheum*. 1994;37:414–423.

36. Jubb RW. Anti-rheumatic drugs and articular cartilage. *Rep Rheum Dis*. 1992;(Ser 2):1.

37. Pelletier JP, Martel-Pelletier J, Cloutier JM, et al. Proteoglycan-degrading metalloprotease activity in human osteoarthritis cartilage and the effect of intraarticular steroid injections. *Arthritis Rheum.* 1987;30(5):541–548.

38. Scott A, Khan KM, Cook JL, et al. What is "inflammation"? Are we ready to move beyond Celsus? *Br J Sports Med.* 2004;38:248–249.

39. Khan KM, Cook JL, Kannus P, et al. Time to abandon the "tendinitis" myth. *BMJ.* 2002;324:626–627.

40. Khan KM, Cook JL, Maffulli N, et al. Where is the pain coming from in tendinopathy? It may be biochemical, not structural in origin. *Br J Sports Med.* 2000;34(2):81–83.

41. Gotoh M, Hamada K, Yamakawa H, et al. Increased substance P in subacromial bursa and shoulder pain in rotator cuff disease. *J Orthop Res.* 1998;16:618–621.

42. Johansson A, Hao J, Sjölund B. Local corticosteroid application blocks transmission in normal nociceptive C-fibres. *Acta Anaesthesiol Scand.* 1990;34(5):335–338.

43. Zulian F, Martini G, Gobber D, et al. Triamcinolone acetonide and hexacetonide intra-articular treatment of symmetrical joints in juvenile idiopathic arthritis: a double-blind trial. *Rheumatology* (Oxford). 2004;43(10):1288–1291.

44. Derendorf H, Mollmann H, Gruner A, et al. Pharmacokinetics and pharmacodynamics of glucocorticoid suspensions after intra-articular administration. *Clin Pharmacol Ther.* 1986;39:313–317.

45. Caldwell JR. Intra-articular corticosteroids: guide to selection and indications for use. *Drugs.* 1996;52:507–514.

46. Eberhard BA, Sison MC, Gottlieb BS, et al. Comparison of the intraarticular effectiveness of triamcinolone hexacetonide and triamcinolone acetonide in treatment of juvenile rheumatoid arthritis. *J Rheumatol.* 2004;31(12):2507–2512.

47. Buchbinder R, Green S, Youd JM, et al. Arthrographic distension for adhesive capsulitis (frozen shoulder). *Cochrane Database Syst Rev.* 2008;(1):CD007005.

48. British Medical Association and Royal Pharmaceutical Society. *British National Formulary No. 72.* London: British Medical Association and Royal Pharmaceutical Society; 2017:610.

49. Piotrowski M, Szczepanski I, Dmoszynska M. Treatment of rheumatic conditions with local instillation of betamethasone and methylprednisolone: comparison of efficacy and frequency of irritative pain reaction. *Rheumatologia.* 1998;36:78–84.

50. British Medical Association and Royal Pharmaceutical Society. *British National Formulary No. 72.* London: British Medical Association and Royal Pharmaceutical Society; 2017:1181.

51. Kannus P, Jarvinen M, Niittymaki S. Long- or short-acting anesthetic with corticosteroid in local injections of overuse injuries? A prospective, randomized, double-blind study. *Int J Sports Med.* 1990;11(5):397–400.

52. Sölveborn SA, Buch F, Mallmin H, et al. Cortisone injection with anaesthetic additives for radial epicondylalgia. *Clin Orthop Relat Res.* 1995;316:99–105.

53. Buchbinder R, Green S, Forbes A, et al. Arthrographic joint distension with saline and steroid improves function and reduces pain in patients with painful stiff shoulder: results of a randomised, double-blind, placebo-controlled trial. *Ann Rheum Dis*. 2004;63:302–309.

54. Gam A, Schydlowsky P, Rossel I, et al. Treatment of "frozen shoulder" with distension and glucorticoid compared with glucorticoid alone: a randomised controlled trial. *Scand J Rheumatol*. 1998;27(6):425–430.

55. Mulcahy KA, Baxter AD, Oni OOA, et al. The value of shoulder distension arthrography with intraarticular injection of steroid and local anaesthetic: a follow-up study. *Br J Radiol*. 1994;67:263–266.

56. Jacobs LGH, Barton MAJ, Wallace WA, et al. Intraarticular distension and steroids in the management of capsulitis of the shoulder. *BMJ*. 1991;302:1498–1501.

57. Ahmed I, Gertner E. Safety of arthrocentesis and joint injection in patients receiving anticoagulation at therapeutic levels. *Am J Med*. 2012;125(3):265–269.

58. Creamer P, Hunt M, Dieppe P. Pain mechanisms in osteoarthritis of the knee: effect of intraarticular anesthetic. *J Rheumatol*. 1996;23:1031–1036.

59. Habib2. GS, Saliba W, Nashashibi M. Local effects of intra-articular corticosteroids. *Clin Rheumatol*. 2010;29(4):347–356.

60. Nichols AW. Complications associated with the use of corticosteroids in the treatment of athletic injuries. *Clin J Sport Med*. 2005;15(5):370–375.

61. Kumar N, Newman RJ. Complications of intra- and peri-articular steroid injections. *Br J Gen Pract*. 1999;49:465–466.

62. Dando P, Green S, Price J. *Problems in General Practice – Minor Surgery*. London: Medical Defence Union; 1997.

63. Lanyon P, Regan M, Jones A, et al. Inadvertent intra-articular injection of the wrong substance. *Br J Rheumatol*. 1997;36:812–813.

64. Avci S, Yilmaz C, Sayli U. Comparison of nonsurgical treatment measures for de Quervain's disease of pregnancy and lactation. *J Hand Surg Am*. 2002;27:322–324.

65. Wallace WA. Injection with methylprednisolone for carpal tunnel syndrome (letter). *Br Med J*. 2000;320:645.

66. Robinson DE, Harrison-Hansley E, Spencer RF. Steroid psychosis after an intra-articular injection. *Ann Rheum Dis*. 2000;59:926.

67. Brinks A, Koes BW, Volkers AC, et al. Adverse effects of extra-articular corticosteroid injections: a systematic review. *BMC Musculoskelet Disord*. 2010;11:206.

68. Gaujoux-Viala C, Dougados M, Gossec L. Efficacy and safety of steroid injections for shoulder and elbow tendonitis: a meta-analysis of randomised controlled trials. *Ann Rheum Dis*. 2009;68(12):1843–1849.

69. Berger RG, Yount WJ. Immediate "steroid flare" from intra-articular triamcinolone hexacetonide injection: case report and review of the literature. *Arthritis Rheum*. 1990;33(8):1284–1286.

70. Pullar T. Routes of drug administration: intra-articular route. *Prescribers J*. 1998;38(2):123–126.

71. Helliwell PS. Use of an objective measure of articular stiffness to record changes in finger joints after intra-articular injection of corticosteroid. *Ann Rheum Dis*. 1997;56:71–73.

72. Kirschke DL, Jones TF, Stratton CW, et al. Outbreak of joint and soft tissue infections associated with injections from a multiple-dose medication vial. *Clin Infect Dis.* 2003;36:1369–1373.

73. Newman RJ. Local skin depigmentation due to corticosteroid injections. *BMJ.* 1984;288:1725–1726.

74. Cassidy JT, Bole GG. Cutaneous atrophy secondary to intra-articular corticosteroid administration. *Ann Intern Med.* 1966;65(5):1008–1018.

75. Basadonna PT, Rucco V, Gasparini D, et al. Plantar fat pad atrophy after corticosteroid injection for an interdigital neuroma: a case report. *Am J Phys Med Rehabil.* 1999;78(3):283–285.

76. Reddy PD, Zelicof SB, Ruotolo C, et al. Interdigital neuroma. Local cutaneous changes after corticosteroid injection. *Clin Orthop Relat Res.* 1995;317:185–187.

77. Salvati G, Punzi L, Pianon M, et al. Frequency of the bleeding risk in patients receiving warfarin submitted to arthrocentesis of the knee. *Reumatismo.* 2003;55(3):159–163.

78. Dunn AS, Turpie AG. Perioperative management of patients receiving oral anticoagulants: a systematic review. *Arch Intern Med.* 2003;163(8):901–908.

79. Thumboo J, O'Duffy JD. A prospective study of the safety of joint and soft tissue aspirations and injections in patients taking warfarin sodium. *Arthritis Rheum.* 1998;41(4):736–739.

80. Goupille P, Thomas T, Noël E. A practice survey of shoulder glucocorticoid injections in patients on antiplatelet drugs or vitamin K antagonists. *Joint Bone Spine.* 2008;75(3):311–314.

81. Nagafuchi Y, Sumitomo S, Soroida Y, et al. The power Doppler twinkling artefact associated with periarticular calcification induced by intra-articular corticosteroid injection in patients with rheumatoid arthritis. *Ann Rheum Dis.* 2013;72:1267–1269.

82. Berthelot JM, Le Goff B, Maugars Y. Side effects of corticosteroid injections: what's new? *Joint Bone Spine.* 2013;80(4):363–367.

83. Clearfield DA, Ruane JJ, Diehl J. Examining the safety of joint injections in patients on warfarin. https://www.practicalpainmanagement.com/ treatments/interventional/injections/examining-safety-joint-inject ions-patients-warfarin.

84. Gray RG, Gottlieb NL. Intra-articular corticosteroids, an updated assessment. *Clin Orthop Relat Res.* 1983;177:235–263.

85. Nanno M, Sawaizumi T, Kodera N, et al. Flexor pollicis longus rupture in a trigger thumb after intrasheath triamcinolone injections: a case report with literature review. *J Nippon Med Sch.* 2014;81(4):269–275.

86. Gray RG, Tenenbaum J, Gottlieb NL. Local corticosteroid injection therapy in rheumatic disorders. *Semin Arthritis Rheum.* 1981;10:231–254.

87. Galloway JB, Hyrich KL, Mercer LK, et al. Risk of septic arthritis in patients with rheumatoid arthritis and the effect of anti-TNF therapy: results from the British Society for Rheumatology Biologics Register. *Ann Rheum Dis.* 2011;70:1810–1814.

88. Cameron G. Steroid arthropathy: myth or reality? *J Orthop Med.* 1995;17(2):51–55.

89. British Medical Association and Royal Pharmaceutical Society. *British National Formulary No. 72*. London: British Medical Association and Royal Pharmaceutical Society; 2017:1000.

90. Cooper C, Kirwan JR. The risks of local and systemic corticosteroid administration. *Baillieres Clin Rheumatol*. 1990;4(2):305–333.

91. Raynauld J, Buckland-Wright C, Ward R, et al. Safety and efficacy of long-term intraarticular steroid injections in osteoarthritis of the knee: a randomized, double-blind, placebo-controlled trial. *Arthritis Rheum*. 2003;48:370–377.

92. Roberts WN, Babcock EA, Breitbach SA, et al. Corticosteroid injection in rheumatoid arthritis does not increase rate of total joint arthroplasty. *J Rheumatol*. 1996;23(6):1001–1004.

93. Smith AG, Kosygan K, Williams H, et al. Common extensor tendon rupture following corticosteroid injection for lateral tendinosis of the elbow. *Br J Sports Med*. 1999;33:423–425.

94. Shrier I, Matheson GO, Kohl HW 3rd. Achilles tendon: are corticosteroid injections useful or harmful? *Clin J Sports Med*. 1996;6:245–250.

95. Mahler F, Fritschy D. Partial and complete ruptures of the Achilles tendon and local corticosteroid injections. *Br J Sports Med*. 1992;26:7–14.

96. Saxena A, Fullem B. Plantar fascia ruptures in athletes. *Am J Sports Med*. 2004;32:662–665.

97. Acevedo JI, Beskin JL. Complications of plantar fascia rupture associated with corticosteroid injection. *Foot Ankle Int*. 1998;19:91–97.

98. Fredberg U. Local corticosteroid injection in sport: review of literature and guidelines for treatment. *Scand J Med Sci Sports*. 1997;7:131–139.

99. Cyriax JH, Cyriax PJ, eds. Principles of treatment. In: *Illustrated Manual of Orthopaedic Medicine*. London: Butterworths; 1983:22.

100. McWhorter JW, Francis RS, Heckmann RA. Influence of local steroid injections on traumatized tendon properties; a biomechanical and histological study. *Am J Sports Med*. 1991;19(5):435–439.

101. Read MT. Safe relief of rest pain that eases with activity in achillodynia by intrabursal or peritendinous steroid injection: the rupture rate was not increased by these steroid injections. *Br J Sports Med*. 1999;33:134–135.

102. Mair SD, Isbell WM, Gill TJ, et al. Triceps tendon ruptures in professional football players. *Am J Sports Med*. 2004;32:431–434.

103. Mottram DR, ed. *Drugs in Sport*. 2nd ed. London: E & FN Spon; 1996.

104. Nanno M, Sawaizumi T, Kodera N, et al. Flexor pollicis longus rupture in a trigger thumb after intrasheath triamcinolone injections: a case report with literature review. *J Nippon Med Sch*. 2014;81(4):269–275.

105. Gill SS, Gelbke MK, Matson SL, et al. Fluoroscopically guided low-volume peritendinous corticosteroid injection for Achilles tendinopathy; a safety study. *J Bone Joint Surg Am*. 2004;86:802–806.

106. Hugate R, Pennypacker J, Saunders M, et al. The effects of intratendinous and retrocalcaneal intrabursal injections of corticosteroid on the biomechanical properties of rabbit Achilles tendons. *J Bone Joint Surg Am*. 2004;86:794–801.

107. Paavola M, Orava S, Leppilahti J, et al. Chronic Achilles tendon overuse injury: complications after surgical treatment. An analysis of 432 consecutive patients. *Am J Sports Med*. 2000;28:77–82.

108. Wiggins ME, Fadale PD, Ehrlich MG, et al. Effects of local injection of corticosteroids on the healing of ligaments; a follow-up report. *J Bone Joint Surg Am*. 1995;77(11):1682–1691.

109. Hughes RA. Septic arthritis. *Rep Rheum Dis*. 1996;(Ser 3):1.

110. Yangco BG, Germain BF, Deresinski SC. Case report: fatal gas gangrene following intra-articular steroid injection. *Am J Med Sci*. 1982;283(2):94–98.

111. Charalambous CP, Tryfonidis M, Sadiq S, et al. Septic arthritis following intra-articular steroid injection of the knee – a survey of current practice regarding antiseptic technique used during intra-articular steroid injection of the knee. *Clin Rheumatol*. 2003;22:386–390.

112. Seror P, Pluvinage P, Lecoq d'Andre F, et al. Frequency of sepsis after local corticosteroid injection (an inquiry on 1160000 injections in rheumatological private practice in France). *Rheumatology* (Oxford). 1999;38:1272–1274.

113. Pal B, Morris J. Perceived risks of joint infection following intra-articular corticosteroid injections: a survey of rheumatologists. *Clin Rheumatol*. 1999;18(3):264–265.

114. Grayson MF. Three infected injections from the same organism. *Br J Rheumatol*. 1998;37:592–593.

115. Jawed S, Allard SA. Osteomyelitis of the humerus following steroid injections for tennis elbow [letter]. *Rheumatology* (Oxford). 2000;39:923–924.

116. von Essen R, Savolainen HA. Bacterial infection following intra-articular injection: a brief review. *Scand J Rheumatol*. 1989;18:7–12.

117. Xu C, Peng H, Chai W, et al. Inadvertent introduction of tissue coring during arthrocentesis: an experimental study. *Med Sci Monit*. 2017;23:3571.

118. Gardner GC, Weisman MH. Pyarthrosis in patient with rheumatoid arthritis: a report of 13 cases and a review of the literature from the past 40 years. *Am J Med*. 1990;88:503–511.

119. Knight DJ, Gilbert FJ, Hutchison JD. Lesson of the week: septic arthritis in osteoarthritic hips. *BMJ*. 1996;313:40–41.

120. Ryan MJ, Kavanagh R, Wall PG, et al. Bacterial joint infections in England and Wales: analysis of bacterial isolates over a four year period. *Br J Rheumatol*. 1997;36:370–373.

121. Gosal HS, Jackson AM, Bickerstaff DR. Intra-articular steroids after arthroscopy for osteoarthritis of the knee. *J Bone Joint Surg Br*. 1999;81:952–954.

122. Geirsson AJ, Statkevicius S, Víkingsson A. Septic arthritis in Iceland 1990–2002: increasing incidence due to iatrogenic infections. *Ann Rheum Dis*. 2008;67:638–643.

123. Sohail MR, Smilack JD. Aspergillus fumigatus septic arthritis complicating intra-articular corticosteroid injection. *Mayo Clin Proc*. 2004;79(4):578–579.

124. Ostensson A, Geborek P. Septic arthritis as a non-surgical complication in rheumatoid arthritis: relation to disease severity and therapy. *Br J Rheumatol*. 1991;30:35–38.

125. Papavasiliou AV, Isaac DL, Marimuthu R, et al. Infection in knee replacements after previous injection of intra-articular steroid. *J Bone Joint Surg Br*. 2006;88:321–323.

126. Kaspar S, de V de Beer J. Infection in hip arthroplasty after previous injection of steroid. *J Bone Joint Surg Br.* 2005;87(4):454–457.

127. Chitre AR, Fehily MJ, Bamford DJ. Total hip replacement after intra-articular injection of local anaesthetic and steroid. *J Bone Joint Surg Br.* 2007;89(2):166–168.

128. Marsland D, Mumith A, Barlow IW. Systematic review: the safety of intra-articular corticosteroid injection prior to total knee arthroplasty. *Knee.* 2014;21(1):6–11.

129. Pang HN, Lo NN, Yang KY, et al. Peri-articular steroid injection improves the outcome after unicondylar knee replacement: a prospective, randomised controlled trial with a two-year follow-up. *J Bone Joint Surg Br.* 2008;90:738–744.

130. Wang JJ, Ho ST, Lee SC, et al. Intraarticular triamcinolone acetonide for pain control after arthroscopic knee surgery. *Anesth Analg.* 1998;87:1113–1116.

131. Beaudouin E, Kanny G, Gueant JL, et al. Anaphylaxis caused by carboxymethylcellulose: report of 2 cases of shock from injectable corticoids. *Allerg Immunol (Paris).* 1992;24(9):333–335.

132. Tsukada S, Wakui M, Hoshino A. The impact of including corticosteroid in a periarticular injection for pain control after total knee arthroplasty: a double-blind randomised controlled trial. *Bone Joint J.* 2016;98(2):194–200.

133. Lane SE, Merry P. Intra-articular corticosteroids in septic arthritis: beneficial or barmy? [letter]. *Ann Rheum Dis.* 2000;59:240.

134. Articular and periarticular corticosteroid injection. *Drugs Ther Bull.* 1995;33(9):67–70.

135. Black DM, Filak AT. Hyperglycemia with non-insulin-dependent diabetes following intra-articular steroid injection. *J Fam Pract.* 1989;28(4):462–463.

136. Younis M, Neffati F, Touzi M, et al. Systemic effects of epidural and intra-articular glucocorticoid injections in diabetic and non-diabetic patients. *Joint Bone Spine.* 2007;74(5):472–476.

137. Wang AA, Hutchinson DT. The effect of corticosteroid injection for trigger finger on blood glucose level in diabetic patients. *J Hand Surg Am.* 2006;31(6):979–981.

138. Mens JMA, De Wolf AN, Berkhout BJ, et al. Disturbance of the menstrual pattern after local injection with triamcinolone acetonide. *Ann Rheum Dis.* 1998;57:700.

139. Weitoft T, Larsson A, Ronnblom L. Serum levels of sex steroid hormones and matrix metalloproteinases after intra-articular glucocorticoid treatment in female patients with rheumatoid arthritis. *Ann Rheum Dis.* 2008;67:422–424.

140. Brook EM, Hu CH, Kingston KA, et al. Corticosteroid injections: a review of sex-related side effects. *Orthopedics.* 2017;40(2):e211–e215.

141. van Tuyl SAC, Slee PH. Are the effects of local treatment with glucocorticoids only local? *Neth J Med.* 2002;60(3):130–132.

142. Lazarevic MB, Skosey JL, Djordjevic-Denic G, et al. Reduction of cortisol levels after single intra-articular and intramuscular steroid injection. *Am J Med.* 1995;99(4):370–373.

SECTION 1

143. Jansen T, van Roon E. Four cases of a secondary Cushingoid state following local triamcinolone acetonide injection. *Neth J Med.* 2002;60(3):151–153.

144. Lansang MC, Farmer T, Kennedy L. Diagnosing the unrecognized systemic absorption of intra-articular and epidural steroid injections. *Endocr Pract.* 2009;15(3):225–228.

145. Kumar S, Singh RJ, Reed AM, et al. Cushing's syndrome after intra-articular and intradermal administration of triamcinolone acetonide in three pediatric patients. *Pediatrics.* 2004;113(6):1820–1824.

146. Weitoft T, Rönnblom L. Glucocorticoid resorption and influence on the hypothalamic-pituitary-adrenal axis after intra-articular treatment of the knee in resting and mobile patients. *Ann Rheum Dis.* 2006;65:955–957.

147. Furtado RN, Oliveira LM, Natour J. Polyarticular corticosteroid injection versus systemic administration in treatment of rheumatoid arthritis patients: a randomized controlled study. *J Rheumatol.* 2005;32(9):1691–1698.

148. Taylor HG, Fowler PD, David MJ, et al. Intra-articular steroids: confounder of clinical trials. *Clin Rheumatol.* 1991;10(1):38–42.

149. Gov UK. Immunisation Against Infectious Disease (The Green Book). www.gov.uk.

150. Ewan PW. Anaphylaxis (ABC of allergies). *BMJ.* 1998;316:1442–1445.

151. Cherasse A, Kahn MF, Mistrih R, et al. Nicolau's syndrome after local glucocorticoid injection. *Joint Bone Spine.* 2003;70(5):390–392.

152. Hajjioui A, Nys A, Poiraudeau S, et al. An unusual complication of intra-articular injections of corticosteroids: tachon syndrome. Two case reports. *Ann Readapt Med Phys.* 2007;50(9):721–723.

153. Boonen S, Van Distel G, Westhovens R, et al. Steroid myopathy induced by epidural triamcinolone injection. *Br J Rheumatol.* 1995;34:385–386.

154. Murphy AD, Lloyd-Hughes H, Ahmed J. Complex regional pain syndrome (type 1) following steroid injection for stenosing tenosynovitis. *J Plast Reconstr Aesthet Surg.* 2010;63(10):e740–e741.

155. Gladman DD, Bombardier C. Sickle cell crisis following intraarticular steroid therapy for rheumatoid arthritis. *Arthritis Rheum.* 1987;30(9):1065–1068.

156. Goldzweig O, Carrasco R, Hashkes PJ. Systemic adverse events following intra-articular corticosteroid injections for the treatment of juvenile idiopathic arthritis: two patients with dermatologic adverse events and review of the literature. *Semin Arthritis Rheum.* 2013;43(1):71–76.

157. Watson DG, Husain S, Brennan S, et al. The chemical stability of admixtures of injectable corticosteroid and local anaesthetics. *CME Orthop.* 2007;4(3):81–83.

158. Tramer MR, Moore RA, Reynolds DJM, et al. Quantitative estimation of rare adverse events which follow a biological progression: a new model applied to chronic NSAID use. *Pain.* 2000;85:169–182.

159. Kerrigan CL, Stanwix MG. Using evidence to minimize the cost of trigger finger care. *J Hand Surg Am.* 2009;34(6):997–1005.

CHAPTER 3: OTHER SUBSTANCES USED FOR INJECTION THERAPY

OVERVIEW

Since the 1930s, an array of substances other than corticosteroids and local anaesthetics has been injected into joints and soft tissues, often with the aim of directly promoting tissue healing. The first injectates, which yielded little benefit, were formalin, glycerine, lipiodol, lactic acid and petroleum jelly.[1,2] Many other agents have been tried since (Box 1.3). For soft tissue lesions in particular, there has long been a clear need for effective conservative therapies and, in recent times, novel agents have been injected specifically to try to promote healing. Depending on your perspective, these treatments exist either on the fringe or the frontier of musculoskeletal therapeutics.

Box 1.3 Examples of substances injected into joints and soft tissues for therapeutic effect

Adalimumab
Actovegin
Air
Anakinra
Aprotinin
Autologous whole blood
Botulinum toxin A
Dextrose
Etanercept
Formalin
Guanethidine
Glycerine
Hyaluronans and their derivatives
Infliximab
Lactic acid
Lipiodol
Methotrexate
Morphine
Nonsteroidal antiinflammatory drugs
Petroleum jelly
Polidocanol
Phenol
Platelet-rich plasma
Osmic acid
Radioactive materials (e.g., [169]erbium, [186]rhenium, [90]yttrium)
Sclerosing agents
Traumeel

OTHER INJECTABLE SUBSTANCES

HYALURONANS Endogenous (naturally occurring) hyaluronan (HA, previously known as hyaluronic acid) is a large, linear glycosaminoglycan that is a major nonstructural component of both the synovial and cartilage extracellular matrices. It is also found in synovial fluid and is produced by the lining layer cells of the joint. These molecules produce a highly viscoelastic solution that is a viscous lubricant at low shear (during slow movement of the joint – e.g., walking) and an elastic shock absorber at high shear (during rapid movement – e.g., running). As well as conferring viscoelasticity, the other key functions of HA in the joint are lubrication and the maintenance of tissue hydration and protein homeostasis through the prevention of large fluid movements by functioning as an osmotic buffer. HA is also considered a physiological factor in the trophic status of cartilage. HA has a very high water-binding capacity; 1 g dissolved in physiological saline occupies 3 L of solution.[3,4] In osteoarthritic joints, the capacity of synovial fluid to lubricate and absorb shock is typically reduced. This is partly because of the production of abnormal HA, with a reduction in the size and concentration of the molecules naturally present in the synovial fluid.[4]

Synthetic HA was isolated from roosters' combs and umbilical cord tissue and developed for clinical use in ophthalmic surgery and arthritis in the 1960s. The rationale for joint injection therapy was to replace the normal physiological properties lost to the osteoarthritic joint as a consequence of the associated reduction in the volume and quality of HA, a concept known as *viscosupplementation*. Commercial preparations of HA have the same structure as endogenous HA, although cross-linked HA molecules (known as hylans) were later engineered by molecular linkage to obtain greater elastoviscosity and intraarticular dwell time.[3]

Osteoarthritic knees may be treated by the intraarticular injection of HA, usually after any effusion is drained.[3-6] The mode of action of exogenous (synthetic) HA and its derivatives is not clear, particularly when an effusion containing endogenous HA is removed and immediately replaced by exogenous HA, which then stays in the joint cavity for only a few days at most. Perhaps these injections stimulate the synthesis of better-quality, more physiologically normal endogenous HA and/or reduce inflammation.[4] Given the relatively short intraarticular residency, any hypothesis for the mechanism of action must account for the long duration of clinical efficacy that has been reported.[3]

A number of commercial preparations are available for injection (Box 1.4), but there is no evidence that any one preparation is superior.[3] The licensed commercial formulations that have been available the longest in the United Kingdom are Hyalgan (sodium hyaluronate) and Synvisc (hylan G-F 20). Hyalgan has a lower molecular weight and is licensed as a medicinal product; it is injected once weekly for 5 weeks and is repeatable at no more than 6-month intervals. Synvisc has a higher molecular weight and is licensed as a medical device; it is injected once weekly for 3 weeks, repeatable once within 6 months, with at least 4 weeks between courses.

The research evidence on the efficacy of HAs is often difficult to interpret because of confounders, including different molecular weights, different injection schedules (ranging from once to a series of five injections) and, despite large

Box 1.4 Hyaluronan preparations available in the United Kingdom 2017

Sodium hyaluronate
   Durolane
   Euflexxa
   Fermathron
   Hyalgan (not available for NHS prescription)
   Orthovisc
   Ostenil
   Suplasyn
   Synocrom
Hylan G-F 20
   Synvisc

NHS, National Health Service.

numbers of studies, generally poor trial design (e.g., lack of intention to treat analyses and limitations in blinding).[6] Intraarticular HA injection for osteoarthritic knees has been endorsed by two authoritative guidelines,[7,8] but was rejected by the UK National Institute for Health and Clinical Excellence (NICE) on the grounds of cost.[3] The European Society for Clinical and Economic Aspects of Osteoporosis and Osteoarthritis (ESCEO) treatment algorithm has recommended intraarticular HA for the management of knee osteoarthritis as second-line treatment in patients who remain symptomatic, despite use of nonsteroidal antiinflammatory drugs. Based on evidence from real-life setting trials and surveys, HA is recommended as a safe and effective component of the multimodal management of knee osteoarthritis (OA).[9]

A systematic review and metaanalysis has concluded that from baseline to week 4, intraarticular corticosteroids appear to be relatively more effective for pain than intraarticular HA. By week 4, both therapies have equal efficacy but, beyond week 8, HA has greater efficacy.[10] A Cochrane review has also suggested that the pain relief with HA therapy is achieved more slowly than with steroid injections, but the effect may be more prolonged.[6] Another metaanalysis of high-quality trials of intraarticular HA versus placebo has shown that this provides a moderate but real benefit for patients with knee OA.[11]

Two prospective double-blind, randomized, placebo-controlled trials with large numbers of osteoarthritic knee patients have reached opposing conclusions. One study of five weekly injections of Hyalgan versus saline after 1 year showed no treatment effect in any outcome measure.[12] The other study compared a single injection of Synvisc with placebo and, after 6 months, showed clinically relevant pain relief. No safety issues were seen in either study.[13] Treatment with three weekly injections of intermediate-molecular-weight HA may be superior to low-molecular-weight HA for knee OA symptoms over 6 months, with similar safety.[14]

Overall, the evidence suggests that HA and hylan derivatives are superior to placebo in terms of pain reduction, efficacy and quality of life outcomes in patients with osteoarthritic knees, although the effect size is generally small. Given this, and the cost of these therapies, together with the increased number of clinician visits required, NICE has concluded that the benefits of HA injection therapy would have to be three to five times higher than current estimates before efficacy reaches the standard threshold for cost-effectiveness to the National Health Service (NHS). NICE also concluded that clinical trials do not suggest that there are subgroups of patients who may have greater benefit from HA treatment, which might improve cost-effectiveness.[3] Limited data are available concerning the effectiveness of multiple courses of HA therapy.[15] Patients older than 65 years and those with the most advanced radiographic stage of osteoarthritis are less likely to benefit.[16]

Some commercial HAs are licensed for use in the hip joint. No significant differences between HA and placebo were reported by a trial evaluating efficacy and function outcomes in patients with hip osteoarthritis[17]; one systematic review has noted methodological limitations in the literature, which were mainly the absence of a control group in most of the studies, overly short follow-up periods and different ways of measuring outcomes. The review concluded that HA injection for hips should only be used under careful supervision and only in those patients for whom other treatments have failed.[18] A second systematic review has concluded that despite the relatively low level of evidence of the included studies, HA injection performed under fluoroscopic or ultrasound guidance seems to be effective and appears to be safe and well tolerated, but cannot be recommended as standard therapy in the wider population.[19] A third review has concluded that this therapy seems to be a valuable technique that may delay the need for surgical intervention, with no difference among products, but further studies are necessary.[20]

The use of HA injections in other joints is being investigated.[21-26] Encouraging, but inconclusive results have been observed for the treatment of shoulder, carpometacarpal and ankle osteoarthritis.[27]

The toxicity of intraarticular HA appears to be negligible. No major safety issues have been identified when compared with placebo, but a definitive conclusion is precluded because of sample size restrictions.[6] HA injections may cause a short-term increase in knee inflammation.[28] A small percentage of patients may experience a transient mild to moderate increase in pain following injection, and some have a flare with marked effusion. Local reactions to hylan G-F-20 occur more often in patients who have undergone more than one course of treatment. Following corticosteroid injection, these reactions abate without apparent sequelae.[29] As with any injection procedure, there is a very small risk of infection.[3]

The synergistic combination of corticosteroid and HA for simultaneous injection is an approach that has been investigated in a small number of studies.[30,31] COR1.1, a 560-patient, international, multicenter, randomized, double-blind study has evaluated the safety and efficacy of Hydros-TA (hyaluronic acid that entraps a low-dose corticosteroid, triamcinolone acetonide [TA], 10 mg) versus the HA component alone and the TA component alone. Hydros-TA met the first of its two primary endpoints, demonstrating a statistically significant improvement from baseline in the WOMAC (Western Ontario and McMaster Universities Osteoarthritis) pain score at week 2 versus Hydros-TA. In addition, Hydros-TA maintained a significant reduction in pain from baseline over 26 weeks. However, patients in the TA component arm continued to show an unexpected significant reduction in pain through 26 weeks. Given the comparable effectiveness at 26 weeks, COR1.1 did not meet its second primary endpoint. Hydros-TA was generally well tolerated, with no treatment-related serious adverse events.[32]

A metaanalysis has indicated that intraarticular HA is an effective and safe alternative therapy for the rheumatoid knee.[33] In another rheumatoid arthritis study, HA and corticosteroid injections generally had similar efficacy rates when patient-perceived satisfaction was used as an index.[34]

PROLOTHERAPY (SCLEROSANTS)

Sclerosing therapy was used by Hippocrates, in the form of cautery at the shoulder, to prevent recurrent dislocation. In current medical practice, sclerosing agents are mainly injected to treat varicose veins, oesophageal varices and piles. This therapy has been used to treat chronic low back pain for almost 70 years[35] and is also known as prolotherapy because it involves injecting a proliferant (i.e., a substance that is intended to stimulate fibroblast proliferation).[36]

Prolotherapy involves the injection of non-biological solutions, typically at soft tissue attachments and within joint spaces, to reduce pain and improve function in painful musculoskeletal conditions. A variety of solutions have been used; dextrose prolotherapy is the most rigorously studied.[37]

The musculoskeletal rationale for prolotherapy is to strengthen inadequate ligaments by exposing them to an irritant that will induce fibroblastic hyperplasia, seeking to stimulate connective tissue growth, and promote the formation of collagen.[35] The treatment aims to cause soft tissue inflammation, the opposite objective to corticosteroid injection therapy,[36] but the histological responses may not be different from those caused by saline injections or needlestick procedures.[38.]

Prolotherapy for musculoskeletal disorders is not widespread but seems to be popular with some patients; a survey of 908 primary care patients receiving opioids for chronic pain in the United States, most commonly for chronic low back pain (38%), has reported that 8% had used prolotherapy in their lifetime, and 6% had used it in the past year.[39] Although this treatment is mostly used for back pain,[35,36,40-42] including the sacroiliac joint (SIJ),[43] it has also been used for those with peripheral instability[41,44] and in elite kicking sport athletes with chronic groin pain from osteitis pubis and/or adductor tendinopathy.[45] Intraarticular dextrose prolotherapy for anterior cruciate ligament laxity has also been reported in a small study.[46]

Prolotherapy has been investigated in Achilles tendinopathy. In a study comparing effectiveness and cost-effectiveness of eccentric loading exercises (ELEs) with prolotherapy or combined treatment, results were better at 12 months for prolotherapy and for combined treatment, which had the lowest incremental cost compared with ELE, but long-term results were similar.[47] Sonographically guided intratendinous injection of 25% hyperosmolar dextrose has also been used to treat chronic Achilles tendinopathy[48] and plantar fasciitis.[49]

The term *prolotherapy* encompasses a variety of treatment approaches rather than a specific protocol, and there are a large number of sclerosants.[42] One of the most common sclerosant solutions consists of a mixture of dextrose, glycerine, phenol and lidocaine (P2G).[42] Some use just dextrose and lidocaine, which may be potentially less neurotoxic, although part of the pain-relieving effect of sclerosant injection may be from a toxic action on nociceptors.

In the most carefully conducted study of prolotherapy for back pain reported so far, there was no difference between the effect of injecting a sclerosant solution or injecting saline at key spinal ligament entheses. However, because both groups of patients improved significantly, it is difficult to decide what the particular effect of sclerosant injections might be.[50]

A critical review has concluded that prolotherapy may be effective at reducing spinal pain, but great variation was found in the protocols used, precluding definite conclusions. It was recommended that future research should focus on those solutions and protocols that are most commonly used in clinical practice, and that have been used in trials reporting effectiveness, to help determine which patients are most likely to benefit.[42]

A Cochrane review has concluded that there is conflicting evidence regarding the efficacy of prolotherapy for chronic low back pain; when used alone, it is not an effective treatment. When combined with spinal manipulation, exercise and other co-interventions, prolotherapy may improve chronic low back pain and disability. Conclusions were confounded by clinical heterogeneity amongst studies and by the presence of co-interventions.[40]

In recent years, there has been a number of studies looking again at this treatment. A systematic review has concluded that the use of dextrose prolotherapy is supported for the treatment of tendinopathies, knee and finger joint OA and spinal or pelvic pain caused by ligament dysfunction, but that efficacy in acute pain, as first-line therapy, and in myofascial pain cannot be determined from the literature.[51] A systematic review and metaanalysis of the comparative effectiveness of dextrose prolotherapy versus control injections and exercise in the management of osteoarthritis pain has concluded that there is decreased pain in OA patients, but this therapy does not exhibit a positive dose-response relationship following serial injections. Dextrose prolotherapy was found to provide a better therapeutic effect than exercise, local anaesthetics and probably corticosteroids when patients were retested 6 months following the initial injection.[52]

Another systematic review and metaanalysis has concluded that overall, prolotherapy confers a positive and significant beneficial effect in the treatment of knee OA, and that adequately powered, longer term trials with uniform endpoints are needed to elucidate the efficacy of prolotherapy better.[53] Yet another systematic review has concluded that current data from trials about prolotherapy for OA should be considered preliminary, but future high-quality trials on this topic are warranted.[54] A descriptive review has concluded that systematic review, including a metaanalysis, and randomized controlled trials suggest that prolotherapy may be associated with symptom improvement in mild to moderate symptomatic knee OA and overuse tendinopathy. The authors commented that although the mechanism of action is not well understood and is likely multifactorial, a growing body of literature has suggested that prolotherapy for knee OA may be appropriate for the treatment of symptoms associated with knee OA in carefully selected patients who are refractory to conservative therapy and deserves further basic and clinical science investigation for the treatment of OA and tendinopathy.[55] A systematic review of prolotherapy for lower limb injections has found limited evidence that this is a safe and effective treatment for Achilles tendinopathy, plantar fasciopathy and Osgood-Schlatter disease.[56] Another systematic review of prolotherapy for chronic painful, Achilles tendinopathy has suggested that this treatment may be effective and can be considered safe, but long-term studies and randomized controlled trials (RCTs), are still needed.[57]

In participants with painful rotator cuff tendinopathy who have undergone physical therapy, injection of hypertonic dextrose onto painful entheses has resulted in superior long-term pain improvement and patient satisfaction compared with blinded saline injection over painful entheses, with intermediate results for entheses injected with saline.[58] Prolotherapy was an easily applicable and satisfying auxiliary method for the treatment of chronic rotator cuff lesions when compared with exercises for chronic rotator cuff lesions.[59] A retrospective case-controlled study has found that prolotherapy improves pain, disability, isometric strength and shoulder range of movement in patients with refractory, chronic, rotator cuff disease and recommended further studies.[60] In a prospective study, prolotherapy resulted in safe and substantial improvement in knee OA specific quality of life measures compared with controls over 52 weeks. Among prolotherapy participants, but not controls, MRI–assessed cartilage volume change and predicted pain severity score change suggested that prolotherapy may have a pain-specific, disease-modifying effect. The authors concluded that further research is warranted.[61]

Our anecdotal experience has been that this treatment may be worth using for conditions in which the symptoms are caused by chronic ligamentous laxity – such as at the ankle, thumb or SIJ – or where other conservative interventions have failed.

POLIDOCANOL   Polidocanol (ethoxysclerol) is a sclerosing local anaesthetic injected to treat tendinopathies. The rationale for its use is that the pain from tendinopathy is related to the growth of new blood vessels (neovascularization) and their closely associated nerves. These vascular changes can be seen on colour Doppler ultrasound examination of tendons. In a pilot study, polidocanol was injected under ultrasound control into the neovessels of patients with Achilles tendinopathy; 8 of 10 subjects had significant reduction in their pain and returned to pain-free, tendon-loading activities, with benefit persisting at 6 months.[62]

An RCT crossover study was conducted to investigate polidocanol in a group of elite athletes with patellar tendinopathy. The treatment group reported a significant improvement after 4 months; there was no change for the control group. After 8 months, when the control group had also undergone active treatment with polidocanol, they had a greater improvement than the treatment group. There was no further improvement in either group at 12-month follow-up.[62a]

Another prospective, double-blind, crossover RCT compared a guided intratendinous single injection with polidocanol with a single injection of local anaesthetic (lidocaine + epinephrine), in patients with tennis elbow. At the 3-month follow-up, additional injections with polidocanol were offered to both groups (crossover for group 2). At 1 year, there was similar pain relief in both groups.[63]

In a retrospective study in which Achilles tendons received polidocanol injections for chronic midportion tendinopathy, pain correlated positively with neovessels on ultrasound. The authors concluded that their study did not confirm the postulated high beneficial value of sclerosing neovascularization injections in patients with this condition; they stressed that polidocanol injection may not be as promising as was first thought.[64]

Larger, longer term, double-blind, randomized placebo-controlled trials of this approach are awaited. It would be especially useful to know how a landmark-guided approach compares with injection using ultrasound guidance.

AUTOLOGOUS BLOOD

It has been postulated that tendon healing and regeneration may be improved by injecting autologous growth factors (AGFs) obtained from the patient's own blood,[65] and there is growing interest in the working mechanisms. The amount and mixture of growth factors produced using different cell-separating systems are largely unknown, however, and it is also uncertain whether platelet activation before injection is necessary. AGF can be injected with autologous whole blood or platelet-rich plasma (PRP) and this therapy is being increasingly used, with high expectations of regenerative effects. Chronic tendinopathies including wrist extensors, flexors, Achilles tendons (and plantar fascia), have been treated with this approach.[66] PRP has also been injected into the knee to encourage the healing of cartilage and relieve pain.[67,68]

In a comparative open study to evaluate the short-term, medium-term, and long-term effects of corticosteroid injection, AGF injection and extracorporeal shock wave therapy in the treatment of tennis elbow, corticosteroid injection gave a high success rate in the short term. However, AGF and shock wave therapy gave better long-term results.[69]

A review of treatments for tennis elbow has concluded that there is strong pilot study level evidence supporting treatment with prolotherapy, polidocanol, AGF and PRP injection, but that rigorous studies of sufficient sample size are needed to determine the long-term effectiveness and safety and whether these techniques can play a definitive role.[70]

In a systematic review, all studies showed that injections of AGF (whole blood and PRP) in chronic tendinopathy had a significant impact on improving pain and/or function over time. However, only three studies using autologous whole blood had a high methodological quality assessment, and none showed any benefit when compared with a control group. The review concluded that there is strong evidence that the use of injections with autologous whole blood should not be recommended. There were no high-quality studies found on PRP treatment and therefore limited evidence to support its use in the management of chronic tendinopathy.[66]

In a subsequent double-blind, randomized, placebo-controlled trial of PRP injection versus eccentric exercises for chronic midportion Achilles tendinopathy, it was found that a PRP injection compared with a saline injection did not result in greater improvement in pain and activity.[71] Achilles tendinopathy in particular remains a frustratingly difficult therapeutic challenge.[72]

According to a Cochrane review, overall, and for individual conditions, there is currently insufficient evidence to support the use of platelet-rich therapies for treating musculoskeletal soft tissue injuries. Researchers contemplating RCTs should consider the coverage of currently ongoing trials when assessing the need for future RCTs on specific conditions. There is a need for standardization of PRP preparation methods.[73]

NICE guidance has stated that current evidence on autologous blood injection for tendinopathy raises no major safety concerns. The evidence on efficacy is inadequate, however, with few studies available that use appropriate comparators; therefore, this procedure should only be used with special arrangements for clinical governance, consent and audit or for research. Clinicians wishing to undertake autologous blood injection for tendinopathy should take the following actions:

- Inform the clinical governance leads in their Trusts.
- Ensure that patients understand the uncertainty about the procedure's efficacy, especially in the long term.
- Make patients aware of alternative treatments, and provide them with clear written information.

Use NICE's information for patients; "Understanding NICE Guidance" is recommended (available from www.nice.org.uk/IPG279publicinfo).

- Audit and review clinical outcomes of all patients having autologous blood injection for tendinopathy.

NICE encourages further research comparing autologous blood injections (with or without techniques to produce PRP) with established nonsurgical methods for managing tendinopathy. Trials should clearly describe patient selection, including the site of tendinopathy, duration of symptoms and any prior treatments, and document whether a dry needling technique is used. Outcomes should include specific measures of pain, quality of life and function and whether subsequent surgical intervention is needed.[74]

APROTININ Aprotinin (Trasylol) is a natural serine proteinase inhibitor obtained from bovine lung. As a broad-spectrum matrix metalloproteinase (MMP) inhibitor, aprotinin is used to treat many conditions, but particularly to prevent blood loss during cardiac surgery; in chronic tendinopathy, injected aprotinin may act as a collagenase inhibitor. Certain MMPs may be present in excessive proportions in patellar and rotator cuff tendinopathy, and it has been postulated that aprotinin could potentially normalize the concentration of MMPs in chronic tendinopathy, which might help healing. There have been many small uncontrolled studies reporting high rates of success in the treatment of tendinopathy.

In a case review and follow-up questionnaire for consecutive patients with tendinopathy treated by aprotinin injection, 76% had improved, 22% reported no change and 2% were worse; 64% found the injections helpful, whereas 36% experienced neither a positive nor negative effect. Achilles patients were more successfully treated than patella tendon patients.[75] In a prospective randomized trial, athletes with patella tendinopathy were injected with aprotinin, methylprednisolone or saline. At 12-month follow-up, there were 72% excellent or good responses in the aprotinin group, 59% in the methylprednisolone group, and 28% in the saline group, with 7%, 12% and 25% poor results, respectively.[76]

Another prospective, randomized, double-blind, placebo-controlled trial compared normal saline plus local anaesthetic injections and eccentric exercises with aprotinin plus local anaesthetic injection and eccentric exercise. It demonstrated no significant benefit over placebo.[77]

Potential side effects include allergy and anaphylaxis, although death has only been reported when injections were given intravenously for cardiac surgery. A delay of 6 weeks between repeat aprotinin injections for tendinopathy reduces the risk of allergic reaction.[78] The test dose of 3 to 5 ml for major procedures is similar to the therapeutic dose for tendinopathy. Injection of aprotinin for tendon injuries is currently an off-label indication.

BOTULINUM TOXIN

Botulinum toxin injection is used to treat various painful conditions, including muscle spasticity, dystonia, headache and myofascial pain. A systematic review to assess the evidence for efficacy of botulinum toxin A (BTA) compared with placebo for myofascial trigger point injection found five clinical trials that met the inclusion criteria. One trial concluded that BTA was effective, and four concluded that it was not. The review concluded that the data are limited and clinically heterogeneous, and current evidence does not support the use of BTA injection in trigger points for myofascial pain.[79]

A randomized, placebo-controlled, crossover trial examined the efficacy of botulinum toxin type A (BoNT-A) injection (Dysport) to the distal vastus lateralis muscle plus an exercise programme for chronic anterior knee pain (AKP) associated with quadriceps muscle imbalance. BoNT-A injection produced a greater reduction in pain and disability than placebo injection in carefully selected patients.[80] Three studies investigated the merits of botulinum toxin for low back pain, but only one had a low risk of bias. There is low-quality evidence that botulinum injections improve pain, function or both better than saline injections and very low-quality evidence that they were better than acupuncture or steroid injections. Further research is very likely to have an important impact on the estimate of effect and our confidence in it. Future trials should standardize patient populations, treatment protocols and comparison groups, enlist more participants and include long-term outcomes, cost-benefit analyses and clinical relevance of findings.[81]

ACTOVEGIN

Actovegin is a deproteinized hemodialysate of calf's blood postulated to improve cellular uptake and utilization of glucose and oxygen. It was initially licensed for intravenous use to improve tissue oxygen transport in patients with arterial disease and has been in use for 60 years.[82] As a gel or cream, it is also used to treat slow-healing skin lesions, such as burns or skin-grafted wounds. Given the popularity of this treatment amongst professional athletes,[83] there is a dearth of clinical trials, with little more than anecdotes in the published literature.[82,84] A Cochrane review of treatments for Achilles tendinopathy[85] has concluded that in the single small trial that compared Actovegin with a control injection, results were promising, but the severity of patient symptoms was questionable.[86] A small study has reported short-term improvement and no adverse effects when Actovegin was injected into OA knees.[87] A pilot study of autologous blood injection for muscle strains used Actovegin plus the homeopathic product Traumeel as a control treatment and found the autologous blood to be superior.[88]

COLLAGENASE

A treatment for Dupuytren's contracture that works as an alternative to surgery, Xiapex is a mixture of two collagenases produced by the bacterium *Clostridium histolyticum*. The two enzymes have complementary substrate specificity; they cleave interstitial collagen at different sites. The product is injected directly into the cord of tissue responsible for the contracture, causing collagen lysis and cord disruption. Two pivotal double-blind studies, CORD I and CORD II, have evaluated the efficacy of collagenase *C. histolyticum* in adults with Dupuytren's contracture with a palpable cord. At study entry, patients had a finger flexion contracture of 20 degrees or more and a positive table top test, defined as the inability to place the affected finger and palm flat against a table top. Patients were randomized to receive up to three injections of collagenase or placebo into the cord at 4-week intervals. If required, a finger extension procedure was performed to facilitate cord disruption. Approximately 4 weeks after the last injection, the percentage of patients who had achieved the primary endpoint, a reduction in contracture to 5 degrees or less, was significantly greater in the collagenase arm than in the placebo arm in both CORD I (64% vs. 6.8%; $p < 0.001$) and CORD II (44.4% vs. 4.8%; $p < 0.001$).[89,90] The treatment is expensive compared with other injectable therapies, but may be cost-effective when compared with surgical fasciectomy.[91]

NORMAL SALINE   Intraarticular normal saline injections have been used as a placebo in a number of RCTs pertaining to the management of knee OA; however, it is believed that these placebo injections may have a therapeutic effect that has not been quantified in the literature. A metaanalysis of randomized, placebo-controlled trials on injection therapy for knee OA between 2006 and 2016 has concluded that the administration of an intraarticular normal saline placebo injection yields a statistically and clinically meaningful improvement in patient-reported outcomes up to 6 months after injection.[92] However, this begs the intriguing questions of how one would perform a placebo-controlled trial of saline injections and how would the mechanism of the therapeutic effects be determined. The potential for a therapy that is low-tech, cheap and readily available, apparently without side effects, and that might be repeatable with impunity demands to be taken seriously.

**RADIOSYN-
OVECTOMY**   Radiosynovectomy (RSV; also known as radiosynoviorthesis) is the local intraarticular injection of radionuclides (beta particle emitters) in colloidal form for radiotherapy. First used in 1952 for medical synovectomy, the technique treats resistant synovitis of individual joints after failure of long-term systemic pharmacotherapy and intraarticular corticosteroid injections. RSV relieves pain and inflammation from rheumatoid arthritis, for which it initially was used, and is accepted as an alternative to surgical synovectomy in cases of this or other inflammatory joint diseases, such as haemophiliac arthropathy. A systematic review and metaanalysis of the effectiveness of [169]erbium–[186]rhenium RSV (used predominantly in small joints) and [90]yttrium RSV (used predominantly in knee joints) has reported that success rates are high, but differences in effect with corticosteroid injection are less evident. However, there is marked heterogeneity in the design of the small number of comparative studies. In comparison with surgical synovectomy, RSV produces equivalent results, costs less, allows the patient to remain ambulatory and is repeatable. RSV has been proposed as the initial procedure of choice for the treatment of patients with haemarthrosis in haemophilia. In addition, the local instillation of radiopharmaceuticals can effectively reduce effusions after implantation of a

prosthesis.[93,94] RSV is recommended for the treatment of chronic or recurrent acute calcium pyrophosphate crystal arthritis (pseudogout).[95]

OTHER INJECTION TREATMENTS

New treatment modalities for arthropathy and tendinopathy and novel potential pharmacological agents have been and are currently being evaluated as joint and soft tissue injection therapies.[96-100] A promising idea is the use of high-volume injections. In a preliminary study, athletes with resistant tendinopathy who failed to improve with an eccentric loading program were injected with 10 ml of 0.5% bupivacaine hydrochloride, 25 mg of hydrocortisone acetate and 40 ml normal saline solution under ultrasound guidance. There was a statistically significant difference between baseline and 3-week follow-up in all the outcome measures, with improved symptoms, reduced neovascularization and decreased maximal tendon thickness.[101]

Finally, it may be useful to bear in mind that a promising treatment is generally just the larval stage of a disappointing one.[102]

REFERENCES

1. Pemberton R. *Arthritis and Rheumatoid Conditions. Their Nature and Treatment.* Philadelphia: Lea and Febiger; 1935.
2. Ropes MW, Bauer W. *Synovial Fluid Changes in Joint Disease.* Cambridge, MA: Harvard University Press; 1953.
3. National Institute for Health and Care Excellence. https://www.nice.org.uk/guidance/cg177.
4. Uthman I, Raynauld JP, Haraoui B. Intra-articular therapy in osteoarthritis. *Postgrad Med J.* 2003;79:449–453.
5. Hyaluronan or hylans for knee osteoarthritis? *Drug Ther Bull.* 1999;37(9):71–72.
6. Bellamy N, Campbell J, Robinson V, et al. Viscosupplementation for the treatment of osteoarthritis of the knee. *Cochrane Database Syst Rev.* 2006;(2):CD005321.
7. Jordan KM, Arden NK, Doherty M, et al. Standing Committee for International Clinical Studies Including Therapeutic Trials ESCISIT. EULAR Recommendations 2003: an evidence- based approach to the management of knee osteoarthritis: report of a Task Force of the Standing Committee for International Clinical Studies Including Therapeutic Trials (ESCISIT). *Ann Rheum Dis.* 2003;62:1145–1155.
8. Recommendations for the medical management of osteoarthritis of the hip and knee: 2000 update. American College of Rheumatology Subcommittee on Osteoarthritis Guidelines. *Arthritis Rheum.* 2000;43:1905–1915.
9. Maheu E, Rannou F, Reginster JY. Efficacy and safety of hyaluronic acid in the management of osteoarthritis: evidence from real-life setting trials and surveys. *Semin Arthritis Rheum.* 2016;45(suppl):S28–S33.
10. Bannuru RR, Natov NS, Obadan IE, et al. Therapeutic trajectory of hyaluronic acid versus corticosteroids in the treatment of knee

osteoarthritis: a systematic review and meta-analysis. *Arthritis Rheum.* 2009;61(12):1704–1711.

11. Richette P, Chevalier X, Ea HK, et al. Hyaluronan for knee osteoarthritis: an updated meta-analysis of trials with low risk of bias. *RMD Open.* 2015;1(1):e000071.

12. Jorgensen A, Stengaard-Pedersen K, Simonsen O, et al. Intra-articular hyaluronan is without clinical effect in knee osteoarthritis: a multicentre, randomised, placebo-controlled, double-blind study of 337 patients followed for 1 year. *Ann Rheum Dis.* 2010;69:1097–1102.

13. Chevalier X, Jerosch J, Goupille P, et al. Single, intra-articular treatment with 6 ml hylan G-F 20 in patients with symptomatic primary osteoarthritis of the knee: a randomised, multicentre, double-blind, placebo-controlled trial. *Ann Rheum Dis.* 2010;69:113–119.

14. Berenbaum F, Grifka J, Cazzaniga S, et al. A randomised, double-blind, controlled trial comparing two intra-articular hyaluronic acid preparations differing by their molecular weight in symptomatic knee osteoarthritis. *Ann Rheum Dis.* 2012;71:1454–1460.

15. Kotz R, Kolarz G. Intra-articular hyaluronic acid: duration of effect and results of repeated treatment cycles. *Am J Orthop.* 1999;29(suppl 11): 5–7.

16. Wang CT, Lin J, Chang CJ, et al. Therapeutic effects of hyaluronic acid on osteoarthritis of the knee; a meta-analysis of randomized controlled trials. *J Bone Joint Surg Am.* 2004;86:538–545.

17. Qvistgaard E, Christensen R, Torp PS, et al. Intra-articular treatment of hip osteoarthritis: a randomized trial of hyaluronic acid, corticosteroid, and isotonic saline. *Osteoarthritis Cartilage.* 2006;14(2):163–170.

18. Fernandez-Lopez JC, Ruano-Ravina A. Efficacy and safety of intraarticular hyaluronic acid in the treatment of hip osteoarthritis: a systematic review. *Osteoarthritis Cartilage.* 2006;14(12):1306–1311.

19. van den Bekerom MP, Lamme B, Sermon A, et al. What is the evidence for viscosupplementation in the treatment of patients with hip osteoarthritis? Systematic review of the literature. *Arch Orthop Trauma Surg.* 2008;128(8):815–823.

20. van den Bekerom MPJ, Rys B, Mulier M. Viscosupplementation in the hip: evaluation of hyaluronic acid formulations. *Arch Orthop Trauma Surg.* 2008;128(3):275–280.

21. Tagliafico A, Serafini G, Sconfienza LM, et al. Ultrasound-guided viscosupplementation of subacromial space in elderly patients with cuff tear arthropathy using a high weight hyaluronic acid: prospective open-label non-randomized trial. *Eur Radiol.* 2011;21(1): 182–187.

22. Brander VA, Gomberawalla A, Chambers M, et al. Efficacy and safety of hylan G-F 20 for symptomatic glenohumeral osteoarthritis: a prospective, pilot study. *PM R.* 2010;2(4):259–267.

23. Blaine T, Moskowitz R, Udell J, et al. Treatment of persistent shoulder pain with sodium hyaluronate: a randomized, controlled trial. A multicenter study. *J Bone Joint Surg Am.* 2008;90(5):970–979.

24. Heyworth BE, Lee JH, Kim PD, et al. Hylan versus corticosteroid versus placebo for treatment of basal joint arthritis: a prospective, randomized, double-blinded clinical trial. *J Hand Surg Am.* 2008;33(1):40–48.

25. Schumacher HR, Meador R, Sieck M, et al. Pilot investigation of hyaluronate injections for first metacarpal-carpal (MC-C) osteoarthritis. *J Clin Rheumatol.* 2004;10(2):59–62.

26. Mei-Dan O, Kish B, Shabat S. Treatment of osteoarthritis of the ankle by intra-articular injections of hyaluronic acid: a prospective study. *J Am Podiatr Med Assoc.* 2010;100(2):93–100.

27. Abate M, Pulcini D, Di Iorio A, et al. Viscosupplementation with intra-articular hyaluronic acid for treatment of osteoarthritis in the elderly. *Curr Pharm Des.* 2010;16(6):631–640.

28. Bernardeau C, Bucki B, Liote F. Acute arthritis after intra-articular hyaluronate injection: onset of effusions without crystal. *Ann Rheum Dis.* 2001;60:518–520.

29. Leopold SS, Warme WJ, Pettis PD, et al. Increased frequency of acute local reaction to intra-articular hylan GF-20 (Synvisc) in patients receiving more than one course of treatment. *J Bone Joint Surg Am.* 2002;84:1619–1623.

30. Rovetta G, Monteforte P. Intraarticular injection of sodium hyaluronate plus steroid versus steroid in adhesive capsulitis of the shoulder. *Int J Tissue React.* 1998;20(4):125–130.

31. Callegari L, Spano E, Bini A, et al. Ultrasound-guided injection of a corticosteroid and hyaluronic acid: a potential new approach to the treatment of trigger finger. *Drugs RD.* 2011;11(12):137–145.

32. http://www.carbylan.com/u/files/cor11_clinical_trial_hydrosta.pdf.

33. Saito S, Momohara S, Taniguchi A, et al. The intra-articular efficacy of hyaluronate injections in the treatment of rheumatoid arthritis. *Mod Rheumatol.* 2009;19(6):643–651.

34. Saito S, Kotake S. Is there evidence in support of the use of intra-articular hyaluronate in treating rheumatoid arthritis of the knee? A meta-analysis of the published literature. *Mod Rheumatol.* 2009;19(5):493–501.

35. Dagenais S, Mayer J, Haldeman S, et al. Evidence-informed management of chronic low back pain with prolotherapy. *Spine J.* 2008;8(1):203–212.

36. Dorman T, Ravin T. *Diagnosis and Injection Techniques in Orthopaedic Medicine.* Baltimore, MD: Williams and Wilkins; 1991:33–34.

37. Reeves KD, Sit RW, Rabago DP. Dextrose prolotherapy: a narrative review of basic science, clinical research, and best treatment recommendations. *Phys Med Rehabil Clin N Am.* 2016;27(4): 783–823.

38. Jensen KT, Rabago DP, Best TM, et al. Early inflammatory response of knee ligaments to prolotherapy in a rat model. *J Orthop Res.* 2008;26(6):816–823.

39. Fleming S, Rabago DP, Mundt MP, et al. CAM therapies among primary care patients using opioid therapy for chronic pain. *BMC Complement Altern Med.* 2007;7:15.

40. Dagenais S, Yelland MJ, Del Mar C, et al. Prolotherapy injections for chronic low-back pain. *Cochrane Database Syst Rev.* 2007;(2): CD004059.

41. Rabago D, Slattengren A, Zgierska A. Prolotherapy in primary care practice. *Prim Care.* 2010;37(1):65–80.

42. Dagenais S, Haldeman S, Wooley JR. Intraligamentous injection of sclerosing solutions (prolotherapy) for spinal pain: a critical review of the literature. *Spine J*. 2005;5(3):310–328.

43. Cusi M, Saunders J, Hungerford B, et al. The use of prolotherapy in the sacroiliac joint. *Br J Sports Med*. 2010;44(2):100–104.

44. Reeves KD, Hassanein K. Randomized, prospective, placebo-controlled double-blind study of dextrose prolotherapy for osteoarthritic thumb and finger (DIP, PIP, and trapeziometacarpal) joints: evidence of clinical efficacy. *J Altern Complement Med*. 2000;6(4): 311–320.

45. Topol GA, Reeves KD, Hassanein KM. Efficacy of dextrose prolotherapy in elite male kicking-sport athletes with chronic groin pain. *Arch Phys Med Rehabil*. 2005;86(4):697–702.

46. Reeves KD, Hassanein KM. Long term effects of dextrose prolotherapy for anterior cruciate ligament laxity. *Altern Ther Health Med*. 2003;9(3):58–62.

47. Yelland MJ, Sweeting KR, Lyftogt JA, et al. Prolotherapy injections and eccentric loading exercises for painful Achilles tendinosis: a randomised trial. *Br J Sports Med*. 2011;45(5):421–428.

48. Maxwell NJ, Ryan MB, Taunton JE, et al. sonographically guided intratendinous injection of hyperosmolar dextrose to treat chronic tendinosis of the achilles tendon: a pilot study. *AJR Am J Roentgenol*. 2007;189:W215–W220.

49. Ryan MB, Wong AD, Gillies JH, et al. Sonographically guided intratendinous injections of hyperosmolar dextrose/lidocaine: a pilot study for the treatment of chronic plantar fasciitis. *Br J Sports Med*. 2009;43(4):303–306.

50. Yelland MJ, Glasziou PP, Bogduk N, et al. Prolotherapy injections, saline injections, and exercises for chronic low-back pain: a randomized trial. *Spine*. 2004;29(1):9–16.

51. Hauser RA, Lackner JB, Steilen-Matias D, et al. A systematic review of dextrose prolotherapy for chronic musculoskeletal pain. *Clin Med Insights Arthritis Musculoskelet Disord*. 2016;9:139–159.

52. Hung CY, Hsiao MY, Chang KV, et al. Comparative effectiveness of dextrose prolotherapy versus control injections and exercise in the management of osteoarthritis pain: a systematic review and meta-analysis. *J Pain Res*. 2016;9:847–857.

53. Sit RW, Chung VCh, Reeves KD, et al. Hypertonic dextrose injections (prolotherapy) in the treatment of symptomatic knee osteoarthritis: a systematic review and meta-analysis. *Sci Rep*. 2016;6:25247.

54. Krstičević M, Jerić M, Došenović S, et al. Proliferative injection therapy for osteoarthritis: a systematic review. *Int Orthop*. 2017;41(4):671–679.

55. Rabago D, Nourani B. Prolotherapy for osteoarthritis and tendinopathy: a descriptive review. *Curr Rheumatol Rep*. 2017;19(6):34.

56. Sanderson LM, Bryant A. Effectiveness and safety of prolotherapy injections for management of lower limb tendinopathy and fasciopathy: a systematic review. *J Foot Ankle Res*. 2015;8:57.

57. Morath O, Kubosch EJ, Taeymans J, et al. The effect of sclerotherapy and prolotherapy on chronic painful Achilles tendinopathy – a

systematic review including meta-analysis. *Scand J Med Sci Sports.* 2018;28(1):4–15.

58. Bertrand H, Reeves KD, Bennett CJ, et al. Dextrose prolotherapy versus control injections in painful rotator cuff tendinopathy. *Arch Phys Med Rehabil.* 2016;97(1):17–25.

59. Seven MM, Ersen O, Akpancar S, et al. Effectiveness of prolotherapy in the treatment of chronic rotator cuff lesions. *Orthop Traumatol Surg Res.* 2017;103(3):427–433.

60. Lee DH, Kwack KS, Rah UW, et al. Prolotherapy for refractory rotator cuff disease: retrospective case-control study of 1-year follow-up. *Arch Phys Med Rehabil.* 2015;96(11):2027–2032.

61. Rabago D, Kijowski R, Woods M, et al. Association between disease-specific quality of life and magnetic resonance imaging outcomes in a clinical trial of prolotherapy for knee osteoarthritis. *Arch Phys Med Rehabil.* 2013;94(11):2075–2082.

62. Ohberg L, Alfredson H. Ultrasound guided sclerosis of neovessels in painful chronic Achilles tendinosis: pilot study of a new treatment. *Br J Sports Med.* 2002;36:173–177.

62a. Hoksrud A, Ohberg L, Alfredson H, et al. Ultrasound-guided sclerosis of neovessels in painful chronic patellar tendinopathy: a randomized controlled trial. *Am J Sports Med.* 2006;34(11):1738–1746.

63. Zeisig E, Fahlström M, Ohberg L, et al. Pain relief after intratendinous injections in patients with tennis elbow: results of a randomised study. *Br J Sports Med.* 2008;42(4):267–271.

64. van Sterkenburg MN, de Jonge MC, Sierevelt IN, et al. Less promising results with sclerosing ethoxysclerol injections for midportion achilles tendinopathy: a retrospective study. *Am J Sports Med.* 2010;38(11):2226–2232.

65. Creaney L, Hamilton B. Growth factor delivery methods in the management of sports injuries: the state of play. *Br J Sports Med.* 2008;42:314–320.

66. de Vos RJ, van Veldhoven PLJ, Moen MH, et al. Autologous growth factor injections in chronic tendinopathy: a systematic review. *Br Med Bull.* 2010;95:63–77.

67. Kon E, Buda R, Filardo G, et al. Platelet-rich plasma: intra-articular knee injections produced favorable results on degenerative cartilage lesions. *Knee Surg Sports Traumatol Arthrosc.* 2010;18(4):472–479.

68. Chen CPC, Cheng CH, Hsu CC, et al. The influence of platelet-rich plasma on synovial fluid volumes, protein concentrations, and severity of pain in patients with knee osteoarthritis. *Exp Gerontol.* 2017;93:68–72.

69. Ozturan KE, Yucel I, Cakici H, et al. Autologous blood and corticosteroid injection and extracorporeal shock wave therapy in the treatment of lateral epicondylitis. *Orthopedics.* 2010;33(2):84–91.

70. Rabago D, Best TM, Zgierska AE, et al. A systematic review of four injection therapies for lateral epicondylosis: prolotherapy, polidocanol, whole blood and platelet-rich plasma. *Br J Sports Med.* 2009;43(7):471–481.

71. de Vos RJ, Weir A, van Schie HT, et al. Platelet-rich plasma injection for chronic Achilles tendinopathy: a randomized controlled trial. *JAMA.* 2010;303(2):144–149.

72. Magnussen RA, Dunn WR, Thomson AB. Nonoperative treatment of midportion Achilles tendinopathy: a systematic review. *Clin J Sports Med*. 2009;19(1):54–64.

73. Moraes VY, Lenza M, Tamaoki MJ, et al. Platelet-rich therapies for musculoskeletal soft tissue injuries. *Cochrane Database Syst Rev*. 2014;(4):CD010071.

74. National Institute for Health and Clinical Excellence. Autologous blood injection for tendinopathy. https://www.nice.org.uk/Guidance/IPG438.

75. Orchard J, Massey A, Brown R. Successful management of tendinopathy with injections of the MMP-inhibitor aprotinin. *Clin Orthop Relat Res*. 2008;466(7):1625–1632.

76. Capasso G, Testa V, Maffulli N, et al. Aprotinin, corticosteroids and normosaline in the management of patellar tendinopathy in athletes: a prospective randomized study. *BMJ Open Sport Exerc Med*. 1997;3:111–115.

77. Brown R, Orchard J, Kinchington M, et al. Aprotinin in the management of Achilles tendinopathy: a randomised controlled trial. *Br J Sports Med*. 2006;40(3):275–279.

78. Orchard J, Massey A, Rimmer J, et al. Delay of 6 weeks between aprotinin injections for tendinopathy reduces risk of allergic reaction. *J Sci Med Sport*. 2008;11(5):473–480.

79. Ho KY, Tan KH. Botulinum toxin A for myofascial trigger point injection: a qualitative systematic review. *Eur J Pain*. 2007;11(5):519–527.

80. Singer BJ, Silbert PL, Song S, et al. Treatment of refractory anterior knee pain using botulinum toxin type A (Dysport) injection to the distal vastus lateralis muscle: a randomised placebo controlled crossover trial. *Br J Sports Med*. 2011;45(8):640–645.

81. Waseem Z, Boulias C, Gordon A, et al. Botulinum toxin injections for low-back pain and sciatica. *Cochrane Database Syst Rev*. 2011;(1):CD008257.

82. Lee P, Rattenberry A, Connelly S, et al. Our experience on Actovegin; is it cutting edge? *Int J Sports Med*. 2011;32(4):237–241.

83. Tsitsimpikou C, Tsiokanos A, Tsarouhas K, et al. Medication use by athletes at the Athens 2004 Summer Olympic Games. *Clin J Sports Med*. 2009;19(1):33–38.

84. Lee P, Kwan A, Nokes L. Actovegin – cutting-edge sports medicine or "voodoo" remedy? *Curr Sports Med Rep*. 2011;10(4):186–190.

85. McLauchlan GJ, Handoll HH. Interventions for treating acute and chronic Achilles tendinitis. *Cochrane Database Syst Rev*. 2001;(2):CD000232.

86. Pförringer W, Pfister A, Kuntz G. The treatment of Achilles paratendinitis: results of a double-blind, placebo-controlled study with a deproteinized hemodialysate. *Clin J Sports Med*. 1994;4(2):92–99.

87. Kuptniratsaikul V, Kuptniratsaikul S. Intra-articular injection of deproteinized hemodialysate in osteoarthritis of the knee: a case-series. *J Med Assoc Thai*. 2004;87(1):100–105.

88. Wright-Carpenter T, Klein P, Schäferhoff P, et al. Treatment of muscle injuries by local administration of autologous conditioned serum:

a pilot study on sportsmen with muscle strains. *Int J Sports Med.* 2004;25(8):588–593.

89. Hurst LC, Badalamente MA, Hentz VR, et al. Injectable collagenase Clostridium histolyticum for Dupuytren's contracture. *N Engl J Med.* 2009;361:968–979.

90. Gilpin D, Coleman S, Hall S, et al. Injectable collagenase Clostridium histolyticum: a new nonsurgical treatment for Dupuytren's disease. *J Hand Surg Am.* 2010;35:2027–2038.

91. Mehta S, Belcher H. A single-centre cost comparison analysis of collagenase injection versus surgical fasciectomy for Dupuytren's contracture of the hand. *J Plast Reconstr Aesthet Surg.* 2014;67:368–372.

92. Saltzman BM, Leroux T, Meyer MA, et al. The therapeutic effect of intra-articular normal saline injections for knee osteoarthritis. *Am J Sports Med.* 2017;45(11):2647–2653.

93. van der Zant FM, Boer RO, Moolenburgh JD, et al. Radiation synovectomy with (90)Yttrium, (186)Rhenium and (169)Erbium: a systematic literature review with meta-analyses. *Clin Exp Rheumatol.* 2009;27(1):130–139.

94. Schneider P, Farahati J, Reiners C. Radiosynovectomy in rheumatology, orthopedics, and hemophilia. *J Nucl Med.* 2005;46(suppl 1):48S–54S.

95. Abhishek A, Doherty M. Update on calcium pyrophosphate deposition. *Clin Exp Rheumatol.* 2016;34(suppl 98):32–38.

96. Maffulli N, Longo UG, Loppini M, et al. New options in the management of tendinopathy. *Open Access J Sports Med.* 2010;1:29–37.

97. Forslund C, Aspenberg P. Improved healing of transected rabbit Achilles tendon after a single injection of cartilage-derived morphogenetic protein-2. *Am J Sports Med.* 2003;31:555–559.

98. Connell D, Datir A, Alyas F, et al. Treatment of lateral epicondylitis using skin-derived tenocyte-like cells. *Br J Sports Med.* 2009;43:293–298.

99. Cui Y, Xiao Z, Shuxia W, et al. Computed tomography guided intra-articular injection of etanercept in the sacroiliac joint is an effective mode of treatment of ankylosing spondylitis. *Scand J Rheumatol.* 2010;39(3):229–232.

100. International Olympic Committee. IOC consensus statement on molecular basis of connective tissue and muscle injuries in sport; 2007. www.olympic.org/en/content/The-IOC/Commissions/Medical/?Tab=2.

101. Humphrey J, Chan O, Crisp T, et al. The short-term effects of high-volume image-guided injections in resistant non-insertional Achilles tendinopathy. *J Sci Med Sport.* 2010;13(3):295–298.

102. Bastian H. Learning from evidence-based mistakes. *Br Med J.* 2004;329:1053.

SECTION 1

CHAPTER 4: LANDMARK- AND IMAGE-GUIDED INJECTION THERAPY

OVERVIEW

The new millennium has seen a great increase in the number of investigations into the accurate placement of musculoskeletal injections. A search on PubMed (May 2017) using the term *accuracy of intraarticular injection* revealed 15 studies before 2000 (1948–1999) and 221 (human) studies between 2000 and 2017.

Traditionally, joint and soft tissue injections have mostly been facilitated via the visualization and palpation of anatomical landmarks to guide appropriate placement. A number of studies have reported on the comparative accuracy of landmark-guided and image-guided joint and soft tissue injection techniques, and some have explored the relationship between the accuracy of these injections and clinical outcomes (see tables on the website that accompanies this book).

Some authors describe landmark-guided injections as *blind*, but we avoid using this term because it undermines and undervalues the skills required for successful application of this technique.

CORRECT INJECTION PLACEMENT

EXPERIENCE The experience and seniority of the injector do not appear to influence the accuracy of injection placement in some studies[1-3] but do in others, with the more experienced injectors being more accurate.[4-8] Experienced injectors may be overconfident about how accurate they are.[9]

NEEDLE SIZE It is important to use a needle that is long enough, especially in obese patients, or the joint cavity may not be reached. For example, in the knee, a 2-inch needle may sometimes be required rather than a standard 1.5-inch needle.[10]

Measured arthroscopically, the mean distance from skin surface to the subacromial bursa with anterior needle placement is 29 ± 6 mm (maximum, 35 mm [1.4 inches]), with lateral needle placement 29 ± 7 mm (maximum, 36 mm [1.4 inches]) and with posterior needle placement 52 ± 11 mm (maximum, 63 mm [2.5 inches]) in a group of patients with a mean body mass index of 27.5 (range, 18.7–42.8). The distance to the subacromial bursa from the anterior and lateral approaches appears to be consistent and within reach of a standard 21 gauge (green, 40 mm) needle.[11]

ENTRY SITE AND POSITIONING

The choice of entry portal and positioning of a joint may affect accurate injection placement. The superolateral approach to the knee appears to be the most accurate, using landmarks.[12,13] In one study, injecting a dry knee in the extended position using a lateral midpatellar approach into the patellofemoral joint was intraarticular more than 90% of the time and more accurate than injecting through the eyes of the knee (anteromedial and anterolateral to the patellar tendon), with the knee in partial flexion.[10] Aspirating the knee with the patient in a supine position is more successful than aspirating the knee with the patient sitting.[14.]

In a systematic review, the posterior landmark approach to glenohumeral joint injection was found to be more accurate than the anterior approach,[8] but other studies support the latter.[5,9,15,16]

PAIN ON INJECTION

"A painful injection is a misplaced injection" is a good rule of thumb. Once through the skin, an injection should be painless unless the needle touches bone.

When injecting hyaluronans (HAs), the small amount of viscous fluid and the resistance to flow in the needle may make it difficult to feel whether the solution is passing into periarticular tissue or into the joint space. Pain during the injection, and increased pain afterwards, is associated with extraarticular needle placement and may be linked to a higher incidence of adverse reactions. Once the instantaneous discomfort of needle placement has subsided, the injection of HA should not be painful.[10]

CONFIRMATION OF NEEDLE PLACEMENT

Needle placement may be confirmed when an effusion is present. During joint aspiration, the appearance of synovial fluid indicates intraarticular placement of the needle.[10] Remarkably, however, even the ability to aspirate fluid is not a perfect predictor of intraarticular placement of a subsequent injection.[1]

In the absence of an effusion, needle placement requires the use of anatomical landmarks and tactile feedback to help the clinician position the needle. Minimal retraction of the needle after "caressing" articular cartilage or bone with the needle tip may help ensure intraarticular placement.[10] Successful placement of an intraarticular knee injection may be confirmed by adding 1 to 2 ml of air to the injection. Immediately following the procedure a squishing sound is audible from the knee when it is passively moved through its range of motion. In one small study, this simple test had a sensitivity of 85% and a specificity of 100%.[17] A similar test has been described in the shoulder.[18] When the needle is correctly sited for a carpal tunnel injection, pulling back on the plunger causes a small bubble of air to be aspirated into the syringe (our observation).

The backflow technique may be used to ascertain the accurate placement of the needle for intraarticular injections in patients with dry osteoarthritic knee – that is, a knee without any clinically detectable effusion. A small volume of normal saline is injected and reaspirated, the premise being that successful reaspiration indicates that the needle is in the joint. In 32 of 33 cases in one osteoarthritic knee study, with obtained backflow, the needle was correctly placed in all 32. In the remaining case, the needle was positioned outside the joint. Further studies are needed to assess the technique for other joint injections.[19] It does not appear to be a reliable technique at the hip.[20]

For trigger finger injections, the synovial space between the tendon and sheath is narrow and often difficult to enter by direct injection. In one study, just before surgical release, 72 patients had methylene blue dye injected percutaneously into the synovial sheaths of the finger. The dye was present within the sheath in only 49% of cases.[21] To facilitate accurate injection, the flexor tendons are palpated over the metacarpal head, with the fingers extended. The patient is then asked to flex the fingers, and the needle is inserted through the sheath and onto the tendon. The patient is then asked to extend the fingers. If the bevel of the needle has penetrated too far and has entered the tendon, it will slip out and remain in the synovial space as the tendon moves distally. Confirmation of synovial space placement occurs when there is no resistance to instillation. The technique may also be used for injection into the synovial space surrounding the thumb (trigger thumb). In this case, the space is entered at the midpoint of the proximal phalanx of the thumb on the volar surface. The needle is aimed at an oblique angle in a proximal direction, with the thumb extended. The patient is asked to flex the thumb that pulls the tendon away from the needle end.[22]

Successful injection of the trapeziometacarpal joint (TMCJ) may be indicated by observing that the thumb extends slightly while being injected, the so-called thumbs-up sign.[23]

The whoosh test may be used to confirm accurate needle placement in caudal epidurals. This involves listening for a whoosh, with a stethoscope placed over the sacrum while a small amount of air is injected before the attempt to inject into the epidural space. In a small study of patients undergoing caudal epidural injection, 19 of 26 patients had correct needle placement as determined by epidurography. All of them had a positive whoosh test, and there were no false-positives.[24]

POSTINJECTION

If local anaesthetic is part of the injection mixture, then postinjection retesting should elicit a significant improvement in pain, sometimes to the extent of temporary total abolition. The physical signs should also improve.

ACCURACY OF LANDMARK TECHNIQUE INJECTIONS

When expert clinicians deliver intraarticular injections, they normally do not need guidance from imaging techniques to place the needle successfully in the target area.[9,13,25,26] For most joint injections, it is sufficient to follow an anatomical landmark.[27] Even the hip, a joint considered relatively inaccessible,[27] may be successfully injected using anatomical landmarks.[28-30] although image guidance is often recommended.[20,31]

However, some studies have reported variable accuracy in placement of the needle in landmark-guided intraarticular injections.[3,32,33] Placing the needle accurately in landmark injections may be challenging in deep joints (e.g., hip or spinal joints). In addition, in conventional landmark routes, the risk of incidental needling or drug delivery to the adjacent nontarget structures, which may include blood vessels, peripheral nerves, muscles, ligaments, intratendinous tissue and subcutaneous fat, cannot be completely avoided.[25]

Studies examining the landmark techniques cited below are summarized in the tables on the website that accompanies this book.

CADAVER STUDIES

Landmark-guided injection techniques have been studied in cadavers. Either dye is injected and then a dissection performed, or radiopaque material is injected and an x-ray is taken to assess how accurately the injectate has been placed. Conclusions from cadaveric studies must be interpreted with caution because they may not be able to be reproduced in a clinical setting.[34]

Based on their findings from these cadaveric studies, some authors have recommended image guidance under certain circumstances. For example, landmark-guided injecting may be too inaccurate in the acromioclavicular and finger joints, so correct positioning of the needle in the joint could be facilitated by fluoroscopy or musculoskeletal ultrasound (MSKUS), thereby guaranteeing an intraarticular injection,[25] particularly in doubtful cases,[27] because an unintended periarticular injection may cause complications, and an unsuccessful aspiration can delay diagnosis.[35,36] Optimized techniques might improve the accuracy and limit the dispersal of landmark-guided injections in clinical situations, benefiting efficacy and safety, but further evaluation is required in these settings.[37] Although further clinical research is warranted, clinicians should consider imaging guidance to optimize injectate placement into areas when optimal accuracy is necessary for diagnostic purposes to assist in surgical decision making or if the joint is abnormal.[38,39]

Choice of portals, such as in knee injection (often cited as one of the technically easier techniques) might depend on the experience of the clinician,[12,13] although 100% accuracy cannot be obtained through any portal. This should be kept in mind when treating knee problems with intraarticular medications.[12,40]

A crossover trial has evaluated the relative success of MSKUS-guided and landmark-guided aspirations of first metatarsophalangeal joint effusions simulated in fresh-frozen cadavers. In this study, MSKUS-guided aspiration did not prove superior to landmark-guided aspiration for first-pass aspiration, and there was no statistically significant time difference to complete a successful aspiration.[41]

A cadaver study of artificially created effusions in the hip, ankle and wrist was unable to detect significant differences in actual procedural success between MSKUS-guided versus landmark-guided arthrocentesis.[42]

A cadaver study of tennis elbow injections resulted in the majority being localized in the elbow joint.[56]

CLINICAL STUDIES

Clinical studies supporting the accuracy of landmark-guided injections

Some studies have reported accuracy of 80% or greater for landmark-guided joint and soft tissue injections at multiple sites,[43] including the subacromial space, knee, TMCJ and shoulder joint.[9,10,19,44-47]

Hip injections by use of the direct anterior approach, from the intersection of the lines drawn from the anterior superior iliac spine and 1 cm distal to the tip of the greater trochanter were found to be safe and reproducible in one study, with 51 correct needle placements and 4 misses, yielding a 93% success rate.[30] In another study, 78% accuracy was reported for hips that were injected from a lateral approach; when unsuccessful, the injected material was not found close to any neurovascular structures. This technique had an acceptable learning curve and, it was suggested, could be used safely in a standard office setting.[28]

In a subacromial injection study, the accuracy of landmark-guided and MSKUS-guided injection was the same; the fluid was injected using landmarks into the bursa in all cases as reliably as with MSKUS-guided injection, and landmark-guided injection was recommended for routine daily use.[44] In another study, landmark-guided injections performed in the subacromial region by experienced individuals were reliably accurate and, the authors concluded, could therefore be given in daily routines.[26] In a systematic review and metaanalysis, MSKUS-guided injections showed greater accuracy for all shoulder girdle injections compared with landmark guidance, with the exception of the subacromial space.[48]

The landmark-guided, superolateral approach to the knee joint is highly accurate.[12,13] One study using real-time fluoroscopic imaging with contrast material investigated landmark- guided needle placement into the intraarticular space of the knee when an effusion was not present. A lateral midpatellar injection into the patellofemoral joint was intraarticular 93% of the time and was more accurate than injections performed by the same orthopaedic surgeon using two other portals. This study highlighted the need for clinicians to refine their injection technique.[10]

In a controlled, prospective, double-blind study, landmark-guided tendon sheath injection for de Quervain tendovaginitis was more than 80% accurate.[49] Landmark-guided injections appear to be particularly accurate in patients with rheumatoid arthritis (RA).[50,51] There was however, a 25% soft tissue extravasation rate for successful intraarticular injection in one study.[47] Some of these studies had very small numbers of subjects, so the results must be treated with caution.

Clinical studies not supporting the accuracy of landmark-guided injections

The glenohumeral joint proved difficult to inject accurately using landmark guidance in three studies, with success rates ranging between 27 and 52%.[2,32,34] In some studies, landmark- guided injection of the subacromial space was also challenging, with success rates between 27 and 70%.[32,52,53] There is a 60% potential for acromioclavicular (AC) joint injections to be out of the joint if performed by landmarks alone, and the routine use of image intensification guidance has been recommended for this injection.[54] Despite the relatively superficial location of the AC joint, the clinical accuracy of AC joint injections remains relatively low.[55]

In another study of landmark-guided TMCJ injections, the needle was incorrectly placed, and its position had to be adjusted using fluoroscopy in 42% of cases to ensure correct intraarticular placement. Entering into an osteoarthritic TMCJ was not straightforward.[57]

In two studies, the success rate of landmark hip injections was from 51 to 65%. Obese patients, patients with severe grade 4 arthritis and no joint space and those with flexion deformities were the majority of failed cases. The authors proposed that hip injections should be carried out by trained specialists under imaging guidance.[20,31] The trochanteric bursa was successfully injected only 45% of the time in one study.[58]

Again, some of these studies had very small numbers of subjects, so the results must be treated with caution.

IMAGE-GUIDED INJECTIONS

Image guided injections have been in use for many years, especially techniques using x-ray guidance (fluoroscopy) for spinal injections. Other imaging techniques, including air and contrast x-ray arthrography, CT and MRI (using a vertically open magnetic resonance unit) have also been used to guide injections and localize needle placement.

In the new millennium, musculoskeletal ultrasound (MSKUS), a safe, noninvasive, patient-friendly and readily repeatable form of imaging has been taken up widely, particularly in Europe. Elsewhere, however, there has been less enthusiasm amongst clinicians who treat musculoskeletal disorders.[59] MSKUS has been enthusiastically advocated as a highly useful tool to guarantee accurate injection delivery and successful aspiration.[25,60-62]

ACCURACY The gold standard for determining the accuracy of any injection technique is an immediate postinjection surgical dissection when the exact location of the injectate can be directly visualized.[21,28] The gold standard imaging test is contrast arthrography with x-rays or MRI. Studies to verify the accuracy of MSKUS using gold standard techniques have been undertaken.[63] Innovative methodologies are continuously being developed, such as the glucocorticoid-air-saline mixture (GAS)–graphy method, as an alternative to the radiographic contrast medium method in verifying successful landmark-guided intraarticular injections.[43]

UTILITY OF MUSCULO-SKELETAL ULTRASOUND The feasibility and accuracy of MSKUS for guided musculoskeletal injections has been demonstrated for many regions of the locomotor system. These include the subacromial bursa,[52] radiocarpal joint,[64] carpal tunnel,[65] trigger finger,[66] hip,[67,68] knee,[69] Achilles and patellar tendons[70] and foot and ankle.[71]

THE FUTURE OF MUSCULO-SKELETAL ULTRASOUND Rheumatologists are being encouraged to introduce MSKUS into their clinical practice.[72]

Benefits

There is accumulating evidence that MSKUS improves clinical diagnosis and intervention skills. High-resolution ultrasound is superior to clinical examination in the diagnosis and localization of joint and bursal effusion and synovitis. MSKUS is the imaging modality of choice for the diagnosis of tendon pathology. It is seven times more sensitive than plain radiography for the detection of rheumatoid erosions, allowing for earlier diagnosis of progressive RA. Ligament, muscle, peripheral nerve and cartilage pathology can also be readily demonstrated by MSKUS. There is evidence that it might be able to be used by rheumatologists to diagnose and monitor not just joint and muscle disease noninvasively, but also nerve compression syndromes, scleroderma, vasculitis and Sjögren syndrome.

Joint aspiration and injection accuracy can be improved by MSKUS, with improved short- term (2–6 weeks) efficacy over landmark-guided injections.[48,63,73-77] As the number of rheumatologists (and other clinicians) performing MSKUS increases, and technical capabilities improve, there is likely to be a growing number of proven clinical indications for its application in rheumatology practice.[72] MSKUS-guided injections may offer a useful alternative in difficult cases, such as patients with altered anatomy postoperatively, or when there is no effective clinical outcome from a landmark-guided injection.[78]

One group of authors is very firmly of the opinion that although landmark-guided intraarticular shoulder injections are inexpensive and easily applicable, injection should be performed under imaging control.[79]

Disadvantages

Although MSKUS is a flexible and promising imaging modality for the future, and is likely to become a routine part of musculoskeletal clinical management, its introduction remains controversial, reflecting the relative infancy of the area. Problems to overcome include the significant investment in time and money required to set up a service and the lack of outcome data.[80]

There is a significant learning curve and time commitment for the acquisition of MSKUS skills that are also highly operator-dependent with moderate to good interobserver reliability.[81] In particular, guided injections of deep anatomical targets require more experience than superficial injections. The oblique direction of the needle to the ultrasound beam in deep injections decreases its visibility during these procedures.[25]

Further consensus on the standardization of scanning techniques and diagnostic criteria is necessary to improve the consistency of MSKUS.[82] There also appears to be a tendency in the current literature to emphasize the positives and highlight marginal benefits, and not to delve too deeply into the duration of any benefits or issues related to cost-effectiveness.[62,83,84]

One group of authors is very firmly of the opinion that image guidance is not necessary for injecting the knee joint. They have therefore continued the use of landmark-guided intraarticular knee injections in an effort to reduce cost, as compared with other injection modalities, with positive results.[85]

IMAGE GUIDANCE AND CLINICAL OUTCOMES

The main question is whether image-guided injections, irrespective of their greater potential for accuracy, produce significantly different clinical outcomes from those using anatomical landmarks.[27] There have been relatively few high-quality, prospective, randomized controlled trials (RCTs) investigating this issue. A central concern in clinical practice is the need for proof of clinical relevance and improved patient care when using guided injections.[85] Although many MSKUS studies have indicated improved accuracy compared with landmark-guided techniques, there is evidence for only short-term benefit (2–6 weeks) for MSKUS over landmark techniques, and the cost-effectiveness is uncertain.[48,62,75-77,86] There has been a paucity of studies investigating important endpoints,[83] and one study indicated no difference in outcomes for MSKUS-guided compared with landmark-guided subacromial injections.[87]

STUDIES THAT CORRELATE EFFECTIVENESS WITH ACCURACY

All these studies used some form of imaging to determine the placement of the injectate. In one study, 148 painful joints were randomized to injection by conventional landmark guidance or MSKUS-guided injection enhanced with a one-handed control syringe (the reciprocating device). Relative to conventional landmark methods, MSKUS guidance resulted in a reduction in procedural pain and absolute pain scores at the 2-week outcome. MSKUS also increased detection of effusion by 200% and volume of aspirated fluid by 337% and, the authors concluded, significantly improved the performance and outcomes of outpatient injections in a clinically significant manner (over 2 weeks) compared with conventional landmark guidance.[60] A small number of shoulder studies have indicated that image-guided intraarticular injections may offer advantages over a landmark-guided technique for the treatment of adhesive capsulitis and may deliver clinical benefits during the first few weeks of treatment. This suggests that the improved targeting to the intraarticular space by using MSKUS may result in better treatment.[88]

In one study of subacromial impingement, 2 weeks after treatment, failure to obtain an accurate placement was associated with return to pretreatment assessment values, whereas significant improvement continued in patients who were accurately injected.[45] In another study, at 2 weeks postinjection of the subacromial space and glenohumeral joint, there were significant positive differences in relation to outcome between the accurately and inaccurately placed groups.[32] In another shoulder study, at 6 weeks postinjection, there was significantly greater improvement with MSKUS versus landmark guidance. The authors suggested that MSKUS-guided injections should at least be indicated for patients with a poor response to a previous landmark-guided injection to ensure accurate medication placement.[89]

Another study compared joint and soft tissue aspiration between a conventional landmark-guided technique and a MSKUS-guided technique. In the landmark group, 32 joints in 30 consecutive patients were aspirated by an experienced consultant rheumatologist. In the image-guided group, 31 consecutive patients were examined by MSKUS to confirm the presence and location of fluid. Following MSKUS examination, aspiration was performed by a second rheumatologist based on the MSKUS localization of fluid or under direct MSKUS guidance. Its use to localize joint and soft tissue fluid collection greatly improved the rate of diagnostic synovial fluid aspiration, particularly in small joints; the authors stated that there were important implications for the accurate administration of local steroid therapy, highlighting the importance of MSKUS as a useful tool in clinical rheumatological practice.[73]

STUDIES THAT DO NOT CORRELATE EFFECTIVENESS WITH ACCURACY

In a study of patients with RA, clinicians who used MSKUS guidance reliably assessed the accuracy of joint injection, whereas those who used landmark guidance did not. One-third of landmark-guided injections were inaccurate, but there was no significant difference in clinical outcome between the group receiving MSKUS-guided injections and the group receiving landmark-guided injections. MSKUS guidance significantly improved the accuracy of joint injection, allowing a trainee to achieve higher accuracy than more experienced rheumatologists rapidly, but did not improve the short-term outcome of joint injection.[50]

In a study of landmark-guided glenohumeral injections, about 50% were not intracapsular. Improvements in all subjects for pain and self-reported function at 4 weeks postinjection occurred irrespective of accuracy, even in light of a wide variance in subject duration of symptoms, multiple injectors with varied training, landmark approach to injection and multiple injection approaches. The accuracy of the injection did not appear to depend on the experience of the physician, and the authors suggested that experience might be irrelevant in treating shoulder pain of multiple origins.[2]

In another study, the accuracy of subacromial injection was 70%. There was significant improvement in shoulder function and pain level at 3 months postinjection, but clinical improvement did not correlate with accuracy, although accurate injections did reliably produce a positive impingement test.[53] No significant differences were found in the clinical outcomes of another study comparing ultrasound-guided subacromial injections with landmark-guided injections for subacromial impingement syndrome.[90]

CT control–guided and landmark-guided approaches to performing suprascapular nerve blocks result in similar significant and prolonged reductions in pain and disability. Both approaches are safe.[91]

During trochanteric bursa injections, one group of investigators found that radiological confirmation of bursal spread is necessary to ensure that the injectate reaches the area of pathology.[92] Subsequently, however, the same group found that this does not improve outcomes compared with landmark-guided injection. They also noted that fluoroscopic guidance dramatically increases treatment costs for greater trochanteric pain syndrome.[58]

In another study, accurate intraarticular injection of corticosteroid did not result in superior outcome in terms of pain compared with inaccurate injection in symptomatic knee OA.[93]

MSKUS-guided injection is effective for the management of plantar fasciitis, but is not more effective than landmark-guided injection. MSKUS may be used as an objective measure of response to treatment in plantar fasciitis.[94,95] In another study, MSKUS-guided, palpation-guided and scintigraphy-guided injections were equally effective in the conservative treatment of plantar fasciitis at 25 months postinjection.[96]

Ultrasound-guided injections were carried out in 20 sacroiliac joints (SIJs) of 14 consecutive patients suffering from active sacroiliitis. Immediately following SIJ injection, MRI scanning was performed to verify the correct placement of the drug. Only 8 injections (40%) were exactly positioned into the SIJ space, whereas the other 12 injections (60%) missed it. However, there were no significant differences observed in the clinical outcome between the accurately injected group and the group injected via the periarticular route. There was similar pain relief observed in both groups 24 hours and 28 days following the intervention, respectively. These results demonstrate that intraarticular SIJ injections remain technically challenging despite ultrasound guidance, but also indicate that periarticular deposition of triamcinolone appears sufficient for pain and symptom control in patients suffering from active sacroiliitis.[63]

Carpal tunnel syndrome responds to injections deliberately given proximal to the tunnel.[97] In one de Quervain study, there were better outcomes associated with more accurate injections,[49] but good outcomes were found in another study when the injection was deliberately placed outside the tendon sheath.[98]

There was no significant difference in clinical outcomes between a group receiving MSKUS-guided injections and a group receiving landmark-guided injections of the distal radioulnar joint (DRUJ). MSKUS-guided injection showed significantly higher accuracy than landmark-guided injection in the DRUJ, and corticosteroid injections were effective in improving the pain of patients with DRUJ disorder during 6 months of follow-up.[99]

Unexpectedly, one study indicated better results for trigger finger with injections outside the sheath; 95 patients with 107 trigger digits were divided into two groups and studied prospectively to evaluate steroid injection placement and efficacy. In one group, an attempt was made to inject into the tendon sheath at the A1 pulley; in the other group, one injection infiltrated the subcutaneous tissues overlying the A1 pulley. Radiopaque dye was added to the injection medium, and postinjection x-rays identified the true delivery site. Of the 52 digits into which intrasheath injection was attempted, 19 digits (37%) received all the injection within the sheath, 24 (46%) into both the sheath and subcutaneous tissues and 9 (17%) received no medication within the tendon sheath. The results were analysed to determine whether injection placement influences the efficacy of steroid injection. The confirmed all-sheath injection group exhibited a 47% good response, the mixed sheath and subcutaneous group had a 50% good response and the all-subcutaneous group had a 70% good response. The results suggest that true intrasheath injection offers no apparent advantage over subcutaneous injection in the treatment of trigger digits.[100]

WHY MIGHT CLOSE ENOUGH BE GOOD ENOUGH?

In some cases, an injection that is outside but close to the target may be effective. A good therapeutic response may be experienced when an attempted joint or tendon sheath injection is periarticular or peritendinous, suggesting that the total accuracy of needle placement may not be essential to a satisfactory outcome.[1,47,100]

The effect of accurate needle placement on the therapeutic response to local corticosteroid injection needs further elucidation.[63] Various explanations have been put forth, but the mechanism of local corticosteroid action is not well understood. Both a systemic effect and a local action by diffusion of the steroid suspension, either into blood vessels or the surrounding anatomical structures, could explain the therapeutic effect, even when the injection does not reach the target tissue.

Systemic corticosteroid administration is certainly effective for some focal musculoskeletal conditions. Oral prednisolone, 30 mg daily for 3 weeks, is superior to placebo for improving pain, function and range of motion in adhesive shoulder capsulitis, with significant short-term benefits, although these are not maintained beyond 6 weeks.[101] In two intriguing studies, no important differences in short-term outcomes were found between local

MSKUS-guided corticosteroid injection and systemic corticosteroid injection in rotator cuff disease.[102,103] Injecting a joint and finding another distant joint significantly improved is a phenomenon familiar to all regular injectors.

It is plausible that precise deposition of a musculoskeletal injection is not always required. If so, we do not yet know in which circumstances absolute precision is critical.

THE FUTURE FOR LANDMARK-GUIDED INJECTIONS

For most, if not all, disorders treated by musculoskeletal injection, the optimum landmark- guided technique has yet to be firmly established. The approaches described in this text are based on our clinical experience and on techniques described in the medical literature. Further studies are needed to verify reproducible and accurate methods of therapeutic delivery into joint and soft tissue lesions without the need for imaging confirmation. Novel approaches should be welcomed and vigorously evaluated.[97,104,105]

There is a need to develop evidence-based criteria for the selection of patients best suited to an image-guided injection. The explicit creation of anatomically accurate schematics of musculoskeletal anatomy that highlight superficial and deep landmarks and sources of potential complications relevant to needle procedures should allow for safer and more accurate nonimage-guided needle procedures.[106]

Studies could be conducted on the accuracy of needle placement in osteoarthritic patients, with the results categorized by radiographic severity, because the approach may need to be modified according to disease severity.[46]

The specific effects of training on the successful application of landmark-guided injections and aspirations have barely been explored. Of note is a study that has clearly demonstrated that nonmedical surgical care practitioners who complete hip aspirations on a regular basis have significantly lower failure rates than surgeons, probably as a result of the impressive learning curve that this study demonstrated.[107] Training on a cadaver model was found to produce significant improvement between the pretest and posttest analyses of third-year medical students in all aspects assessed in a study of elbow, knee and wrist arthrocentesis.[108] Furthermore, the utility and potential of MSKUS as a training tool to optimize landmark-guided procedures need to be fully explored and exploited.

CONCLUSION

It remains for proponents of image-guided injections to demonstrate that this approach does more than improve short-term outcomes and makes a real difference over the longer term, sufficient to justify the extra cost.[27,58,62] MSKUS guidance can maximize injection accuracy in the intended target area and minimize adverse effects, but benefits are seen only over 2 to 6 weeks (see tables on the website that accompanies this book). There is a tendency in the current literature to emphasize the positives in MSKUS-guided techniques and not consider the length of the therapeutic effects or their cost-effectiveness.

One must not forget that peripheral joint and soft tissue injection, whether image-guided or landmark-guided, is a skill, and there will be inherent differences among physicians, regardless of the level of their training or experience. This is an important confounding factor in all studies that can never be fully accounted for. Although many studies have supported improvements with image guidance, important shortcomings in study power and methodology make definitive conclusions difficult.[109,110]

The hypothesis that precise localization is always necessary for successful injection therapy is also one that needs to be tested. Until there is sufficient evidence from both participant and outcome-assessor blinded, randomized trials documenting a real difference between image- guided needle placement and the anatomical landmark-guided approach over the longer term – sufficient to justify the extra cost – the requirement for precise localization remains speculative.[59]

Image-guided injection should be reserved for specific indications (see Practice point: When image guidance may be particularly useful).[46,78,89] These indications are currently based on expert opinion. For example, there is as yet no prospective trial in which patients who have failed a landmark-guided injection have been randomized to a further landmark-guided or image-guided injection, so this indication, as with most of the others, is not currently evidence-based.

Before the use of image-guided techniques can be considered as superior or even mandatory, we need to be certain that the potential for landmark-guided techniques has been fully exploited and optimized, and that the superiority of MSKUS or other imaging techniques in daily clinical practice, particularly their cost-effectiveness, has been firmly established. We must resist replacing a nonstandardized, relatively straightforward, inexpensive approach with an equally nonstandardized, complex and expensive one. Novel treatments, especially those involving advanced technology, are seductive.[111] Before clinicians who inject invest their money in hardware, and their time and money in training and the acquisition and maintenance of a new skill, they needs to be sure that they have not fallen for the lure of technology, and that the emperor is actually wearing some clothes. Physicians are also at times driven to use the newest technology and perform many diagnostic tests for fear of litigation if they do not. This practice is often independent of the best evidence we need to provide cost-effective treatments.[112]

Therefore, until we have good evidence that image-guided injections in routine therapeutic practice are both more clinically effective and cost-effective, it seems reasonable to conclude that most injections can be given using an anatomical landmark-guided approach.

Practice point: When image guidance may be particularly useful

Diagnosis remains secure but landmark-guided injection or aspiration has failed
Purpose is primarily diagnostic, rather than therapeutic (e.g., surgical planning)
Very obese patients
Highly anatomically abnormal joints
Spinal injections
When training clinicians to inject
Verification of correct placement in research studies[113]
When monitoring the effect of injection therapy[114-118]

REFERENCES

1. Jones A, Regan M, Ledingham J, et al. Importance of placement of intra-articular steroid injection. *BMJ*. 1993;307:1329–1330.
2. Hegedus EJ, Zavala J, Kissenberth M, et al. Positive outcomes with intra-articular glenohumeral injections are independent of accuracy. *J Shoulder Elbow Surg*. 2010;19(6):795–801.
3. Pichler W, Weinberg AM, Grechenig S, et al. Intra-articular injection of the acromioclavicular joint. *J Bone Joint Surg Br*. 2009;91(12):1638–1640.
4. Heidari N, Kraus T, Fischerauer S, et al. Do the presence of pathologic changes and the level of operator experience alter the rate of intra-articular injection of the first metatarsophalangeal joint? A cadaver study. *J Am Podiatr Med Assoc*. 2013;103(3):204–207.
5. Mattie R, Kennedy DJ. Importance of image guidance in glenohumeral joint injections: comparing rates of needle accuracy based on approach and physician level of training. *Am J Phys Med Rehabil*. 2016;95(1):57–61.
6. Maricar N, Parkes MJ, Callaghan MJ, et al. Where and how to inject the knee – a systematic review. *Semin Arthritis Rheum*. 2013;43(2):195–203.
7. Curtiss HM, Finnoff JT, Peck E, et al. Accuracy of ultrasound-guided and palpation-guided knee injections by an experienced and less-experienced injector using a superolateral approach: a cadaveric study. *PM R*. 2011;3(6):507–515.
8. Daley EL, Bajaj S, Bison LJ, et al. Improving injection accuracy of the elbow, knee, and shoulder: Does injection site and imaging make a difference? A systematic review. *Am J Sports Med*. 2011;39(3):656–662.
9. Sidon E, Velkes S, Shemesh S, et al. Accuracy of non assisted glenohumeral joint injection in the office setting. *Eur J Radiol*. 2013;82(12):e829–e831.
10. Jackson DW, Evans NA, Thomas BM. Accuracy of needle placement into the intra-articular space of the knee. *J Bone Joint Surg Am*. 2002;84:1522–1527.
11. Sardelli M, Burks RT. Distances to the subacromial bursa from 3 different injection sites as measured arthroscopically. *Arthroscopy*. 2008;24(9):992–996.
12. Hermans J, Bierma-Zeinstra SM, Bos PK, et al. The most accurate approach for intra-articular needle placement in the knee joint: a systematic review. *Semin Arthritis Rheum*. 2011;41(2):106–115.
13. Maricar N, Parkes MJ, Callaghan MJ, et al. Where and how to inject the knee – a systematic review. *Semin Arthritis Rheum*. 2013;43(2):195–203.
14. Zhang Q, Zhang T, Lv H, et al. Comparison of two positions of knee arthrocentesis: how to obtain complete drainage. *Am J Phys Med Rehabil*. 2012;91(7):611–615.
15. Tobola A, Cook C, Cassas KJ, et al. Accuracy of glenohumeral joint injections: comparing approach and experience of provider. *J Shoulder Elbow Surg*. 2011;20(7):1147–1154.

16. Jo CH, Shin YH, Shin JS. Accuracy of intra-articular injection of the glenohumeral joint: a modified anterior approach. *Arthroscopy*. 2011;27(10):1329–1334.

17. Glattes RC, Spindler KP, Blanchard GM, et al. A simple, accurate method to confirm placement of intra-articular knee injection. *Am J Sports Med*. 2004;32:1029–1031.

18. Jacobs LGH, Barton MAJ, Wallace WA, et al. Intra-articular distension and steroids in the management of capsulitis of the shoulder. *BMJ*. 1991;302:1498–1501.

19. Luc M, Pham T, Chagnaud C, et al. Placement of intra-articular injection verified by the backflow technique. *Osteoarthritis Cartilage*. 2006;14(7):714–716.

20. Diraçoğlu D, Alptekin K, Dikici F, et al. Evaluation of needle positioning during blind intra-articular hip injections for osteoarthritis: fluoroscopy versus arthrography. *Arch Phys Med Rehabil*. 2009;90(12):2112–2115.

21. Kahmin M, Engel J, Heim M. The fate of injected trigger fingers. *Hand*. 1983;15:218–220.

22. Platt AJ, Black MJM. Injection into the synovial space of the flexor tendons of the hand. *Ann R Coll Surg Engl*. 1996;78:392.

23. Erpelding JM, Shnayderman D, Mickschl D, et al. The "Thumbs-up" sign and trapeziometacarpal joint injection: a useful clinical indicator. *Hand (N Y)*. 2015;10(2):362–365.

24. Lewis MP, Thomas P, Wilson LF, et al. The 'whoosh' test; a clinical test to confirm correct needle placement in caudal epidural injections. *Anaesthesia*. 1992;47(1):57–58.

25. Iagnocco A, Naredo E. Ultrasound-guided corticosteroid injection in rheumatology: accuracy or efficacy? *Rheumatology* (Oxford). 2010;49(8):1427–1428.

26. Dogu B, Yucel SD, Sag SY, et al. Blind or ultrasound-guided corticosteroid injections and short-term response in subacromial impingement syndrome: a randomized, double-blind, prospective study. *Am J Phys Med Rehabil*. 2012;91(8):658–665.

27. Hall S, Buchbinder R. Do imaging methods that guide needle placement improve outcome? *Ann Rheum Dis*. 2004;63:1007–1008.

28. Ziv YB, Kardosh R, Debi R, et al. An inexpensive and accurate method for hip injections without the use of imaging. *J Clin Rheumatol*. 2009;15(3):103–105.

29. Hoeber S, Aly AR, Ashworth N, et al. Ultrasound-guided hip joint injections are more accurate than landmark-guided injections: a systematic review and meta-analysis. *Br J Sports Med*. 2016;50(7):392–396.

30. Mei-Dan O, McConkey MO, Petersen B, et al. The anterior approach for a non-image-guided intra-articular hip injection. *Arthroscopy*. 2013;29(6):1025–1033.

31. Kurup H, Ward P. Do we need radiological guidance for hip joint injections? *Acta Orthop Belg*. 2010;76(2):205–207.

32. Eustace JA, Brophy DP, Gibney RP, et al. Comparison of the accuracy of steroid placement with clinical outcome in patients with shoulder symptoms. *Ann Rheum Dis*. 1997;56:59–63.

SECTION 1

33. Sethi PM, El Attrache N. Accuracy of intra-articular injection of the glenohumeral joint: a cadaveric study. *Orthopedics*. 2006;29:149–152.

34. Sethi PM, Kingston S, Elattrache N. Accuracy of anterior intra-articular injection of the glenohumeral joint. *Arthroscopy*. 2005;21(1):77–80.

35. Pichler W, Grechenig W, Grechenig S, et al. Frequency of successful intra-articular puncture of finger joints: influence of puncture position and physician experience. *Rheumatology* (Oxford). 2008;47(10):1503–1505.

36. Partington PF, Broome GH. Diagnostic injection around the shoulder: hit and miss? A cadaveric study of injection accuracy. *J Shoulder Elbow Surg*. 1998;7(2):147–150.

37. Hanchard N, Shanahan D, Howe T, et al. Accuracy and dispersal of subacromial and glenohumeral injections in cadavers. *J Rheumatol*. 2006;33(6):1143–1146.

38. Wisniewski SJ, Smith J, Patterson DG. Ultrasound-guided versus nonguided tibiotalar joint and sinus tarsi injections: a cadaveric study. *PM R*. 2010;2(4):277–281.

39. Kirk KL, Campbell JT, Guyton GP, et al. Accuracy of posterior subtalar joint injection without fluoroscopy. *Clin Orthop Relat Res*. 2008;466(11):2856–2860.

40. McGarry JG, Daruwalla ZJ. The efficacy, accuracy and complications of corticosteroid injections of the knee joint. *Knee Surg Sports Traumatol Arthrosc*. 2011;19(10):1649–1654.

41. Naylor JF, Dekay KB, Donham BP, et al. Ultrasound versus landmarks for great toe arthrocentesis. *Mil Med*. 2017;182(S1):216–221.

42. Berona K, Abdi A, Menchine M, et al. Success of ultrasound-guided versus landmark-guided arthrocentesis of hip, ankle, and wrist in a cadaver model. *Am J Emerg Med*. 2017;35(2):240–244.

43. Koski JM, Hermunen HS, Kilponen VM, et al. Verification of palpation-guided intra-articular injections using glucocorticoid-air-saline mixture and ultrasound imaging (GAS-graphy). *Clin Exp Rheumatol*. 2006;24(3):247–252.

44. Rutten MJ, Collins JM, Maresch BJ, et al. Glenohumeral joint injection: a comparative study of ultrasound and fluoroscopically guided techniques before MR arthrography. *Eur Radiol*. 2009;19(3):722–730.

45. Esenyel CZ, Esenyel M, Yeşiltepe R, et al. The correlation between the accuracy of steroid injections and subsequent shoulder pain and function in subacromial impingement syndrome. *Acta Orthop Traumatol Turc*. 2003;37(1):41–45.

46. Toda Y, Tsukimura N. A comparison of intra-articular hyaluronan injection accuracy rates between three approaches based on radiographic severity of knee osteoarthritis. *Osteoarthritis Cartilage*. 2008;16(9):980–985.

47. Pollard MA, Cermak MB, Buck WR, et al. Accuracy of injection into the basal joint of the thumb. *Am J Orthop*. 2007;36(4):204–206.

48. Aly AR, Rajasekaran S, Ashworth N. Ultrasound-guided shoulder girdle injections are more accurate and more effective than landmark-guided injections: a systematic review and meta-analysis. *Br J Sports Med*. 2015;49(16):1042–1049.

49. Zingas C, Failla JM, Van Holsbeeck M. Injection accuracy and clinical relief of de Quervain's tendinitis. *J Hand Surg Am*. 1998;23:89–96.

50. Cunnington J, Marshall N, Hide G, et al. A randomized, double-blind, controlled study of ultrasound-guided corticosteroid injection into the joint of patients with inflammatory arthritis. *Arthritis Rheum.* 2010;62(7):1862–1869.
51. Lopes RV, Furtado RN, Parmigiani L, et al. Accuracy of intra-articular injections in peripheral joints performed blindly in patients with rheumatoid arthritis. *Rheumatology* (Oxford). 2008;47(12):1792–1794.
52. Yamakado K. The targeting accuracy of subacromial injection to the shoulder: an arthrographic evaluation. *Arthroscopy.* 2002;18(8): 887–891.
53. Kang MN, Rizio L, Prybicien M, et al. The accuracy of subacromial corticosteroid injections: a comparison of multiple methods. *J Shoulder Elbow Surg.* 2008;17(suppl 1):61S–66S.
54. Bisbinas I, Belthur M, Said HG, et al. Accuracy of needle placement in ACJ injections. *Knee Surg Sports Traumatol Arthrosc.* 2006;14(8): 762–765.
55. Wasserman BR, Pettrone S, Jazrawi LM, et al. Accuracy of acromioclavicular joint injections. *Am J Sports Med.* 2013;41(1):149–152.
56. Keijsers R, van den Bekerom MP, Koenraadt KL, et al. Injection of tennis elbow: hit and miss? A cadaveric study of injection accuracy. *Knee Surg Sports Traumatol Arthrosc.* 2017;25(7):2289–2292.
57. Helm AT, Higgins G, Rajkumar P, et al. Accuracy of intra-articular injections for osteoarthritis of the trapeziometacarpal joint. *Int J Clin Pract.* 2003;57(4):265–266.
58. Cohen SP, Strassels SA, Foster L, et al. Comparison of fluoroscopically guided and blind corticosteroid injections for greater trochanteric pain syndrome: multicentre randomised controlled trial. *BMJ.* 2009;338:b1088.
59. Naredo E, Cabero F, Cruz A, et al. Ultrasound guided musculoskeletal injections. *Ann Rheum Dis.* 2005;64:341.
60. Sibbitt WL Jr, Peisajovich A, Michael AA, et al. Does sonographic needle guidance affect the clinical outcome of intraarticular injections? *J Rheumatol.* 2009;36(9):1892–1902.
61. Sofka CM, Collins AJ, Adler RS. Use of ultrasonographic guidance in interventional musculoskeletal procedures: a review from a single institution. *J Ultrasound Med.* 2001;20(1):21–26.
62. Huang Z, Du S, Qi Y, et al. Effectiveness of ultrasound guidance on intraarticular and periarticular joint injections: systematic review and meta-analysis of randomized trials. *Am J Phys Med Rehabil.* 2015;94(10):775–883.
63. Hartung W, Ross CJ, Straub R, et al. Ultrasound-guided sacroiliac joint injection in patients with established sacroiliitis: precise IA injection verified by MRI scanning does not predict clinical outcome. *Rheumatology* (Oxford). 2010;49(8):1479–1482.
64. Lohman M, Vasenius J, Nieminen O. Ultrasound guidance for puncture and injection in the radiocarpal joint. *Acta Radiol.* 2007;48(7):744–747.
65. Grassi W, Farina A, Filippucci E, et al. Intralesional therapy in carpal tunnel syndrome: a sonographic-guided approach. *Clin Exp Rheumatol.* 2002;20(1):73–76.

66. Bodor M, Flossman T. Ultrasound-guided first annular pulley injection for trigger finger. *J Ultrasound Med.* 2009;28:737–743.
67. Micu MC, Bogdan GD, Fodor D. Steroid injection for hip osteoarthritis: efficacy under ultrasound guidance. *Rheumatology* (Oxford). 2010;49(8):1490–1494.
68. Smith K, Hurdle MB, Weingarten TN. Accuracy of sonographically guided intra-articular injections in the native adult hip. *J Ultrasound Med.* 2009;28:329–335.
69. Im SH, Lee SC, Park YB, et al. Feasibility of sonography for intra-articular injections in the knee through a medial patellar portal. *J Ultrasound Med.* 2009;28(11):1465–1470.
70. Fredberg U, Bolvig L, Pfeiffer-Jensen M, et al. Ultrasonography as a tool for diagnosis, guidance of local steroid injection and, together with pressure algometry, monitoring of the treatment of athletes with chronic jumper's knee and Achilles tendinitis: a randomized, double-blind, placebo-controlled study. *Scand J Rheumatol.* 2004;33(2):94–101.
71. Reach JS, Easley ME, Chuckpaiwong B, et al. Accuracy of ultrasound guided injections in the foot and ankle. *Foot Ankle Int.* 2009;30(3):239–242.
72. Kang T, Lanni S, Nam J, et al. The evolution of ultrasound in rheumatology. *Ther Adv Musculoskeletal Dis.* 2012;4(6):399–411.
73. Balint PV, Kane D, Hunter J, et al. Ultrasound-guided versus conventional joint and soft tissue fluid aspiration in rheumatology practice: a pilot study. *J Rheumatol.* 2002;29:2209–2213.
74. Raza K, Lee CY, Pilling D, et al. Ultrasound guidance allows accurate needle placement and aspiration from small joints in patients with early inflammatory arthritis. *Rheumatology* (Oxford). 2003;42(8):976–979.
75. Finnoff JT, Hall MM, Adams E, et al. American Medical Society for Sports Medicine Position Statement: interventional musculoskeletal ultrasound in sports medicine. *Clin J Sport Med.* 2015;25(1):6–22.
76. Gilliland CA, Salazar LD, Borchers JR. Ultrasound versus anatomic guidance for intra-articular and periarticular injection: a systematic review. *Phys Sportsmed.* 2011;39(3):121–131.
77. Wu T, Dong Y, Song HX, et al. Ultrasound-guided versus landmark in knee arthrocentesis: a systematic review. *Semin Arthritis Rheum.* 2016;45(5):627–632.
78. Rutten MJ, Maresch BJ, Jager GJ, et al. Injection of the subacromial-subdeltoid bursa: blind or ultrasound-guided? *Acta Orthop.* 2007;78(2):254–257.
79. Ağırman M, Leblebicier MA, Durmuş O, et al. Should we continue to administer blind shoulder injections? *Eklem Hastalik Cerrahisi.* 2016;27(1):29–33.
80. Wakefield RJ, Brown AK, O'Connor PJ, et al. Musculoskeletal ultrasonography: What is it and should training be compulsory for rheumatologists? *Rheumatology* (Oxford). 2004;43(7):821–822.
81. Le Corroller T, Cohen M, Aswad R, et al. Sonography of the painful shoulder: role of the operator's experience. *Skeletal Radiol.* 2008;37(11):979–986.

82. Naredo E, Möller I, Moragues C, et al. Interobserver reliability in musculoskeletal ultrasonography: results from a "Teach the Teachers" rheumatologist course. *Ann Rheum Dis.* 2006;65:14–19.

83. Soh E, Li W, Ong KO, et al. Image-guided versus blind corticosteroid injections in adults with shoulder pain: a systematic review. *BMC Musculoskelet Disord.* 2011;12:137.

84. Raeissadat SA, Rayegani SM, Langroudi TF, et al. Comparing the accuracy and efficacy of ultrasound-guided versus blind injections of steroid in the glenohumeral joint in patients with shoulder adhesive capsulitis. *Clin Rheumatol.* 2017;36(4):933–940.

85. Bloom JE, Rischin A, Johnston RV, et al. Image-guided versus blind glucocorticoid injection for shoulder pain. *Cochrane Database Syst Rev.* 2012;(8):CD009147.

86. Lee HJ, Lim KB, Kim DY, et al. Randomized controlled trial for efficacy of intra-articular injection for adhesive capsulitis: ultrasonography-guided versus blind technique. *Arch Phys Med Rehabil.* 2009;90(12):1997–2002.

87. Dávila-Parrilla A, Santaella-Santé B, Otero-López A. Does injection site matter? A randomized controlled trial to evaluate different entry site efficacy of knee intra-articular injections. *Bol Asoc Med P R.* 2015;107(2):78–81.

88. Lee HJ, Lim KB, Kim DY, et al. Randomized controlled trial for efficacy of intra-articular injection for adhesive capsulitis: ultrasonography-guided versus blind technique. *Arch Phys Med Rehabil.* 2009;90(12):1997–2002.

89. Naredo E, Cabero F, Beneyto P, et al. A randomized comparative study of short-term response to injection versus sonographic-guided injection of local corticosteroids in patients with painful shoulder. *J Rheumatol.* 2004;31:308–314.

90. Cole BF, Peters KS, Hackett L, et al. Ultrasound-guided versus blind subacromial corticosteroid injections for subacromial impingement syndrome: a randomized, double-blind clinical trial. *Am J Sports Med.* 2016;44(3):702–707.

91. Shanahan EM, Smith MD, Wetherall M, et al. Suprascapular nerve block in chronic shoulder pain: Are the radiologists better? *Ann Rheum Dis.* 2004;63(9):1035–1040.

92. Cohen SP, Narvaez JC, Lebovits AH, et al. Corticosteroid injections for trochanteric bursitis: Is fluoroscopy necessary? A pilot study. *Br J Anaesth.* 2005;94(1):100–106.

93. Hirsch G, O'Neill TW, Kitas G, et al. Accuracy of injection and short-term pain relief following intra-articular corticosteroid injection in knee osteoarthritis – an observational study. *BMC Musculoskelet Disord.* 2017;18(1):44.

94. Kane D, Greaney T, Shanahan M, et al. The role of ultrasonography in the diagnosis and management of idiopathic plantar fasciitis. *Rheumatology.* 2001;40:1002–1008.

95. Kane D, Greaney T, Bresnihan B, et al. Ultrasound-guided injection of recalcitrant plantar fasciitis. *Ann Rheum Dis.* 1998;57:383–384.

96. Yucel I, Yazici B, Degirmenci E, et al. Comparison of ultrasound-, palpation-, and scintigraphy-guided steroid injections in the treatment of plantar fasciitis. *Arch Orthop Trauma Surg.* 2009;129(5):695–701.

97. Dammers JW, Veering MM, Vermeulen M. Injection with methylprednisolone proximal to the carpal tunnel: randomised double blind trial. *BMJ.* 1999;319(7214):884–886.

98. Apimonbutr P, Budhraja N. Suprafibrous injection with corticosteroid in de Quervain's disease. *J Med Assoc Thai.* 2003;86(3):232–237.

99. Nam SH, Kim J, Lee JH, et al. Palpation versus ultrasound-guided corticosteroid injections and short-term effect in the distal radioulnar joint disorder: a randomized, prospective single-blinded study. *Clin Rheumatol.* 2014;33(12):1807–1814.

100. Taras JS, Raphael JS, Pan WT, et al. Corticosteroid injections for trigger digits: Is intrasheath injection necessary? *J Hand Surg Am.* 1998;23:717–722.

101. Buchbinder R, Green S, Youd JM, et al. Oral steroids for adhesive capsulitis. *Cochrane Database Syst Rev.* 2006;(4):CD006189.

102. Koes BW. Corticosteroid injection for rotator cuff disease. *BMJ.* 2009;338:a2599.

103. Ekeberg OM, Bautz-Holter E, Tveita EK, et al. Subacromial ultrasound-guided or systemic steroid injection for rotator cuff disease: randomised double-blind study. *BMJ.* 2009;338:a3112.

104. Sawaizumi T, Nanno M, Ito H. De Quervain's disease: efficacy of intra-sheath triamcinolone injection. *Int Orthop.* 2007;31(2): 265–268.

105. Bankhurst AD, Nunez SE, Draeger HT, et al. A randomized controlled trial of the reciprocating procedure device for intraarticular injection of corticosteroid. *J Rheumatol.* 2007;34(1):187–192.

106. Harrell JS, Chiou-Tan FY, Zhang H, et al. Procedure-oriented sectional anatomy of the shoulder. *J Comput Assist Tomogr.* 2009;33(5): 814–817.

107. Tingle SJ, Marriott A, Partington PF, et al. Performance and learning curve of a surgical care practitioner in completing hip aspirations. *Ann R Coll Surg Engl.* 2016;98(8):543–546.

108. Kay RD, Manoharan A, Nematollahi S, et al. A novel fresh cadaver model for education and assessment of joint aspiration. *J Orthop.* 2016;13(4):419–424.

109. Hall MM. The accuracy and efficacy of palpation versus image-guided peripheral injections in sports medicine. *Curr Sports Med Rep.* 2013;12(5):296–303.

110. Kane D, Koski J. Musculoskeletal interventional procedures: with or without imaging guidance? *Best Pract Res Clin Rheumatol.* 2016;30(4):736–750.

111. Lehoux P. The power of technology; resisting the seduction through rationality. *Healthc Pap.* 2005;6(1):32–39.

112. Weinstein J. Threats to scientific advancement in clinical practice. *Spine.* 2007;32(11):S58–S62.

113. Bliddal H. Placement of intra-articular injections verified by mini air-arthrography. *Ann Rheum Dis.* 1999;58:641–643.

114. Filippucci E, Farina A, Carotti M, et al. Grey scale and power Doppler sonographic changes induced by intra-articular steroid injection treatment. *Ann Rheum Dis.* 2004;63:740–743.

115. Terslev L, Torp-Pedersen S, Qvistgaard E, et al. Estimation of inflammation by Doppler ultrasound: quantitative changes after intra-articular treatment in rheumatoid arthritis. *Ann Rheum Dis.* 2003;62:1049–1053.
116. Bliddal H, Torp-Pedersen S. Use of small amounts of ultrasound-guided air for injections [letter]. *Ann Rheum Dis.* 2000;59:926–927.
117. Kamel M, Kotob H. High frequency ultrasonographic findings in plantar fasciitis and assessment of local steroid injection. *J Rheumatol.* 2000;27:2139–2141.
118. Koski JM. Ultrasound-guided injections in rheumatology. *J Rheumatol.* 2000;27:2131–2138.

CHAPTER 5: ASPIRATION AND MISCELLANEOUS INJECTIONS

OVERVIEW

A number of conditions may be associated with a joint effusion. Fluid may also accumulate in bursae and synovial sheaths. If fluid is present, then aspiration (arthrocentesis) is useful both diagnostically and therapeutically.[1] Aspiration may rapidly relieve pain by reducing intraarticular hypertension and may be particularly helpful in reaching a diagnosis when a patient presents with an acute hot, red, swollen joint.[1,2] Diagnostic arthrocentesis is associated with a low frequency of adverse events; septic arthritis rarely occurs afterwards.[3]

An effusion in a joint is known to result in loss of muscle strength (arthrogenic muscle inhibition), so rehabilitation is unlikely to be successful unless any effusion is suppressed.[4-6] In rheumatoid arthritis (RA) of the knee, aspiration of synovial fluid before steroid injection significantly reduces the risk of relapse.[7] In inflammatory arthritis, the effect of an injection may be prolonged by 24 hours of bed rest immediately after the procedure,[8,9] but the benefit of this in osteoarthritis (OA) is less certain.[10] In OA of the knee, there is controversy as to whether the presence of an effusion predicts a better response to joint injection than if the knee is dry.[11,12]

Aspiration guidelines have been published by the Italian Society of Rheumatology (Box 1.5).[13]

Box 1.5 Italian Society of Rheumatology Arthrocentesis Guidelines, 2007[a]

- This is indicated when synovial effusion of unknown origin is present, especially if septic or crystal arthritis is suspected.
- The patient should be clearly informed of the benefits and risks of the procedure to give informed consent.
- Fluid evacuation often has a therapeutic effect and facilitates the success of the intraarticular injection that follows.
- Careful skin disinfection and the use of sterile disposable material are mandatory for avoiding septic complications.
- Disposable nonsterile gloves should always be used by the operator, mainly for his or her own protection.
- Contraindications include the presence of skin lesions or infections in the area of the puncture.
- Anticoagulant treatment is not a contraindication, providing the therapeutic range is not exceeded.
- Joint rest after arthrocentesis is not indicated.
- Ultrasonography should be used to facilitate arthrocentesis in difficult joints.

[a]Several of these recommendations were based on experts' opinions rather than on published evidence.
Modified from Punzi L, Cimmino MA, Frizziero L, et al. Italian Society of Rheumatology (SIR) recommendations for performing arthrocentesis. *Reumatismo.* 2007;59(3):227–234.

ASPIRATION

EQUIPMENT   Joint fluid may be loculated, very viscous and contain debris, all of which may prevent complete aspiration. With a small-bore needle it may be impossible to aspirate anything, so use at least a 21 gauge or even a 19 gauge needle. Disposable gloves are recommended to protect the clinician,[14] and absorbent towels are recommended to protect the treatment area.

Often, when aspirating a joint, the syringe fills up but there is still fluid to be removed. When the full syringe is disconnected from the in-situ needle fluid tends to drip out of the open end of the needle – hence the need for gloves and absorbent towels to catch the drips – so another syringe should be ready to connect immediately. A three-way connector between needle and syringe is useful to prevent having to disconnect everything. If the needle is left in the joint, and the syringe is disconnected, the pressure between the inside and outside of the joint will equalize, which may make aspiration more difficult.

A novel double-barrelled, one-handed reciprocating procedure syringe has been compared with a conventional syringe for aspiration and injection in a randomized trial. The reciprocating syringe prevented significant pain, reduced procedure time and improved physician performance of arthrocentesis. We await a cost-effectiveness analysis.[15] (See a demonstration at www.youtube.com/watch?v=wrcedExWgJE.)

TECHNIQUE   Using a landmark technique, once the needle is thought to be positioned within the fluid, hold the barrel of the syringe with the index finger and thumb of the nondominant hand while bracing the back of the same hand against the patient. This helps maintain the needle position while gently pulling on the plunger of the syringe with the dominant hand.

The flow of synovial fluid might become intermittent or stop as a result of temporary obstruction by synovial fronds, blockage by fibrin or debris, loculation of synovial fluid or displacement of the needle outside the joint cavity. Moving the tip of the needle a few millimetres or rotating it through 90 degrees may improve the flow into the syringe. Alternatively, a small amount of fluid could be injected back into the joint to clear the needle of debris or overlying fronds, allowing the aspiration to continue.[1]

In the knee it may be helpful, while maintaining position with the braced nondominant hand, to use the other hand to massage fluid towards the needle.

Emptying a large effusion may require more than one syringe. Increasing syringe size is associated with the undesirable characteristic of loss of control

---

Practice point: Local anaesthetic for knee aspiration?

Before aspiration of the knee with a large-bore (19 gauge) needle, should you inject local anaesthetic into the aspiration site to make the procedure more comfortable? Only one randomized trial (RCT) has studied this and found that it makes no difference to patient comfort.

Modified from Kirwan JR, Haskard DO, Higgens CS. The use of sequential analysis to assess patient preference for local skin anaesthesia during knee aspiration. *Br J Rheumatol*. 1984;23:210–213.

of the needle in the forward or reverse direction. Two-handed operation of a syringe results in greater control than one-handed operation.[16]

Clinical assessment

After aspiration, the fluid should be immediately examined for colour, clarity and viscosity. The clinical context will usually accurately predict the nature of the aspirate. The gross appearance of the fluid can provide a quick bedside orientation about the amount of inflammation present. Totally transparent serous fluid originates in noninflammatory conditions, of which OA is the most common, and the amount of turbidity grossly relates to the amount of inflammation.[17]

Laboratory assessment

Ideally, any aspirate should be examined in the laboratory within 4 hours of aspiration. If analysis is delayed, there will be a decrease in cell count and crystal dissolution, and artefacts will start to appear. Storage at $4\,°C$ will delay but not prevent these changes. The requirement for all aspirates to be sent for microscopy and culture to exclude crystal arthritis[18] and infection has been challenged.[19]

An estimated one-third of rheumatologists routinely send aspirated synovial fluid samples for culture, irrespective of the underlying diagnosis. This is done even when sepsis is not suspected. A review of 507 synovial fluid culture requests[20] has revealed that positive bacterial growth was rare, even when sepsis was queried on the request forms, but none was positive in any of the routine samples, throwing doubt on the value of routine synovial fluid culture. One recommended policy is that such cultures are undertaken only when infection is a possibility and in immunocompromised patients. This approach would be very cost-effective. Clinicians need to develop local policies in consultation with their colleagues.[20]

Although many laboratory tests may be performed on synovial fluid, only the white blood cell count (and percentage of polymorphonuclear lymphocytes), presence or absence of crystals, Gram staining and bacterial culture are helpful in routine clinical practice.[19,21] A critical appraisal of the relevant literature has concluded that given the importance of synovial fluid tests, rationalization of their use, together with improved quality control, should be immediate priorities. Further investigation was recommended regarding the contribution of synovial fluid inspection and white cell counts to diagnosis, as well as of the specificity and sensitivity of synovial fluid microbiological assays, crystal identification and cytology.[21]

The white cell count offers quantitative information, but the boundaries between noninflammatory and inflammatory synovial fluid, and between this and septic fluid, are very hazy, and figures have to be interpreted in the clinical setting.[17] Priority for joint aspirations with limited fluid volumes should be given instead to Gram staining, culture and crystal analysis.[22] The future may lie with innovative technological devices such as Synovial Chip (JC Krebs et al., Case Western Reserve University, Cleveland, OH, USA), a microfluidic platform that allows standardized synovial fluid cytological analysis based on specific cell surface markers in miniscule volumes of patient synovial fluid samples in the clinic.[23]

The percentage of polymorph leucocytes in synovial fluid aspirated from rheumatoid knees may have a modest predictive value for the medium-term effectiveness of subsequent intraarticular steroid injection.[24] Synovial fluid centrifugation may be of additional value in reducing the number of false-negative analyses in select patients with suspected calcium pyrophosphate deposition disease (pseudogout) and, to a lesser extent, for gout.[25]

DIAGNOSIS OF SEPSIS

Synovial fluid analysis is of major diagnostic value in acute arthritis when septic arthritis is suspected.[20] Direct microscopy with Gram staining is performed on the fluid as soon as possible. To exclude tuberculosis (TB), Ziehl-Neelsen (Z-N) staining must be specifically requested. Prolonged culture, usually 6 weeks, may be necessary. TB is more common in immunosuppressed patients, recent immigrants, Asians and alcoholics. Special cultures are also needed if fungal infection is suspected.

Inoculation of the aspirate from joints and bursae into liquid media bottles (blood culture bottles) increases sensitivity in the detection of sepsis.[26,27] *Staphylococcus aureus* is the most common organism in cases of septic arthritis (see the section on sepsis in Chapter 2). A systematic review has identified features associated with septic arthritis (Box 1.6).[28]

When done properly under sterile technique, cultures taken from knee arthrocentesis in patients without prosthetic joints should not yield a false-positive result with a perceived contaminant species. A positive specimen finding on culture should raise a strong suspicion of bacterial septic arthritis.[29]

There is a significantly high false-negative rate associated with joint aspiration in patients who have had prior administration of empirical antibiotic therapy. These patients are significantly less likely to demonstrate an organism on microscopy and culture of their initial aspirate, and their management may be compromised.[30]

In patients who have had a joint replacement, the diagnosis of periprosthetic joint infection is easily made in 90% of patients by carrying out erythrocyte sedimentation rate (ESR) and C-reactive protein (CRP) blood tests. These tests

---

Box 1.6 Predictive features for the diagnosis of nongonococcal bacterial arthritis

Risk factors that significantly increase the probability of septic arthritis
Age
Diabetes mellitus
Rheumatoid arthritis
Joint surgery
Hip or knee prosthesis
Skin infection
Human immunodeficiency virus type 1 infection

Clinical features (in order of sensitivity)
Joint pain, history of joint swelling, fever – the only findings that occur in >50% of patients
Sweats, rigors – less common findings in septic arthritis
(Sensitivity means that the condition is less likely if the feature is *not* present.)

Synovial fluid examination
The likelihood increases as the synovial fluid white blood cell count increases.

may be followed by selective aspiration of the joint for synovial fluid analysis if these values are elevated or if the clinical suspicion is high.[31]

DIAGNOSIS OF CRYSTAL ARTHROPATHY

Synovial fluid analysis is of major diagnostic value in acute arthritis when crystal arthropathy is suspected.[21] Detection of monosodium urate (MSU) and calcium pyrophosphate dihydrate (CPPD) crystals in synovial fluid, even from uninflamed joints during intercritical periods, allows a precise diagnosis of gout and of calcium pyrophosphate crystal–related arthritis (pseudogout).[1]

The identification of crystals in synovial fluids and joint tissues is the most rapid and accurate method of diagnosing the common forms of crystal-associated arthritis. Although there are numerous methods available for identifying and characterizing crystals in biological specimens, including x-ray crystallography and Fourier transform infrared spectroscopy, polarizing light microscopy is used almost exclusively for articular crystals in practice. Unfortunately, problems with reliability and reproducibility undercut the usefulness of this simple procedure.[32] When examined using polarized microscopy, MSU crystals are negatively birefringent. CPPD crystals are positively birefringent but only one in five CPPD crystals have sufficient birefringence for easy detection, and they are easily missed if searched for only using a polarized microscope.[17] For trained observers, the detection and identification of crystals in synovial fluid is a consistent procedure.[33]

The incidence of concurrent septic and crystal arthritis may be higher than previously thought. Synovial fluid samples in concomitant septic and crystal arthritis are significantly less likely to have a positive Gram stain at microscopy than in cases of an isolated septic arthritis. Clinicians should maintain a high index of suspicion for septic arthritis in these patients.[34]

One study has found that early management of patients with hot swollen joint(s), including synovial fluid aspiration and blood cultures, is not being done in accordance with guidelines. The authors of this study suggested that medical trainee curricula should incorporate joint aspiration skills as an "essential procedure" to improve trainee doctors' confidence and competence at managing acute hot swollen joint(s), adherence to guidelines and consequently, patient outcomes.[35]

IMAGE-GUIDED ASPIRATION

In joints that are difficult to aspirate (e.g., small joints in the hand), ultrasound guidance may improve the accuracy and frequency of joint aspiration, and a performance checklist has been created[36]. Ultrasonography may also be useful in revealing the presence of synovial fluid before the joint aspiration and, subsequently, distinguishing some aspects characteristic of crystal-induced arthropathies.[37] Overall, musculoskeletal ultrasound (MSKUS)–guided arthrocentesis may be superior to arthrocentesis guided by anatomical landmarks and palpation, and may result in significantly less procedural pain, improved arthrocentesis success, greater synovial fluid yield, more complete joint decompression and improved clinical outcomes.[38-40] However, a cadaver study of artificially created effusions in the hip, ankle and wrist was unable to detect significant differences in procedural success between ultrasound-guided versus landmark-guided arthrocentesis.[41]

A continental survey has highlighted the relatively low prevalence of MSKUS-guided joint aspiration and injection by rheumatologists compared with their high rate (>80%) of performing conventional joint injection in most of the European countries surveyed. The reported variations in practice and the lack of available structured training programmes for trainees in most countries indicate the need for standardized training guidelines.[42]

WHAT THE ASPIRATE MIGHT BE AND WHAT TO DO

FRANK BLOOD   Usually, there is a history of recent trauma, with the joint or bursa swelling up rapidly afterwards. Aspiration gives pain relief, allows joint movement and removes an irritant that causes synovitis. Blood often means a significant traumatic lesion, so an x-ray is mandatory. Haemarthrosis of the knee is caused by anterior cruciate ligament (ACL) rupture in up to 40% of cases (Fig. 1.2A). Joint aspiration in acute ACL injury of the knee with a suspected haemarthrosis, could be considered as a diagnostic procedure. As well as relieving pain, early joint aspiration might also improve the sensitivity of the physical examination for diagnosing an acute ACL injury.[43]

If there is a lipid layer on top of the blood, this suggests an intraarticular fracture. It may not be advisable to inject into a joint from which blood has been aspirated because there is unlikely to be a lesion that will respond, and injection may encourage further bleeding. There may also be rapid intravascular drug absorption from a bleeding surface. This view, however, has been challenged, and it has been suggested that steroid injection following aspiration of a haemarthrosis may prevent a subsequent chemical synovitis and accelerate recovery.[44] Recommended practice may change if and when more evidence becomes available. Further management depends on the cause of the haemarthrosis.

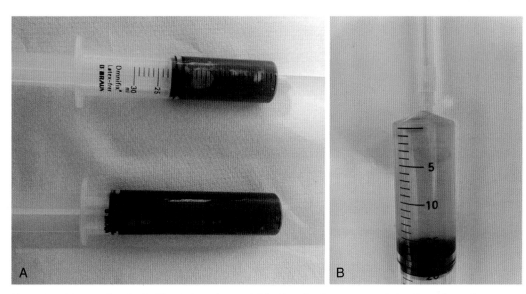

Fig. 1.2 A, Haemarthrosis. **B,** Blood-tinged synovial fluid, reflecting trauma at the time of needle insertion.

Rarely, haemarthrosis may be caused by a bleeding disorder, anticoagulant treatment or a vascular lesion in the joint (e.g., a haemangioma).

SEROUS FLUID OF VARIABLE VISCOSITY

Normal or noninflammatory synovial fluid is a viscous, colourless or pale yellow (straw-coloured) substance normally present in small amounts in joints, bursae and tendon sheaths that is often found in larger amounts when synovium is irritated (e.g., in osteoarthritis; Fig. 1.3). It has mechanical and physiological functions (see Chapter 3: Hyaluronan). It contains few cells (mainly mononuclear) and little debris and therefore appears clear. It does not clot and is very viscous because of its high hyaluronan content. This high viscosity can be demonstrated in the drip test; a small amount of aspirated fluid is gently expelled from the end of a horizontal syringe and forms a string 2-5 cm long before separating.

Greatly increased viscosity may be attributed to a recent steroid injection into that joint or to hypothyroidism.

OTHER FLUIDS

Serous fluid streaked with fresh blood

This is not uncommon and is usually related to the trauma of the aspiration. It may occur at the end of the procedure when the tap becomes dry or during the procedure if the needle tip is moved (see Fig. 1.2B).

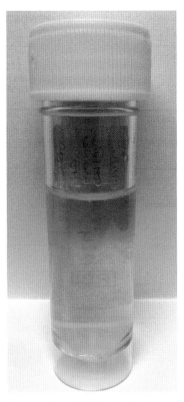

Fig. 1.3 Synovial fluid aspirated from an osteoarthritic knee.

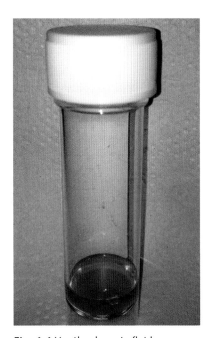

Fig. 1.4 Xanthochromic fluid.

Blood mixed with serous fluid

The terms *haemoserous* (predominantly blood) and *serosanguineous* (predominantly serous fluid) describe different types of mixed effusions.

Xanthochromic fluid

This is old blood that has broken down and appears orange in colour (Fig. 1.4). Its presence implies old trauma.

Turbid fluid

Inflammatory fluid tends to be less viscous than normal joint fluid, so it forms drops in the drip test. It also looks darker and more turbid, often with an opaque lemon colour caused by the increase in debris, cells and fibrin, and clots may form. It is impossible to determine the inflammatory process from the gross appearance, so *do not* inject but await results of direct microscopy and culture studies (Fig. 1.5A).

Increasing joint inflammation is associated with an increased volume of synovial fluid, reduced viscosity, increasing turbidity and cell count and an increasing ratio of polymorphonuclear to mononuclear cells, but such changes are nonspecific and must be interpreted in the clinical setting.[1]

Frank pus

This is rare in practice. The patient is likely to be very ill and in need of urgent hospital admission. The aspirate may have a foul smell (see Fig. 1.5B).

Other aspirates

Uniformly milky white fluid may result from plentiful cholesterol or urate crystals. Rice bodies are small shiny white objects composed of sloughed microinfarcted synovial villi.

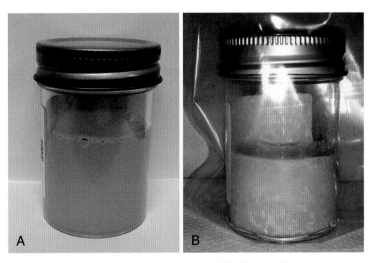

Fig. 1.5 Naked eye appearances of synovial fluids. **A,** Inflammatory synovial fluid. **B,** Pyarthrosis.

UNEXPECTED ASPIRATION

Sometimes, when performing a landmark-guided injection into a joint presumed to be dry, drawing back on the syringe to confirm that the needle is not in a blood vessel may unexpectedly aspirate joint fluid, which then contaminates the injection solution. Using gloves and towels, carefully disconnect the loaded syringe from the needle, taking care not to displace the needle tip or desterilize the tip of the syringe. Attach a fresh empty 10 ml to 20 ml syringe, lock it tightly onto the needle without displacement and aspirate.

If the aspirate is suspect, do not inject. If it remains appropriate to inject, you may use the original solution providing that it is not too heavily contaminated and that the end of the syringe is kept sterile, such as by attaching it to a sterile needle. If in doubt, draw up a fresh solution, and be sure to lock the syringe tightly onto the needle.

Very rarely, you may puncture a blood vessel, such as an artery at the wrist in a carpal tunnel injection. Fresh bright red arterial blood will pump into the syringe, which should be withdrawn, and firm pressure applied over the puncture site for several minutes.

ASPIRATING GANGLIA

Ganglion cysts account for approximately 60% of soft tissue, tumour-like swellings affecting the hand and wrist. They usually develop spontaneously in adults 20 to 50 years of age, with a female-to-male preponderance of 3 : 1. The dorsal wrist ganglion arises from the scapholunate joint and constitutes about 65% of ganglia of the wrist and hand. The volar wrist ganglion arises from the distal aspect of the radius and accounts for about 20 to 25% of ganglia. Flexor tendon sheath ganglia make up the remaining 10 to 15%. These cystic structures are found near or are attached to tendon sheaths and joint capsules. The cyst is filled with soft, gelatinous, sticky and mucoid fluid.[45]

Most ganglia resolve spontaneously and do not require treatment. If the patient has symptoms, including pain or paraesthesia, or is disturbed by the appearance, aspiration without injection of a corticosteroid may be effective[45] (Fig. 1.6). In a study comparing aspiration of wrist ganglia with aspiration

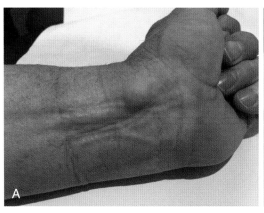 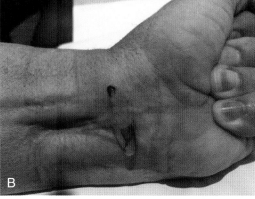

Fig. 1.6 A, Typical volar wrist ganglion. **B,** Clear viscous gel released after ganglion puncture.

plus steroid injection, both treatments had a 33% success rate. Almost all ganglia that recurred after one aspiration did not resolve with further aspirations. After aspiration and explanation of the benign nature of ganglia, only 25% of patients requested surgery.[46]

> **Practice point: Ganglia – should you aspirate?**
>
> Many untreated ganglia resolve spontaneously, with 50% of patients "ganglion-free" at 6 years. Higher rates of spontaneous resolution (70 to 80%) are reported for ganglia in children. Despite this, a large number are referred to hand surgeons for advice and treatment. Patients seek advice mainly for cosmetic reasons or because of concern about malignancy or pain. For patients who remain concerned about malignancy, seeing the aspiration fluid can reinforce verbal reassurance and reduce the demand for surgical intervention.

Modified from Burke FD, Melikyan EY, Bradley MJ, Dias JJ. Primary care referral protocol for wrist ganglia. *Postgrad Med J.* 2003;79:329–331.

MISCELLANEOUS INJECTIONS

GOUT Joint aspiration in acute gout can ease pain and facilitate diagnosis. Aspiration of joints in the intercritical period (the interval between acute attacks) can also help make the diagnosis of gout. Intraarticular injection of steroid is an effective treatment; a single dose of triamcinolone acetonide, 40 mg, may resolve symptoms within 48 hours. Smaller doses (e.g., 10 mg in knee joints or 8 mg in smaller joints) may also be effective. Intraarticular injection requires a precise diagnosis and should not be used if there is a suspicion of joint infection. The two may coexist.[47,48]

MUCOID CYSTS Mucoid cysts are small swellings typically found on the distal interphalangeal joints of patients with osteoarthritis. They are a form of ganglion and communicate directly with the joint. On the affected finger, they are often associated with nail ridging or deformity, which frequently resolves after successful injection treatment. In one study, 60% of mucoid cysts had not recurred 2 years after receiving multiple punctures with a 25 gauge needle and a small volume (<1 ml) injection of steroid and local anaesthetic.[49]

RHEUMATOID NODULES In one small study, superficial rheumatoid nodules injected with steroid and local anaesthetic disappeared or significantly reduced in volume compared with nodules injected with placebo, with no significant complications.[50]

TRIGGER POINTS Trigger points are discrete, focal, hyperirritable areas located in a taut band of skeletal muscle. They produce pain locally and in a referred pattern and often accompany chronic musculoskeletal disorders. Trigger points may manifest as regional persistent pain, tension headache, tinnitus, temporomandibular joint pain, and decreased range of motion in the legs and low back pain. Palpation of a hypersensitive bundle or nodule of muscle of harder than normal consistency is typical and may elicit pain locally and/or cause radiation of pain towards a zone of reference and a local twitch response. The commonly encountered locations of trigger points and their pain reference zones are consistent.[51]

Injection of 1% lidocaine without steroid appears to be effective.[52] The trigger point is fixed by pinching it between the thumb and index finger; the needle is then inserted 1 to 2 cm away from the trigger point and advanced into the trigger point at an angle of 30 degrees to the skin. Warn the patient of the possibility of sharp pain, muscle twitching or an unpleasant sensation as the needle contacts the taut muscular band. A small amount (0.2 ml) of local anaesthetic is injected once the needle is inside the trigger point. The needle is then withdrawn to the level of the subcutaneous tissue and redirected superiorly, inferiorly, laterally and medially, repeating the needling and injection process in each direction until the local twitch response is no longer elicited or resisting muscle tautness is no longer perceived. Repeated injections are not recommended if two or three previous attempts have been unsuccessful. Patients are encouraged to remain active, putting muscles through their full range of motion in the week following trigger point injections.[52]

DUPUYTREN DISEASE

Intralesional injection of nodules of Dupuytren disease with corticosteroid may modify progression of the disease. Over a 4-year period, 63 patients with Dupuytren nodules (75 hands) were treated with a series of injections with triamcinolone acetonide directly into the area of disease. The purpose of the study was to determine whether intralesional injections of triamcinolone acetonide could produce softening and flattening in nodules of Dupuytren disease, as seen in the intralesional injections of hypertrophic scars and keloids. After an average of 3.2 injections per nodule, 97% of the hands showed regression of disease, as exhibited by a softening or flattening of the nodule(s). Although some patients had complete resolution of the nodules, most experienced definite but incomplete resolution of the nodules, in the range of 60 to 80%. Although a few patients did not experience recurrence or reactivation of the disease in the injected nodules or the development of new nodules, 50% of patients did experience reactivation of disease in the nodules 1 to 3 years after the last injection, necessitating one or more injections.[53]

JOINT LAVAGE

Joint lavage is a technique to wash out any loose tissue or debris from inside the joint space. It involves temporally inserting small tubes into one or more entry points into the knee and running normal saline into the joint. The fluid may run out of a tube on the other side of the knee or a bag of saline may be run into the knee and then drained back into the same bag under gravity. A Cochrane review has concluded that joint lavage does not result in a relevant benefit for patients with knee osteoarthritis in terms of pain relief or improvement of function.[54]

REFERENCES

1. Courtney P, Doherty M. Joint aspiration and injection and synovial fluid analysis. *Best Pract Res Clin Rheumatol.* 2013;27(2):137–169.

2. Abhishek A, Roddy E, Doherty M. Gout – a guide for the general and acute physicians. *Clin Med (Lond)*. 2017;17(1):54–59.

3. Taylor WJ, Fransen J, Dalbeth N, et al. Diagnostic arthrocentesis for suspicion of gout is safe and well tolerated. *J Rheumatol*. 2016;43(1):150–153.

4. Reeves ND, Maffulli N. A case highlighting the influence of knee joint effusion on muscle inhibition and size. *Nat Clin Pract Rheumatol*. 2008;4(3):153–158.

5. Fahrer H, Rentsch HV, Gerber NJ, et al. Knee effusion and reflex inhibition of the quadriceps. A bar to effective retraining. *J Bone Joint Surg Br*. 1988;70:635–637.

6. Spencer JD, Hayes KC, Alexander IJ. Knee joint effusion and quadriceps reflex inhibition in man. *Arch Phys Med Rehabil*. 1984;65:171–177.

7. Weitoft T, Uddenfeldt P. Importance of synovial fluid aspiration when injecting intra-articular corticosteroids. *Ann Rheum Dis*. 2000;59:233–235.

8. Chakravarty K, Pharoah PD, Scott DG. A randomized controlled study of post-injection rest following intra-articular steroid therapy for knee synovitis. *Br J Rheumatol*. 1994;33:464–468.

9. Richards AJ. Post-injection rest following intra-articular steroid therapy for knee synovitis. *Br J Rheumatol*. 1994;33:993–994.

10. Berthelot JM, Le Goff B, Maugars Y. Side effects of corticosteroid injections: what's new? *Joint Bone Spine*. 2013;80(4):363–367.

11. Jones A, Doherty M. Intra-articular corticosteroid injections are effective in osteoarthritis but there are no clinical predictors of response. *Ann Rheum Dis*. 1996;55:829–832.

12. Gaffney K, Ledingham J, Perry JD. Intra-articular triamcinolone hexacetonide in knee osteoarthritis: factors influencing the clinical response. *Ann Rheum Dis*. 1995;54:379–381.

13. Punzi L, Cimmino MA, Frizziero L, et al. Italian Society of Rheumatology (SIR) recommendations for performing arthrocentesis. *Reumatismo*. 2007;59(3):227–234.

14. UK Departments of Health. *Guidance for Clinical Health Care Workers: Protection Against Infection with Blood-borne Viruses*. London: HMSO; 1998. http://www.open.gov.uk/doh/chcguid1.htm.

15. Draeger HT, Twining JM, Johnson CR, et al. A randomised controlled trial of the reciprocating syringe in arthrocentesis. *Ann Rheum Dis*. 2006;65(8):1084–1087.

16. Michael AA, Moorjani G, Peisajovich A. Syringe size: does it matter in physician-performed procedures? *J Clin Rheumatol*. 2009;15(2):56–60.

17. Pascual E, Jovaní V. Synovial fluid analysis. *Best Pract Res Clin Rheumatol*. 2005;19(3):371–386.

18. Dieppe P, Swan A. Identification of crystals in synovial fluid. *Ann Rheum Dis*. 1999;58:261–263.

19. Shmerling RH, Delbanco TL, Tosteson AN, et al. Synovial fluid tests – what should be ordered? *JAMA*. 1990;264:1009–1014.

20. Pal B, Nash EJ, Oppenheim B, et al. Routine synovial fluid culture: is it necessary? Lessons from an audit. *Br J Rheumatol*. 1997;36:1116–1117.

21. Swan A, Amer H, Dieppe P. The value of synovial fluid assays in the diagnosis of joint disease: a literature survey. *Ann Rheum Dis.* 2002;61:493–498.

22. Jennings JD, Zielinski E, Tosti R, et al. Septic arthritis of the wrist: incidence, risk factors, and predictors of infection. *Orthopedics.* 2017;40(3):e526–e531.

23. Krebs JC, Alapan Y, Dennstedt BA, et al. Microfluidic processing of synovial fluid for cytological analysis. *Biomed Microdevices.* 2017;19(2):20.

24. Luukkainen R, Hakala M, Sajanti E, et al. Predictive value of synovial fluid analysis in estimating the efficacy of intra-articular corticosteroid injections in patients with rheumatoid arthritis. *Ann Rheum Dis.* 1992;51:874–876.

25. Boumans D, Hettema ME, Vonkeman HE, et al. The added value of synovial fluid centrifugation for monosodium urate and calcium pyrophosphate crystal detection. *Clin Rheumatol.* 2017;36(7):1599–1605.

26. Stell IM, Gransden WR. Simple tests for septic bursitis: comparative study. *BMJ.* 1998;316:1877.

27. Von Essen R, Holtta A. Improved method of isolating bacteria from joint fluids by the use of blood culture bottles. *Ann Rheum Dis.* 1986;45:454–457.

28. Margaretten ME, Kohlwes J, Moore D, et al. Does this adult patient have septic arthritis? *JAMA.* 2007;297(13):1478–1488.

29. Jennings JM, Dennis DA, Kim RH, et al. False-positive cultures after native knee aspiration: true or false. *Clin Orthop Relat Res.* 2017;475(7):1840–1843.

30. Hindle P, Davidson E, Biant LC. Septic arthritis of the knee: the use and effect of antibiotics prior to diagnostic aspiration. *Ann R Coll Surg Engl.* 2012;94(5):351–355.

31. Ting NT, Della Valle CJ. Diagnosis of periprosthetic joint infection – an algorithm-based approach. *J Arthroplasty.* 2017;32(7):2047–2050.

32. Rosenthal AK, Mandel N. Identification of crystals in synovial fluids and joint tissues. *Curr Rheumatol Rep.* 2001;3(1):11–16.

33. Lumbreras B, Pascual E, Frasquet J, et al. Analysis for crystals in synovial fluid: training of the analysts results in high consistency. *Ann Rheum Dis.* 2005;64(4):612–615.

34. Stirling P, Tahir M, Atkinson HD. The limitations of Gram-stain microscopy of synovial fluid in concomitant septic and crystal arthritis. *Curr Rheumatol Rev.* 2017;Mar 29. doi:10.2174/157339711366661703291 23308. [Epub ahead of print].

35. Farah Z, Reddy V, Matthews W, et al. Poor adherence to guidelines on early management of acute hot swollen joint(s): an evaluation of clinical practice and implications for training. *Int J Clin Pract.* 2015;69(5):618–622.

36. Kunz D, Pariyadath M, Wittler M, et al. Derivation of a performance checklist for ultrasound-guided arthrocentesis using the modified Delphi method. *J Ultrasound Med.* 2017;36(6):1147–1152.

37. Punzi L, Oliviero F. Arthrocentesis and synovial fluid analysis in clinical practice: value of sonography in difficult cases. *Ann N Y Acad Sci.* 2009;1154:152–158.

38. Sibbitt WL Jr, Kettwich LG, Band PA, et al. Does ultrasound guidance improve the outcomes of arthrocentesis and corticosteroid injection of the knee? *Scand J Rheumatol.* 2012;41(1):66–72.

39. Wiler JL, Costantino TG, Filippone L, et al. Comparison of ultrasound-guided and standard landmark techniques for knee arthrocentesis. *J Emerg Med.* 2010;39(1):76–82.

40. Berona K, Abdi A, Menchine M, et al. Success of ultrasound-guided versus landmark-guided arthrocentesis of hip, ankle, and wrist in a cadaver model. *Am J Emerg Med.* 2017;35(2):240–244.

41. Naylor JF, Dekay KB, Donham BP, et al. Ultrasound versus landmarks for great toe arthrocentesis. *Mil Med.* 2017;182(S1):216–221.

42. Mandl P, Naredo E, Conaghan PG. Practice of ultrasound-guided arthrocentesis and joint injection, including training and implementation, in Europe: results of a survey of experts and scientific societies. *Rheumatology* (Oxford). 2012;51(1):184–190.

43. Wang JH, Lee JH, Cho Y, et al. Efficacy of knee joint aspiration in patients with acute ACL injury in the emergency department. *Injury.* 2016;47(8):1744–1749.

44. Leadbetter W. Anti-inflammatory therapy in sports injury. The role of nonsteroidal drugs and corticosteroid injection. *Clin Sports Med.* 1995;14(2):353–410.

45. Tallia AF, Cardone DA. Diagnostic and therapeutic injection of the wrist and hand region. *Am Fam Physician.* 2003;67(4):745–751.

46. Varley GW, Needoff M, Davis TR, et al. Conservative management of wrist ganglia: aspiration versus steroid infiltration. *J Hand Surg [Br].* 1997;22(5):636–637.

47. Gout in primary care. *Drug Ther Bull.* 2004;42(5):37–40.

48. Pascual E. Management of crystal arthritis. *Rheumatology* (Oxford). 1999;38:912–916.

49. Rizzo M, Beckenbaugh RD. Treatment of mucous cysts of the fingers: review of 134 cases with minimum 2-year follow-up evaluation. *J Hand Surg Am.* 2003;28(3):519–525.

50. Ching DW, Petrie JP, Klemp P, et al. Injection therapy of superficial rheumatoid nodules. *Br J Rheumatol.* 1992;31:775–777.

51. Simons DG, Travell JG, Simons LS. *Travell & Simons' Myofascial Pain And Dysfunction: The Trigger Point Manual.* 2nd ed. Baltimore: Williams & Wilkins; 1999:94–173.

52. Alvarez D, Rockwell PG. Trigger points: diagnosis and management. *Am Fam Physician.* 2002;65(4):653–661.

53. Ketchum LD, Donahue TK. The injection of nodules of Dupuytren's disease with triamcinolone acetonide. *J Hand Surg.* 2000;25:1157–1162.

54. Reichenbach S, Rutjes AW, Nüesch E, et al. Joint lavage for osteoarthritis of the knee. *Cochrane Database Syst Rev.* 2010;(5):CD007320.

CHAPTER 6: SAFETY, DRUGS AND SPORT, MEDICOLEGAL ISSUES

IMMEDIATE ADVERSE REACTIONS

Adverse reactions to corticosteroid are extremely rare: the drug most likely to provoke a serious reaction is a local anaesthetic, but reactions may also occur with other injectable substances. Always ask the patient if they have ever had a reaction to an injection. Bear in mind the guidelines in Section 2.

The most important immediate adverse reactions to injection therapy are as follows:

- Acute anaphylaxis
- Toxicity from local anaesthetic
- Syncope

ACUTE ANAPHYLAXIS

Anaphylaxis is a severe, life-threatening, generalized or systemic hypersensitivity reaction.[1] Patients who have an anaphylactic reaction have rapidly developing life-threatening airway and/or breathing and/or circulation problems usually associated with skin and mucosal changes.[1]

Acute systemic anaphylaxis results from widespread mast cell degranulation triggered by a specific allergen. Clinically, it is characterized by laryngeal oedema, bronchospasm and hypotension.[2] The true incidence of anaphylaxis is unknown; fatal anaphylaxis is rare, but probably underestimated. A register established in 1992 recording fatal reactions gave an incidence of only 20 cases per year in the United Kingdom, of which 50% were iatrogenic, mainly occurring in hospital, 25% were related to food allergy, and 25% were related to venom allergy.[3] In a published series of suspected triggers for fatal anaphylactic reactions in the United Kingdom between 1992 and 2001, only one was caused by local anaesthetic.[4]

True allergic reactions to local anaesthetic occur very rarely,[5] mainly with the ester types such as procaine and less frequently with the amide types, such as lidocaine and bupivacaine.[6] The pathomechanism of immediate hypersensitivity reactions to local anaesthetic is largely unknown; it is commonly regarded as pseudoallergic or nonimmune-type anaphylaxis. Immunologically mediated reactions have rarely been observed with positive skin prick tests. Other ingredients in local anaesthetic preparations have to be considered as elicitors – for example, preservatives such as benzoates or sulfites or latex contaminants in injection bottles.[7]

A patient may be allergic to local anaesthetic and be unaware of this. A previous uneventful injection is not a guarantee that they will not be allergic this time, although it does provide some reassurance.

Recognition of an anaphylactic reaction

A diagnosis of an anaphylactic reaction is likely if a patient who is exposed to a trigger (allergen) develops a sudden illness (usually within minutes of exposure), with rapidly progressing skin changes and life-threatening airway, breathing and/or circulation problems.[1] The reaction is usually unexpected.

Anaphylactic reactions begin rapidly. The time taken for a full reaction to evolve varies. In a fatal reaction following an intravenous drug injection or insect sting, the interval between exposure and collapse from cardiovascular shock is usually 5 to 15 minutes.[1] There are no data specifically relating to injection therapy.

The lack of any consistent clinical manifestation and a range of possible presentations cause diagnostic difficulties. Many patients with a genuine anaphylactic reaction are not given the correct treatment. Patients have been given injections of adrenaline inappropriately for allergic reactions just involving the skin or for vasovagal reactions or panic attacks.[8] Guidelines for the treatment of an anaphylactic reaction must therefore take into account some inevitable diagnostic errors, with an emphasis on the need for safety.

A single set of criteria will not identify all anaphylactic reactions. There is a range of signs and symptoms, none of which are entirely specific; however, certain combinations of signs make the diagnosis more likely.

Skin or mucosal changes alone are not a sign of an anaphylactic reaction; skin and mucosal changes may be subtle or absent in up to 20% of reactions.

The features of an allergic reaction may be any of the following – onset is usually abrupt, and the patient feels and looks ill (Table 1.4). Circulatory collapse, cardiac arrest and death may follow.

Table 1.4 Features of anaphylaxis	Symptoms	Signs
	Nervousness	Skin – blotches, urticaria (nettle rash), decreased capillary filling, clammy, (cyanosis, late sign)
	Feeling of impending catastrophe	Eyes – puffy, watering, red, sore
	Feeling drunk or confused	Nose – runny, sneezing
	Metallic taste, difficulty swallowing	Mouth – swelling of lips, tongue, throat (angiooedema), noisy breathing
	Abdominal or back pain	Voice – stridor, difficulty talking, hoarse voice
	Nausea, vomiting, diarrhoea	Chest – tachypnoea, wheezing, coughing
	Itching	Pulse – tachycardia
	Chest tightness	Blood pressure – profound hypotension
	Difficulty breathing	Neurological – loss of consciousness, convulsions

Anaphylaxis is likely when all of the following three criteria are met:[1]

- Sudden onset and rapid progression of symptoms
- Life-threatening airway, breathing and/or circulation problems
- Skin and/or mucosal changes (e.g., flushing, urticaria, angioedema)

Remember the following:

- Skin or mucosal changes alone are not a sign of an anaphylactic reaction.
- Skin and mucosal changes can be subtle or absent in up to 20% of reactions (some patients may have only a decrease in blood pressure).
- There may also be gastrointestinal symptoms (e.g., vomiting, abdominal pain, incontinence)

TREATMENT OF SEVERE ALLERGIC REACTIONS

Patients having an anaphylactic reaction should be recognized and treated using the airway, breathing, circulation, disability, exposure (ABCDE) approach, with life-threatening problems treated as they are recognized.[1] The exact treatment will depend on the patient's location, the equipment and drugs available and the skills of those treating the reaction.[1] Clinicians will give injection therapy in a variety of settings, including hospitals with and without crash teams, and various community premises, including primary care and private facilities. Every clinician must prepare for the worst case scenario in their setting and have a well thought-out plan of action that is regularly reviewed in the light of current guidelines and individual experience. Basic life support skills should be acquired and maintained. Written protocols may be laminated and mounted in consulting rooms. The immediate action to take in the presence of severe anaphylaxis is detailed in Box 1.7.

Box 1.7 Immediate action in the presence of severe anaphylaxis[a]

- Stop injecting.
- Summon help.
- Maintain the airway.
- Administer adrenaline intramuscularly.
- Administer oxygen if necessary.
- Give cardiopulmonary resuscitation if necessary.
- Transfer the patient to hospital as quickly as possible if in the community.

[a]That is, hypotension, laryngeal oedema and/or bronchospasm

Adrenaline (epinephrine)

Adrenaline reverses the immediate symptoms of anaphylaxis by its effects on alpha and beta adrenoceptors. It reverses peripheral vasodilation, reduces oedema, induces bronchodilation, has positive inotropic and chronotropic effects on the myocardium and suppresses further mediator release. It may be harmful if given outside the context of life threatening anaphylaxis.[8]

In a study of a series of deaths related to anaphylaxis, two deaths occurred after adrenaline overdose in the absence of anaphylaxis, three deaths after adrenaline overdose in the management of allergic reactions and two fatal myocardial infarctions after adrenaline administration for mild iatrogenic reactions (for which less aggressive treatment may have been appropriate).[3] Administering the doses recommended in the guidelines via the intramuscular route should avoid serious problems.

For further details on the current guidelines for the management of anaphylaxis, visit www.resus.org.uk.

TOXICITY FROM LOCAL ANAESTHETIC

Toxic effects from a local anaesthetic are usually a result of excessive plasma concentrations. Care must be taken to avoid accidental intravascular injection. The main toxic effects are excitation of the central nervous system (CNS), followed by CNS depression (Table 1.5).[6]

With an intravenous injection, convulsions and cardiovascular collapse may occur very rapidly. Significant toxic reactions to a local anaesthetic are very unlikely with the dosages recommended in this text.

Table 1.5
Features of local anaesthetic toxicity

Symptoms	Signs
Lightheadedness Feeling drunk	Sedation Circumoral paraesthesia Twitching Convulsions in severe reactions

SYNCOPE

A few people may experience syncope – that is, fainting, not as a reaction to what was injected, but to being injected – the result of pain or needle phobia (Table 1.6). Patients who express apprehension before having an injection should lie down for the procedure; the clinician may be so intent on placing the needle correctly that the warning features are missed. Unlike an anaphylactic reaction, which appears abruptly following the procedure, there are usually warning features before or during the procedure. There may be a history of fainting with previous invasive procedures, so do ask.

Table 1.6
Features of syncope

Symptoms	Signs
Anxiety before the procedure Lightheadedness, dizziness Patient tells you they are going to faint Nausea Ringing in the ears Vision "going grey"	Apprehension Pallor Sweating Slight swaying Pulse – bradycardia Blood pressure – hypotension

Syncope must be distinguished from an adverse drug reaction; it is treated by the following:

- Reassuring patients that they will recover shortly
- Lying them down in the recovery position
- Protecting the airway and giving 35% oxygen if loss of consciousness occurs

Syncope may be accompanied by brief jerking or stiffening of the extremities and may be mistaken for a convulsion by the inexperienced. Distinguishing a simple faint from a fit is helped by the presence of precipitating factors (e.g., painful stimuli, fear), and the other features described above. Incontinence is rare with syncope, and recovery of consciousness usually occurs within 1 minute.[9]

PREVENTION OF ADVERSE REACTIONS

The clinician must be prepared for any adverse reaction. Take the following precautions:

- Ask the patient about any known allergies to drugs, especially local anaesthetic.
- If in doubt, use steroid alone or diluted with normal saline.
- Lie the patient on a treatment table for the procedure.
- Control the amount of local anaesthetic given (see individual dosage recommendations).
- Always aspirate before injecting to check that the needle is not in a blood vessel.
- Ask the patient to wait for 30 minutes after the injection.
- Anyone with a suspected anaphylactic reaction should be referred to an allergy specialist.

ADVERSE REACTION REPORTING

In the United Kingdom, any severe adverse reaction to any drug treatment should be reported to the Committee on Safety of Medicines (CSM) using the Yellow Card Scheme. Yellow Card report forms can be found in the back of the *British National Formulary* (BNF).

HEALTH AND SAFETY

The clinician should be vaccinated against hepatitis B and have had a blood test to confirm immunity.[10] You should refer to your local recommendations regarding the policy on booster dosages. If in doubt, a doctor or hospital occupational health department specialist should be consulted.

Local policies on needlestick injuries must be observed. In the United Kingdom, there are national guidelines on the occupational exposure to HIV available via NHS employers (nhsemployers.org) and the Health and Safety Executive (hse.gov.uk). The best way to avoid a needlestick injury is to be well organized and never rush an injection.

EMERGENCY SUPPLIES FOR THE TREATMENT ROOM

Have a supply of emergency equipment and medications available.

ESSENTIAL EMERGENCY KIT

- Disposable plastic airways
- An Ambu bag and mask for assisted ventilation
- Adrenaline, 1:1000 (1 mg/1 ml) strength or EpiPen or Anapen device
- Oxygen with masks and tubing

ADDITIONAL EMERGENCY KIT FOR MEDICAL PERSONNEL

- Chlorpheniramine (Piriton) for injection
- Hydrocortisone for injection
- Nebulized salbutamol
- A selection of intravenous cannula and fluid-giving sets

- Normal saline for infusion
- Plasma substitute for infusion

All drugs and fluids should be checked regularly to ensure that they are in date.

DRUGS AND SPORT

Clinicians are advised to consult the latest World Anti-Doping Agency (WADA) World Anti-Doping Code and annually updated Prohibited List (International Standard) before prescribing or administering any therapeutic substance to a competitive athlete (www.wada-ama.org).

CORTICO-STEROIDS

In competition, corticosteroids come under section Section 9 of the WADA 2017 Prohibited List. All glucocorticosteroids are prohibited when administered by an oral, intravenous, intramuscular or rectal route. In accordance with the International Standard for Therapeutic Use Exemptions, a Declaration of Use must be completed by the athlete for glucocorticosteroids administered by an intraarticular, periarticular, peritendinous, epidural, intradermal and inhalation route.

Local anaesthetics

The local anaesthetics mentioned in Chapter 2 are not on the WADA prohibited list.

WORLD ANTI-DOPING AGENCY RULES

Athletes are warned that they are subject to the rule of strict liability, which means that they are responsible for any prohibited substance found in their body. It is each athlete's personal duty to ensure that no prohibited substance enters his or her body. Athletes are responsible for any prohibited substance or its metabolites or markers found to be present in their samples. Accordingly, it is not necessary that intent, fault, negligence or knowing use on the athlete's part be demonstrated to establish an antidoping violation under Article 2.1 of the WADA World Anti-Doping Code with effect from 1st April 2018.

It is expected that most athletes competing in the Olympic Games who require a therapeutic use exemption (TUE) would have already received it from their international federation. Under the WADA code, corticosteroids are one of a number of specified substances that are particularly susceptible to unintentional antidoping rule violations because of their general availability in medicinal products. Doctors and athletes should seek specific advice about drug restrictions with their own sport's governing body. In some sports, such as Australian Rules Football, corticosteroids used by a nonsystemic routes – namely, intraarticular, periarticular, peritendinous, epidural, intradermal injections and inhaled routes – are subject to a declaration of use to the sport's own medical officer (Australian Football League Anti-Doping Code).

If you are not the team doctor and wish to use injection therapy for an athlete, it would be good practice to discuss this with the team doctor. The athlete should be provided with a letter describing the rationale for treatment and the names and doses of drugs prescribed. If selected for a drug test, the athlete should declare the treatment on the doping control form. Virtually insoluble corticosteroids may be detectable months after the injection, although it is difficult to say just how many months.

Therapeutic use exemption

Athletes, like all others, may have illnesses or conditions that require them to take a particular medication. If the medication an athlete is required to take to treat an illness or condition happens to fall under the prohibited list, a TUE may give that athlete the authorization to take the needed medicine.

The criteria for granting a TUE are as follows:

- The athlete would experience significant health problems without taking the prohibited substance or method.
- The therapeutic use of the substance would not produce significant enhancement of performance.
- There is no reasonable therapeutic alternative to the use of the otherwise prohibited substance or method.

Under the World Anti-Doping Code, WADA has issued an international standard for TUEs. The standard states that all international federations (IFs) and national antidoping organizations (NADOs) must have a process in place whereby athletes with documented medical conditions can request a TUE. This request should be dealt appropriately with by a panel of independent physicians, called a therapeutic use exemption committee (TUEC). IFs and NADOs, through their TUECs, are then responsible for granting or declining such applications.

Declaration of use

A declaration of use must be made for glucocorticosteroids administered by localized injection (but intramuscular injection requires a TUE).

The UK Anti-Doping website (www.ukad.org.uk) has useful resources and links to the following:

- Declaration of Use Form
- Therapeutic Use Exemption Form
- Global Drug Reference online (www.globaldro.com)

The status of medications and substances may also be checked in the United Kingdom by calling the Drug Enquiry Line, 0800 528 0004, or by emailing at drug-free@uksport.gov.uk.

USE OF LOCAL ANAESTHETICS IN COMPETITION
The use of local anaesthetic injections to block pain temporarily and allow athletes to compete while suffering from a painful injury is a contentious issue. In professional football, the use of local anaesthetic pain-killing injections can counter the performance-reducing impact of injury and lower the rate of players missing matches through injury. In most cases, however, these injections are probably safe, although scientific evidence in this area is scant, particularly regarding long-term follow-up. The known long-term

injury sequelae of professional football injuries, such as increased rates of osteoarthritis of the knee (in particular), hip, ankle and lumbar spine, do not generally relate to the injuries for which local anaesthetic is commonly used. The most commonly injected injuries (e.g., acromioclavicular joint sprains, finger and rib injuries and iliac crest haematomas) are probably the safest to inject.[11]

Local anaesthetic injections as painkillers are to be given as follows:[11]

- They should only be used when both the doctor and player consider that the benefits clearly outweigh the anticipated possible risks.
- Intraarticular injections to the knee, ankle, wrist, joints of the foot, pubic symphysis and major tendons of the lower limb are best avoided in most circumstances.

To enable the benefit and risk profile of local anaesthetic injections to be better understood, it is recommended that professional football competitions make local anaesthetics legal only with compulsory notification.[11]

Clinicians looking after athletes who request such interventions are recommended to read John Orchard's balanced, detailed and pragmatic description of his experience in Australian professional football.[11-13] His conclusion was that local anaesthetic for pain relief can be used for certain injuries, although complications can be expected. The use of local anaesthetic in professional football may reduce the rate of players missing matches through injury, but there are risks of worsening injuries and known specific complications when local anaesthetic is used. Players requesting injections should be made fully aware of these risks and complications.

ILLICIT USE OF PERFORMANCE-ENHANCING DRUGS

Beware the athlete who is taking performance-enhancing drugs. They will probably not admit this, but if they develop complications from the use of anabolic steroids, for example, they might blame your injection. Look out for the very muscular athlete with bad skin. Otherwise healthy people, especially those who seem excessively dedicated to developing their physique, need to be asked specifically about their use of illicit drugs.[14]

MEDICOLEGAL CONSIDERATIONS

CONSENT

The courts require information to be disclosed to the patient in a discussion with the clinician. Thus, simply handing patients an explicit consent form may not be considered enough unless the issues are discussed with patients and they have an opportunity to ask further questions.[15]

1. The aim of obtaining consent should be to enable the patient to determine whether or not to undergo the proposed intervention.
2. Information should be provided in a form and manner that help patients understand the condition and treatment options available.
3. This information needs to be appropriate to the patient's circumstances, personality, expectations, fears, beliefs, values and cultural background.

What are material risks?

A risk is material if the following is involved:

- A reasonable person in the patient's position, if warned of the risk, would be likely to attach significance to it.
  or
- If the medical practitioner is or should reasonably be aware that the particular patient, if warned of the risk, would be likely to attach significance to it (Rogers v Whitaker).[16]

In general terms, a known risk should be disclosed when the following is involved:

- An adverse outcome is a common event, even though the detriment is slight.
- An outcome is severe, even though its occurrence is rare.

Summary of important points

- A competent adult patient has a right to give (or withhold) consent to a medical examination, investigation, procedure or treatment.
- A patient should be informed of the material risks associated with an intervention. A clinician who fails to provide this information risks a medical negligence claim for failure to warn.

Excellent advice about consent is also available from the UK General Medical Council at gmc-uk.org.

In the United Kingdom, the law on informed consent changed following a Supreme Court judgment in the case of Montgomery v Lanarkshire Health Board, 2015.[17] The change, however, simply enshrines in law consent practices previously recommended by the General Medical Council and UK medical defence organizations. Doctors must now ensure that patients are aware of any "material risks" involved when undergoing a proposed treatment and of reasonable alternatives. This replaces the Bolam test, which asked whether a doctor's conduct would be supported by a responsible body of medical opinion. "The test of materiality is whether, in the circumstances of the particular case, a reasonable person in the patient's position would be likely to attach significance to the risk, or the doctor is or should reasonably be aware that the particular patient would be likely to attach significance to it" (Duffy J. A year on from Montgomery. mdujournal.themdu.com).

In the context of joint and soft tissue injections, the patient must be informed about the relevant risks and benefits of the injection. The clinician should document that such a discussion has taken place and that the patient has consented to the treatment. In England, the patient is not required to sign a consent form, and this may be less medicolegally robust than clear and reasonable documentation of the discussion in the notes. According to the Medical Protection Society website, 'The notes do not need to be exhaustive, but should state the nature of the proposed procedure or treatment and itemize the risks, benefits and alternatives brought to the attention of the patient. Any particular fears or concerns raised by the patient should also be noted'.[18]

USE OF DRUGS BEYOND LICENCE

The following is adapted from "The Use of Drugs Beyond Licence in Palliative Care and Pain Management; Recommendations of the Association for Palliative Medicine and the Pain Society" (rcoa.ac.uk). This statement should be seen as reflecting the views of a responsible body of opinion in these clinical specialties.

- The Medicines Control Agency in the United Kingdom grants a product licence for a medical drug. The purpose of the licence is to regulate the activity of the pharmaceutical company when marketing the drug; this does not restrict the prescription of the drug by properly qualified medical practitioners.

- Licensed drugs can be used legally in clinical situations that fall outside the remit of the licence (referred to as off-label drugs), such as a different age group, indication, dose, route or method of administration. Sometimes off-label drugs are used because manufacturers have not sought to extend the terms of the licence for economic reasons, where costs are likely to exceed financial return.

- Unlicensed drugs refers to those products that have no licence for any clinical situation or may be in the process of evaluation.

- Injection therapy may involve the use of unlicensed drugs such as sclerosants or off-label usage of licensed drugs (e.g., Kenalog is not licensed to be mixed with lidocaine, and lidocaine is not licenced for intraarticular injection [although it is for surface infiltration and the caudal route]).

- The risks presented to clinicians when using drugs beyond licence are best managed through clinical governance. Organizations should encourage staff to educate themselves and take responsibility for their own decisions within the framework of a corporate policy.

- The use of drugs beyond licence should be seen as a legitimate aspect of clinical practice and, in pain management practice, is currently both necessary and common.

- Choice of treatment requires partnership between patients and health care professionals, and informed consent should be obtained, whenever possible, before prescribing any drug.

- Patients should be informed of any identifiable risks, and details of any information given should be recorded. It is often unnecessary to take additional steps when recommending drugs beyond licence.

- Health care professionals involved in prescribing, dispensing and administering drugs beyond licence should select those drugs that offer the best balance of benefit against harm for any given patient. They should inform, change and monitor their practice in the light of evidence from audit and published research.

- Organizations providing pain management services should support therapeutic practices that are underpinned by evidence and advocated by a responsible body of professional opinion.

The Faculty of Pain Medicine of the Australian and New Zealand College of Anaesthetists has issued similar guidance (fpm.anzca.edu.au).

SECTION 1

REFERENCES

1. Resuscitation Council (UK). Emergency treatment of anaphylactic reactions. Guidelines for healthcare providers. https://www.resus.org.uk/anaphylaxis/emergency-treatment-of-anaphylactic-reactions.
2. Johnston SL, Unsworth J. Gompels MM. Adrenaline given outside the context of life threatening allergic reactions. *BMJ*. 2003;326:589–590.
3. Pumphrey RSH. Lessons for management of anaphylaxis from a study of fatal reactions. *Clin Exp Allergy*. 2000;30:1144–1150.
4. Pumphrey RS. Fatal anaphylaxis in the UK, 1992-2001. *Novartis Found Symp*. 2004;257:116–128.
5. Gall H, Kaufmann R, Kalveram CM. Adverse reactions to local anesthetics: analysis of 197 cases. *J Allergy Clin Immunol*. 1996;97(4):933–937.
6. British Medical Association and Royal Pharmaceutical Society. *British National Formulary No. 72*. London: British Medical Association and Royal Pharmaceutical Society; 2017:1181.
7. Ring J, Franz R, Brockow K. Anaphylactic reactions to local anesthetics. *Chem Immunol Allergy*. 2010;95:190–200.
8. Johnston SL, Unsworth J. Adrenaline given outside the context of life threatening allergic reactions. *BMJ*. 2003;326:589–590.
9. Sander JW, O'Donaghue MF. Epilepsy: getting the diagnosis right. *BMJ*. 1997;314:158–159.
10. Snashall D. Occupational infections. ABC of work related disorders. *BMJ*. 1996;313:551–554.
11. Orchard JW. Is it safe to use local anaesthetic painkilling injections in professional football? *Sports Med*. 2004;34(4):209–219.
12. Orchard JW. Benefits and risks of using local anaesthetic for pain relief to allow early return to play in professional football. *Br J Sports Med*. 2002;36(3):209–213.
13. Orchard J. The use of local anaesthetic injections in professional football. *Br J Sports Med*. 2001;35:212–213.
14. Medical aspects of drug use in the gym. *Drug Ther Bull*. 2004;42(1):1–5.
15. Mazur DJ. Influence of the law on risk and informed consent. *BMJ*. 2003;327:731–734.
16. Rogers v. Whitaker. *Aust Law J*. 1993;67(1):47–55.
17. Chan SW, Tulloch E, Cooper ES, et al. Montgomery and informed consent: where are we now? *BMJ*. 2017;357:j2224.
18. Douglas L, Primary Care Rheumatology Society. Joint and soft tissue injection guidelines. https://www.pcrsociety.org/resources/other/joint-injections-guidelines.

PRACTICAL GUIDELINES FOR INJECTION THERAPY IN MUSCULOSKELETAL MEDICINE

DIAGNOSIS

Giving injections is easy; it is selection of the suitable patient that is difficult. It is possible to learn how to administer injections in a weekend, but becoming a successful diagnostician can take a lifetime. Competence in injection therapy requires practical knowledge in the *science* of applied anatomy, physiology and pathology, together with experience in the *art* of diagnosis – the most challenging and satisfying aspect of treating musculoskeletal pain.

Nothing can replace the wisdom of the experienced clinician well versed in clinical diagnosis, but in this section we attempt to guide new practitioners with some simple hints on how to clearly assess and clarify the often-conflicting information obtained from the history and physical examination to achieve the ultimate goal of a correct diagnosis.

The distinguished British cardiologist Sir Thomas Lewis (1881–1945), defined diagnosis as "a system of more or less accurate guessing – where the end point achieved is a name." Before using an invasive treatment such as injection therapy, we should ensure that, whenever possible, this name describes the genuine pathology and its correct anatomical site.

Common conditions really do occur commonly: if you hear hoof beats in the night, it is probably a horse, not a zebra. However, rare conditions also exist and should be expected. All diagnoses are provisional, and we should guard against emotional attachment to one; keep an open mind, and do not try to hammer square pegs into round holes to make the facts fit a favoured diagnosis.

THE SCREENING PROCESS

The screening process is divided into four parts: observation, history, inspection and examination.

Observation

The patient is observed as soon as they present for the interview, and the following points should be considered:

- Face – signs of pain or fatigue, general health
- Posture – protective or defensive
- Gait – limping, antalgic, exaggerated

Observing the patient globally can assist in determining the psychological state and in selecting a mode of communication to inspire trust. Are they in severe pain, nervous, clearly unwell? Do they appear to be angry about their situation? Does the patient sound or look depressed? Chronic pain is often accompanied by significant mood disturbance.

History

The patient is asked questions about the following:

- Age – some conditions occur more commonly in certain age groups
- Occupation – heavy manual or repetitive work, prolonged static postures
- Sports and hobbies – injuries, physical contact, endurance, repetitive movements
- Site – location of the main pain

- Spread – where did it start? where has it been? dermatomal reference?
- Onset – gradual, sudden, traumatic, insidious
- Duration – recent or long term
- Behaviour – constant, intermittent, fluctuating, increasing; is there a pattern?
- Signs and symptoms – colour changes, swelling, locking, clicking, stiffness, paraesthesia, anaesthesia, weakness, disturbances to or loss of function, fatigue, fever, loss of appetite and weight, rigors, sweats, musculoskeletal pain elsewhere
- Impact – affected physically, psychologically, emotionally, socially, financially
- Past history – previous episodes, allergies, operations, illnesses, investigations, treatments
- Family history – any conditions that may be linked
- Medications – prescription drugs that might cause musculoskeletal symptoms (e.g., statins, quinolone, antibiotics);over-the-counter drugs (e.g., ibuprofen); drugs the patient may not mention (beware the young person with a great physique and bad skin who may be using anabolic steroids)

By this time, the clinician has usually formulated a working diagnosis but the following physical examination will test the validity of this hypothesis. The examination entails a simple, logical and well-drilled flow performed in an efficient sequence that causes the least discomfort and disturbance to the patient. The more frequently the examiner follows this set routine, the easier the process becomes, and unusual findings should immediately stand out.

Inspection

The patient exposes the relevant part of their anatomy. For some presentations, it may be useful if initially the patient stands with the back to the clinician facing a full-length mirror; this enables the clinician to be less physically threatening while observing both the patient's movements and facial expression from behind. Discreetly observing the patient's actions while undressing also helps decide how much the pain affects normal activities. The lower limb and spine are best examined with the patient lying, but the upper limb can easily be assessed with the patient standing.

Check the following:

- General posture, shape and bony deformity
- Muscle wasting
- Swelling
- Colour changes, bruising, scars, features of ischaemia

The patient is then asked how they feel while standing absolutely still to establish whether there are constant symptoms or not. Often, a patient confuses constant pain at rest with pain produced only on movement.

Examination

The following examination process outlines the minimum number of tests that should be performed; this enables the busy clinician to reach a provisional diagnosis swiftly. If there is still some doubt, there are many other manual tests that could be done but that may be time consuming and not particularly helpful; routinely including additional tests can lead to confusion rather than

SECTION 2

clarity. Equally, routinely ordering expensive investigations should be carefully justified (see "Additional tests" on following page).

The examination routines in each section for upper and lower limbs, lumbar spine and sacroiliac joint are outlined and illustrated later in this textbook.

Active movements

These test ability and willingness to move. The patient is asked to move the part actively in certain directions – for example, extension and rotation at the neck, flexion at the lumbar spine, active elevation of the arm at the shoulder.

Reluctance or inability to perform these tasks may indicate too much pain, too much weakness or just an unwillingness to move the part. There are certain areas of the body that are prone to dysfunction as a manifestation of underlying distress, particularly the neck, lower back, shoulder and groin. Dr James Cyriax (1904–1985), known as "the father of orthopaedic medicine," named these the "emotional areas of the body." At other areas, such as the elbow – where distress is less likely to manifest – performing active tests are time consuming and may not be particularly helpful.

Passive movements

These test pain, range, end feel and presence or absence of a capsular pattern. The capsular pattern was described by Cyriax as a repeatable set pattern of loss of joint range for each joint, consistent with tightening of the capsule. It is one of the most useful diagnostic physical tests and indicates that there is some degree of joint capsulitis caused by degeneration, systemic arthritis or trauma. There may also be a hard end feel in advanced capsulitis. Remembering the typical limited passive movements of older patients is helpful when deciding if the capsular pattern is present. Details of these patterns are found at the beginning of each section.

These tests are carried out with the patient as relaxed as possible so that no muscle action is involved. If pain is produced, is it at the end of normal range, and is the end feel normal for that movement at that joint? End feels are described as follows:

- Soft end feel compresses muscle against muscle – as in normal elbow flexion
- Hard end feel implies bone against bone – as in normal elbow extension
- Elastic end feel tests ligamentous tension – as in full forearm supination

Resisted movements

These test contractile tissue (muscle and tendon complex) for pain and power. The patient is asked to resist movement, with the joint held in a static and midrange position. It is important to prevent any joint movement during these tests.

The outcomes may be as follows:

- No pain at all – not a contractile lesion
- Pain on contraction – a contractile complex lesion
- Pain and weakness – a severe contractile lesion or unwillingness to perform the test
- Weakness with no pain – total rupture or neurological cause

Bear in mind that a fracture or bone disease can present with apparent contractile tissue signs on resisted testing; tensing of the attached muscle can pull on the affected bone. A traumatic or insidious onset should give rise to suspicion of bone involvement.

Additional tests

Manual tests such as repeated movements, individual passive joint play movements and neurological or vascular tests can be performed where indicated. There are also certain special tests typically associated with certain conditions, such as Phalen's test in carpal tunnel syndrome and Finkelstein's test in de Quervain's tenosynovitis. However, confidence in the diagnosis can be sometimes confused by too much examination; there are currently more than 120 physical examination tests described at the shoulder.

Further objective diagnostic tests such as x-rays, blood tests or scans need to be used judiciously when there is doubt about the diagnosis, or it is important to exclude unlikely but serious disorders from the differential diagnoses. A low threshold for investigation is appropriate for a patient who is systemically unwell. The cost of these investigations should always be considered; is additional information something that you need to know or something that would be nice to know, and, if so, is it worth the extra expense?

Practice point 2.1: Diagnostic imaging

Just because an abnormality is present on imaging does not necessarily mean this is the source of the symptoms. It is not uncommon for a patient with shoulder pain to have a scan showing subacromial bursal thickening with impingement and for the clinical examination to reveal a clear-cut capsular pattern of a frozen shoulder. "Treat the man, not the scan."

Incidental and unexpected findings are common with investigations. The great thing about magnetic resonance imaging (MRI) scans, for example, is that they show you everything; the problem with MRI scans is that they show you everything. Incidental findings often cause anxiety (for the patient and the clinician) and lead to further invasive, expensive, worrying tests. A patient can easily become a VOMIT – a victim of medical imaging technology.

Differential diagnoses

After this detailed and sometimes time-consuming assessment (which may need to be spread over more than one attendance, depending on the circumstances in which the clinician practices), the diagnosis may be considered under four headings:

- Local causes – anatomical structures, such as bone, capsule, ligament, muscle, tendon, bursa, nerves, blood vessels
- Referred causes – from areas usually proximal to the site of pain, such as neck or lumbar spine
- Systemic causes – inflammatory conditions, such as rheumatoid arthritis, spondyloarthropathy, gout, infection, tumours, neurological disorders
- Distress causes – more prevalent in the shoulder, cervical or lumbar spine or, rarely, the groin area

Distress

There are many reasons why patients consult with pain. They may be seeking a cure or symptomatic relief, diagnostic clarification, reassurance, legitimization of symptoms, certification for work absence or to express distress, frustration or anger. Outright invention of pain is rare, but distress may lead to disproportionate pain behaviour in some patients, especially in association with chronic pain in the low back, neck or shoulder for which there is often scant objective evidence of a significant underlying organic disorder.

The experienced clinician is familiar with this scenario, but the novice may be initially confused when dealing with patients who are distressed or dysfunctional. To provide effective treatment, the caring clinician needs to have an appropriate assessment and management strategy and to maintain a balance between total naivety and cynical disbelief.[1]

Some helpful points to consider are as follows:

- Face – depressed or angry
- Body language – exaggerated movements or posture
- Use of emotional descriptors – such as torture, agonizing, unbearable.
- Grading pain in high ratios out of 10
- Extreme reluctance to move the area
- Giving way or "juddering" on resisted testing
- Limited, painful straight leg raise, but able to sit up with legs straight
- Movements painful or limited when observed, normal when not

Treatment of these patients is challenging, and we do not have space to discuss it in depth here, but there are many options, such as psychological, chemical or physical factors or a combination of these. Injection therapy is relatively contraindicated in these cases but can be considered if the clinician thinks that the somatic pain element justifies it. Because systemic corticosteroids may precipitate or aggravate a psychotic episode in a patient with a psychotic illness, discuss this with the patient's psychiatrist before giving an injection.

Be sympathetically aware of both the patient's physical and mental state and adjust the approach accordingly. Being too nice may make the patient overdependent; conversely, being too tough may cause distress and the perceived pain to increase. There is a delicate balance to be achieved in the approach to these challenging patients, and referral to a specialist in this field may be the best action. Further reading is recommended.

HOW TO USE THIS BOOK

Please study the following guidelines carefully before using any of the techniques. For ease of practical application, we have simplified each technique and present only the essential facts. In the three sections that follow, each double page covers one anatomical structure showing an injection technique for the most common lesion found there; the text is on the left-hand page, and on the right-hand page is a drawing of the anatomical site and a photograph of the injection position. Each anatomical area begins with joint injections, followed by soft tissue injections and the information is presented under the following headings:

- Anatomical structure and positive examination findings
- Equipment
- Anatomy
- Technique
- Aftercare

There is usually more than one way to give an injection. We have selected the techniques we find to be the safest, least uncomfortable for the patient and easiest for the injector, but we also occasionally describe some equally effective or alternative ways.

Where applicable, we have inserted boxes with Practice points. These are based on our own (hard-won) clinical experience and that of our colleagues. We have also introduced some clinical case histories into Sections 3 and 4, which are designed to test your diagnostic skills. Practice point 2.2 presents the conditions most likely to respond well to a corticosteroid injection.

> **Practice point 2.2: Conditions most likely to respond well to corticosteroid injections**
>
> - Acute and chronic bursitis
> - Acute capsulitis
> - Chronic tendinitis
> - Inflammatory arthritis
> - Nerve root entrapment

GUIDELINES TO TECHNIQUES

A brief outline and illustrations of the minimal examination procedures are presented at the beginning of each section, together with descriptions of the typical capsular patterns of limitation of the joints. The cause of the capsulitis could be osteoarthritis, systemic arthritis or trauma, but the ratio of limitation remains the same.

ANATOMICAL STRUCTURE/ DIAGNOSIS

Taking an appropriate history and performing a thorough physical examination, followed by careful consideration of the potential differential diagnoses, is essential to ensure that the patient is suitable for injection. Give plenty of time to this part.

> **Practice point 2.3: Scheduling injections**
>
> Do not rush or perform an injection if you have to leave the consulting room immediately afterwards. Although things very rarely go wrong, you are tempting fate if you squeeze in an extra patient just before you have to leave promptly for an important engagement. This patient will possibly be the one who faints.

To aid patient selection and establish a diagnosis, the following points are presented:

- Hx – usual history of symptoms
- OE – common findings on examination, such as pain, limitation or paraesthesia; results of active, passive or resisted tests
- DD – some differential diagnoses to consider

Practice point 2.4: Is signed consent necessary before an injection?

No, it is not necessary but you need to document the consent discussion. A standardized checklist (printed or electronic) and a patient information leaflet may assist this (see Appendices 2 and 3).

Practice point 2.5: Accompanying persons

Ask the patient if they are nervous about needles and prepare for the possibility that they might faint (the patient should lie down for the injection, if possible). Also, ask any accompanying family member or friend the same question, or you might suddenly find yourself dealing with two patients.

EQUIPMENT TABLE

The equipment table gives the recommended sizes of syringe and needle, dosage and volume of corticosteroid and local anaesthetic and total volume for the average-sized patient. Larger patients may require greater volumes and longer needles. See Table 2.1.

Syringes

All needles and syringes must be of the single-use, disposable type, and the packing must be checked to ensure that they are in date. Have available 1, 2, 5, 10 and 20 ml sterile syringes; occasionally, a 30 or 50 ml syringe might be necessary for a knee aspiration. All syringes have space that enables extra volume to be introduced; for example, a 2 ml syringe will almost always be capable of holding up to 3 ml total volume.

Needles

Use a large-bore needle, such as a 21 gauge, sterile, in-date needle for drawing up the drug(s). The size of the infiltrating needle depends on the size of the individual patient; select the finest needle of the appropriate length to reach the lesion. Even on a slim person, it is often necessary to use a 3.5 inch (90 mm) or longer needle to infiltrate deep structures successfully, such as the hip joint or psoas bursa. It is better to use a longer needle than might appear necessary than one that is too short, which could necessitate withdrawing and starting again.[2]

When injecting with a long fine spinal needle it is helpful to keep the trochar in place to help control the needle as it passes through tissue planes, then remove the trochar and attach the syringe when the needle is in place.

Table 2.1 Common UK needle sizes and colours[a]	Colour	Gauge	Width (mm)	Length (imperial, metric)
	Orange	25	0.5	0.5 to $\frac{5}{8}$ inch (13–20 mm)
	Blue	23	0.6	1–1.25 inches (25–30 mm)
	Green	21	0.8	1.5–2 inches (39–50 mm)
	White	19	1.1	1.5 inches (40 mm)
	Black	Spinal, 21 or 22	0.7–0.8	3–4 inches (75–100 mm)

[a]Other countries may use different colours.

Practice point 2.6: Needlestick injuries

Attach a laminated copy of your employer's (or other relevant authority's) written policy for managing needlestick injuries to the wall of your work area. The best way to avoid a needlestick injury is to have a well-organized routine for giving injections – not to rush, to dispose of used sharps directly into a sharps box and never resheath needle after use.

DRUGS   See Section 1, Chapter 2.

Corticosteroids

In our practices, we normally use Kenalog 40 (triamcinolone acetonide, 40 mg/ml) for these musculoskeletal injections. This is a remarkably safe drug but any appropriate corticosteroid can be used. The advantage of Kenalog is that it can be used in both small and large areas.

Adcortyl (triamcinolone acetonide, 10 mg/ml) is useful where the total volume to be injected is over 5 ml. This allows greater volume for the same dose and avoids the need to dilute the local anaesthetic further with normal saline, which is helpful when injecting hip or knee joints.

Lederspan (triamcinolone hexacetonide, 20 mg/ml) is currently (2018) UK-licensed to be mixed with 1% or 2% lidocaine hydrochloride. It is manufactured by Intrapharm Laboratories (Maidenhead, United Kingdom) and has recently been approved; it is now back on the market after some years out of production.[4] It is appropriate for use by UK allied health professionals who may be constrained about mixing two drugs. It is known as Aristospan in the United States.

In our experience, Depo-Medrone (methylprednisolone) gives more postinjection flare than Kenalog, particularly in tendinous injections. We have also found that it is prone to precipitation in the syringe when mixed with a local anaesthetic. Depo-Medrone premixed with lidocaine is commonly used in the United Kingdom, but the dosage is more difficult to adjust for the individual lesion.

In thin, dark-skinned patients, hydrocortisone (Hydrocortistab) may be used, especially when injecting superficial soft tissue lesions to avoid the potential risk of fat atrophy or depigmentation (e.g., in tennis elbow or de Quervain's tenosynovitis).

Practice point 2.7: Storing injectable drugs

Follow the manufacturer's recommendations about storage. Keep your drugs for joint and soft tissue injection stored in a separate place from any other injectables. Write the expiry date on the box with a thick marker pen to allow you to keep track of use-by dates, but always check the name, strength and individual expiry date of individual bottles or vials before use.

The effect of the corticosteroid does not usually begin until about 48 hours after the injection, so patients should be warned that they may not see any relief of pain until then. There is great variation in the time to onset, with some experiencing almost immediate improvement and others taking several days. The drug action normally continues for about 3 to 6 weeks.

SECTION 2

Local anaesthetic

Although it is not absolutely necessary to add a local anaesthetic to a corticosteroid injection, there are four good reasons for using it:

> **Practice point 2.8: Benefits of adding local anaesthetic to a corticosteroid injection**
>
> - Analgesia
> - Diagnosis
> - Dilution
> - Distension

The analgesic effect makes the injection more comfortable for the patient and, if the pain is reduced on retesting, the diagnosis is confirmed. In spaces such as joints and bursae, dilution of the fluid enables the drugs to reach more areas, and slight distension of the structure helps prevent friction of the synovial surfaces.

We suggest the use of lidocaine (lignocaine) hydrochloride throughout, but any suitable short-acting local anaesthetic can be used. Because of the risk of a severe allergic reaction, the patient should be carefully questioned about possible allergy to local anaesthetics. Where any doubt exists, do not use it. Normal saline can be used to dilute the corticosteroid, if necessary.

Lidocaine with epinephrine, which comes in ampoules or vials clearly marked in red, should not be used because of the risk of ischaemic necrosis in appendages. Because of its potential half-life of 8 hours or more, we do not recommend the routine use of Marcaine (bupivacaine) but it can be used occasionally when a longer anaesthetic effect is needed. Some practitioners like to mix short-acting and long-acting anaesthetics to gain both the immediate diagnostic effect and the longer therapeutic effect.[5,6]

> **Practice point 2.9: Previous exposure to local anaesthetics**
>
> Always ask about allergy or sensitivity to local anaesthetic. Have you had a joint or soft tissue injection before? Or an injection for stitches? Or to enable a dentist to fill or remove a tooth? Was there any adverse reaction?

Mixing of drugs for UK physiotherapists and other allied health professionals

In 1995, we designed a structured course to enable UK Chartered Physiotherapists (PTs) to undertake training in injection therapy in musculoskeletal medicine and, on passing a comprehensive examination, to practise this skill in the National Health Service and private practice. Gradually, podiatrists, osteopaths and other allied health professionals (AHPs) also were permitted to use injection therapy and many took our training courses.

In 2011, the rules under which these AHPs could mix corticosteroids with local anaesthetic were changed, and the Chartered Society of Physiotherapy (CSP), the governing body for PTs in the United Kingdom, issued a document laying out clear guidelines for their members. Essentially, they were no longer permitted to premix the two drugs in a syringe.[7]

Drug manufacturers specify the conditions under which their drugs may be administered. The manufacturers of the most commonly used injectable steroids in the United Kingdom – Depo-Medrone (Pfizer) and Kenalog 40 and Adcortyl 10 mg (Bristol-Myers Squibb) – do not permit mixing of any suspending agent or solution; legally, this is considered to be manufacturing a new drug, for which a licence is required. To mix these corticosteroids with another agent – for example, local anaesthetic – is deemed to be off-label use of the drug. Doctors and dentists frequently use drugs off label; for example, over 90% of paediatric drugs are not licensed for delivery to children, but are universally administered.

Under current 2018 guidelines in the United Kingdom, an AHP who wishes to mix these drugs in a syringe has to undertake and pass a course on prescribing, thus becoming a registered prescriber, or work under a patient-specific directive (PSD) given by a person who has prescribing rights. AHPs who wish to practise injection therapy and do not have prescribing rights could consider the suggestions listed under frequently asked questions (see Appendix 4).

In this text, we continue to include directions for mixing any suitable injectable corticosteroid with a short-acting local anaesthetic together in the syringe before injecting the patient for the reasons listed in Practice point 2.10.

Practice point 2.10: Mixing corticosteroid and local anaesthetic in the syringe

- It makes the injection less painful.
- It is safer than changing needles or using two syringes.
- It has been common practice since the 1940s.
- It mixes in the tissues anyway.
- There is no current evidence to suggest this practice is detrimental.

We do not recommend adding a local anaesthetic to a corticosteroid when injecting around peripheral nerves – for example, when injecting for carpal tunnel syndrome. This is because the additional volume could increase symptoms, and paraesthesia, rather than pain, is the main complaint. The nerve itself must never be injected because permanent damage might ensue.

Dosages

The corticosteroid doses suggested are what we use for the average-sized adult and are governed by the individual patient's age, size, general health and clinical history. These are guidelines only, and none are cast in stone; it is up to the clinician to decide on variants, depending on individual preference and patient presentation. At all times, however, the minimum effective dose should be given; this will help prevent the appearance of adverse side effects such as facial flushing, intermenstrual bleeding, hyperglycaemia, skin atrophy and depigmentation. See Table 2.2.

The maximum dose we use is 40 mg. This would be indicated in large areas such as the shoulder, knee or hip joints and for the subacromial bursa.

Keep within the recommended maximum doses of local anaesthetic to avoid toxicity. The safe maximum doses we suggest are given in Practice point 2.11. These doses are less than half the maximum published in pharmacological texts, so are they are well within safety limits.[8]

SECTION 2

Practice point 2.11: Suggested safe maximum dosages of local anaesthetic

- Lidocaine 2%, up to a maximum volume of 5 ml
- Lidocaine 1%, up to a maximum volume of 10 ml
- Dilute 1% lidocaine with normal saline (0.9%) for volumes larger than 5 ml, or use Adcortyl, 10 mg/ml, to create more volume (4 ml Adcortyl = 1 ml Kenalog).

Table 2.2
Joint injections: Suggested average doses and total volumes

Joint	Dose (mg)	Volume (ml)
Shoulder	40	5
Elbow	30	4
Wrist	20	2
Thumb	10	1
Fingers	5	0.5
Hip	40	5
Knee	40	5–10
Ankle	30	4
Foot	20	2
Toes	10	1

Volumes

Joints and bursae appear to respond best when sufficient volume of fluid to bathe the internal surfaces is introduced. Possibly the slight distension splints the structure, or perhaps breaks down or stretches out adhesions. In a small patient, the amounts are decreased, and in a large patient they may be increased. Greater volume can be obtained by using normal saline and, especially in the case of the knee joint, where the synovial folds encompass a large total area, greater volume is recommended.

The volumes suggested in Table 2.2 are well within the safe capacity of the joints and will not cause the joint capsule to rupture, as indicated by the observation that it is not unusual to aspirate over 100 ml of blood from an injured knee joint. In the case of attempted overdistension, the back pressure created by too large a volume of injectate would almost certainly blow the syringe off the needle long before the capsule was compromised.

Conversely, tendon entheses should have small volumes injected. This avoids painful distension of the structure and minimizes the risk of rupture. See Practice point 2.12.

Practice point 2.12: Tendon enthesis injections: suggested average doses and volumes

- Small tendons: 10 mg of steroid plus local anaesthetic in a total volume of 1 ml
- Large tendons: 20 mg of steroid plus local anaesthetic in a total volume of 2 ml

ANATOMY

As stated previously, giving the injection is the easy part; the difficult part is the diagnosis, but also placing the drug in the correct affected structure can be tricky. To accomplish this successfully, it is essential to have a high level of anatomical knowledge and can best be obtained by visiting an anatomy department and practising needle placement. This is an essential part of our course, and students are often surprised to find where their needle tip has ended.

This section gives tips for useful ways to localize and imagine size of anatomical structures, based on functional and surface anatomy. Finger sizes refer to the patient's fingers, not the clinician's.

TECHNIQUE   Here we describe a logical sequence for administration of the solution and ways of performing a safe and relatively painless injection. The simple precautions shown in Practice point 2.14 should be taken to prevent the occurrence of sepsis.

Wet hands carry more risk of infection, so hands must be well dried before injecting (see the technique recommended by the World Health Organization).[9] While we do not routinely wear gloves when injecting, their use is mandatory in some countries. We do recommend wearing gloves when aspirating, but they do not need to be sterile.[10]

Injections should not be painful. Skin is very sensitive, especially on the flexor surfaces of the body, as is bone. Muscles, tendons and ligaments are less sensitive, and cartilage is virtually insensitive. Pain caused at the time of the injection is invariably the result of poor technique – 'hitting bone' with the needle instead of 'caressing' it. Afterpain can be caused by a traumatic periostitis because of damaging bone with the needle or possibly by flare caused by the type of steroid used.

Practice point 2.13: Allay patient's fears

Maintain a calm confident approach throughout the procedure and keep a conversation going. Avoid letting the needle phobic patient see the needle as you draw up.

Useful things to say before or while giving an injection:

- Small jab coming now.
- You may feel a tingling or numb sensation.

Don't say the following:

- This may, will, hurt, sting, a little, a lot.
- You will feel a sharp sting, scratch (it feels more like a jab).
- This may, will make you feel (negative experience).

Success does not depend on a painful flare after the infiltration. This is a myth.

Practice point 2.14: Aseptic technique – see Preparation Protocol and Flow Chart pp. 122–123

- Remove watches and jewellery.
- Mark injection site with closed end of the sterile needle guard and discard.
- Clean the injection site with an appropriate cleanser.
- Allow to dry.
- Wash hands for 1 minute; dry well with a disposable paper towel.
- Use prepacked, in-date, sterile disposable needles and syringes.
- Use single-dose ampoules or vials and then discard them.
- Change needles after drawing up the solution.
- Do not touch the skin after marking and cleansing the injection site.
- Do not guide the needle with your finger.
- When injecting joints, aspirate first to check that any fluid does not look infected.

Placing the ulnar side of the operating hand on the patient near to the injection site controls any potential tremor. The secret of giving a reasonably comfortable injection depends on using the needle as an extension of the finger. Once through the skin, slowly and gently pass the needle through the tissues, monitoring the texture of the structures.

Following these three simple rules helps make the procedure relatively painless.

Practice point 2.15: Needle insertion

- Strongly stretch the skin between the forefinger and thumb.
- Hold the needle perpendicular and very close to the skin.
- Rapidly insert needle a perpendicularly short way into the epidermis.

Are vapocoolants before injection useful?

Moderate-quality evidence has indicated that use of a vapocoolant (e.g., ethyl chloride) immediately before intravenous cannulation reduces pain during the procedure. It does not increase the difficulty of cannulation nor cause serious adverse effects, but it is associated with mild discomfort during application. This technique has not been formally assessed for joint and soft tissue injections, but it is quick, simple and cheap and might be considered as a technique to improve patient comfort.[11]

In addition to its local anaesthetic properties, ethyl chloride may be an effective disinfectant alone and may improve skin disinfection when used with povidone-iodine compared with povidone-iodine alone.[12]

Practice point 2.16: Anaesthetic cream

Applying a local anaesthetic cream (e.g., Emla cream [lidocaine and prilocaine]) under occlusion to the target site for an hour before the procedure may help make the injection less painful for the nervous patient. Once the needle has reached the correct structure, always attempt to aspirate; this enables you to see if the needle tip is in a blood vessel or if there is any fluid that should be removed.

Practice point 2.17: The usual "feel" of different tissues

- Muscle – spongy, soft
- Tendon or ligament – fibrous, tough
- Capsule – sometimes slight resistance to needle
- Cartilage – sticky, toffee-like
- Bone – hard and extremely sensitive

Bolus and peppering procedures

Bursae and joint capsules are hollow structures that require the solution to be deposited in one amount, a bolus technique. No resistance to the introduction of fluid indicates that the needle tip is within a space. Chronic bursitis, especially at the shoulder, may result in loculation of the bursa. This gives the sensation of pockets of free flow and then resistance within the bursa, rather like injecting a sponge, so the needle must be slowly and gently moved around to infiltrate these pockets.

Tendons and ligaments require a peppering technique which helps disperse the solution throughout the structure and decreases the possibility of rupture. The needle is gently inserted to caress the bone at the enthesis, and the solution is then introduced in little droplets, as if into all parts of a cube (Fig. 2.1). Knowing the three-dimensional anatomical size of the structure is essential because this indicates the volume of fluid required and how much the needle tip has to be moved around. There is only one skin puncture; this is not multiple acupuncture.

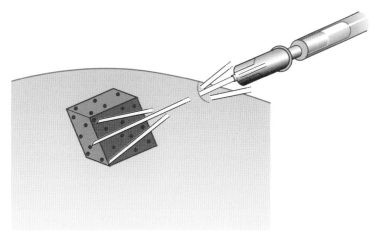

Fig. 2.1 'Peppering' technique.

When injecting tendons in sheaths, after inserting the needle perpendicular to the skin, angle the needle alongside the tendon within the sheath and introduce the fluid. The fluid should flow easily; resistance indicates that the needle tip is within the tendon itself. Often, a small bulge is observed indicating that the fluid is contained within the sheath.

Avoid puncturing a large blood vessel. If this occurs, apply firm pressure over the site for 5 minutes (vein) or 10 minutes (artery).

Practice point 2.18: Prevention of blowback

Use a small-bore, 1 ml tuberculin syringe for small tendons and ligaments because the resistance of the structure can require a certain amount of pressure. Considerable back pressure can cause a syringe to blow off the needle, thus causing both the clinician and patient to be sprayed with the solution, an embarrassing situation. Always ensure that the needle is tightly attached to the syringe by slightly twisting the needle and syringe in opposite directions as you firmly push them together.

Aspiration

See Section 1, Chapter 5. Aspiration can be planned or unplanned. Planned aspirations are common for the knee joint, olecranon bursa, Baker's cyst and ganglia. If the area – for example, the knee joint – looks swollen or feels warm, fluid may be present and aspiration may be necessary, so the appropriate aspiration equipment should be prepared (Practice point 2.19). Gloves should always be worn when aspirating in order to protect the clinician.

SECTION 2

Practice point 2.19: Aspiration equipment

- 20 ml or 50 ml syringe
- 18 gauge needle
- Absorbent towels to cover surface
- Gloves
- Kidney bowl
- Sterile labelled container for sample

Occasionally, an unplanned aspiration may occur. Having placed the needle into the target site and drawn back on the plunger as usual, unexpected aspiration of blood, joint or bursal fluid may occur. To be ready for this, it is useful to have a large syringe and bowl to hand, especially when injecting large joints.

Aspirate steadily, so as not to move the needle tip from the target area, and check any aspirated fluid; if the aspiration is unexpected and sepsis is suspected, detach the syringe containing the injectate from the needle, aspirate with a fresh syringe, deposit a sample of the fluid into a sterile container and send this for microscopy, sensitivity and culture. Abandon the injection.

In a planned aspiration, if the fluid looks like normal serous fluid – clear, with the viscous consistency of runny honey – continue to aspirate while pressing with the flat hand on the area. The fluid should be disposed of according to local policy.

Practice point 2.20: Detaching the needle in situ when aspirating

When aspirating a joint, getting the syringe off the needle without moving the position of the needle tip in the joint (e.g., to allow injection of a freshly aspirated knee) can be tricky. In this situation, when assembling, do not attach them with a twisting motion. To get them apart, hold the needle hub firmly between the index finger and thumb while bracing the back or side of the same hand against the patient's skin to maintain the position of the needle tip. Hold the main body of the syringe (not the plunger) firmly with the other hand, and twist gently in one direction. If that doesn't work, twist in the opposite direction and then to and fro until the syringe detaches.

Should the aspirated joint be injected after an aspiration, or should you await the result of the fluid analysis? This depends on the experience of the aspirating clinician, the clinical context and the appearance of the fluid. If confident that the aspirate is normal serous fluid, and the clinical circumstances warrant it, injection of corticosteroid, with or without local anaesthetic, can continue. If fresh blood is removed, nothing should be injected until a fracture is eliminated.[9,10] If in doubt, do not inject. See Section 1, Chapter 5.

Practice point 2.21: Immediate post injection care

The patient should wait for about 30 minutes within sight and hearing distance in case there is an unusual delayed adverse reaction to the drug/s. It pays to be cautious.

AFTERCARE Many studies have shown that injections give demonstrable relief in the short term but there is not much difference between other treatments or no treatment at all in the long term. To obtain a more successful long-term result, it is essential to address the causes of the pain once the symptoms have been relieved by the injection. In our experience, nearly all common musculoskeletal lesions benefit from a few sessions of some sort of rehabilitative programme. Recurrence of symptoms is common in bursitis and tendinitis, so appropriate advice on prevention is a vital part of the care package.

The ideal outcome is total relief of pain with normal power, a full range of motion and a return to previous function. When local anaesthetic is used, there should be a significant immediate improvement to encourage both patient and clinician that the correct diagnosis has been made and the injection accurately placed.

The patient should be told that the relief of pain will be temporary, depending on the strength and type of anaesthetic used, and the pain may return when this effect wears off. Occasionally, patients may describe this pain as greater than their original pain: this might be as a result of the flare effect of cortisone microcrystal deposition, or because of poor injection technique (e.g., hitting bone). However, it is also possible that pain recurring after some temporary relief might *appear* to be worse to the patient. Any afterpain is usually transient and can be eased by the application of ice or taking simple analgesia.

The anti-inflammatory effect of the corticosteroid is not usually apparent until about 48 hours after the infiltration and can continue for 3 to 6 weeks, depending on the drug used. Therefore, patients should optimize the benefit of the drug action during this period by avoiding aggravating activities.

Arrange to review the patient about 7 to 10 days later. If the pain is severe or begins to return, as might occur in acute capsulitis of the shoulder, arrange an earlier review. In this case, warn patients that it is possible that they will need more than one injection so they are prepared for this and do not consider the treatment a failure.

> **Practice point 2.22: Reassess before repeating an injection**
>
> After a successful treatment, patients may return, requesting a repeat injection for a recurrence. Always fully reassess to make sure that the original problem has indeed recurred and discuss the appropriateness of further injection, as well as alternative treatment modalities

Advise the patient on what to do and what to avoid in the intervening period. Joint conditions usually benefit from a programme of early gentle movement within the pain-free range.

Overuse conditions in tendons and bursae require relative rest. This means that normal activities of daily living can be followed, provided they are not too painful, but return to sport or strenuous repetitive activity and resisted exercises should be postponed until the patient is as pain-free as possible.

When the symptoms have been relieved, patients should be advised about rehabilitation and prevention of recurrence. This is particularly relevant in overuse conditions and might involve correction of posture, ergonomic advice,

SECTION 2

adaptation of movement patterns, mobilization or manipulation, deep friction massage, stretching and/or strengthening regimens. The input of a professional coach in their sport or an expert in orthotics might also be required.

Neurological impingement conditions such as carpal tunnel, Morton's metatarsalgia and meralgia parasthetica usually may need temporary splinting and advice on the avoidance of aggravating compression situations.

Practice point 2.23: Driving after an injection

Ask patients if they have driven (or will drive) to the clinic for the injection. There is no clear consensus among rheumatologists regarding driving following an intraarticular injection. There is no absolute medicolegal bar to driving following an intraarticular injection, and guidance points to clinicians' own judgment as to the safety of driving.[2]

CONTRAINDICATIONS TO INJECTIONS

ABSOLUTE CONTRA-INDICATIONS

See Chapter 6 in Section 1 for further information on safety precautions. NEVER inject under the following conditions:

- Hypersensitivity or allergy to any of the drugs used – risk of anaphylaxis
- Sepsis – local or systemic
- Reluctant patient or no informed consent given – medicolegal implications
- Children younger than 18 years of age (except juvenile arthritis) – children usually heal spontaneously, and injection near an end plate is contraindicated
- Recent fracture site – might delay fusion
- Prosthetic joint – risk of infection
- Gut feeling – when in doubt, don't inject

Practice point 2.24: Anaphylaxis

Anaphylaxis after a joint or soft tissue injection is an extremely rare event (probably less than once in a clinical lifetime) that needs to be prepared for by keeping resuscitation skills up to date. Attach a laminated copy of your employer's (or other relevant authority's) written policy for managing anaphylaxis to the wall of your work area, and have a protocol for regularly checking that the appropriate drugs and equipment are present, in date and that you know how to use them. Keep your resuscitation skills up to date by attending an annual training update course.

RELATIVE CONTRA-INDICATIONS

Injections should be undertaken only after careful consideration of the pros and cons. When in doubt, hesitate to inject if any of the following conditions is present:

- Bleeding risks – anticoagulant therapy, haemophyllia
- Haemarthrosis – this is disputed; pain relief from aspiration can be dramatic.
- Diabetes – greater risk of sepsis; blood sugar levels may rise temporarily
- Immunosuppressed – by disease (e.g., leukaemia) or drugs (e.g., systemic steroids)
- Large tendinopathies – e.g., Achilles or infrapatellar tendons (image first as greater risk of rupture)
- Impending joint replacement surgery – discuss with surgeon and be prepared for a range of replies.
- Pregnancy – medicolegal considerations
- Distressed patient – pain may be perceived to be aggravated by an injection.

Practice point 2.25: Patients on warfarin

In patents taking warfarin, make sure that the international normalized ratio (INR) is in the therapeutic range for the condition being treated and that the patient is not currently experiencing any unexplained bleeding or bruising.

SECTION 2

PREPARATION PROTOCOL

1. **Prepare patient:**
   - Take history and carefully examine patient
   - Check for absolute or relative contraindications
   - Discuss other treatment options, injection procedure and possible side effects
   - Obtain informed consent and record this
   - Place patient in a comfortable supported position, with injection site accessible

2. **Select drugs:**
   - Decide first on total volume based on size of structure
   - Choose dose of drug(s); use minimal effective amount
   - Select corticosteroid vials and/or single-use local anaesthetic ampoules
   - Check names, strengths and expiration dates

3. **Assemble following equipment and place close to patient:**
   - Appropriate-sized, sterile, in-date syringe
   - Sterile, in-date, 21 gauge needle for drawing up
   - Sterile in-date appropriate-sized needle for infiltrating
   - Alcohol swab or iodine skin preparation
   - Cotton wool or gauze and skin plaster – check for allergy
   - Waste bin and sharps box
   - Spare syringe and sterile container if aspiration likely

4. **Prepare site:**
   - Identify structure and stretch skin strongly between finger and thumb
   - Mark injection site with end of a fresh needle cap, then discard
   - Clean skin with a suitable preparation in an outward spiral motion

5. **Prepare injection:**
   - Wash hands with cleanser for 1 minute and dry well with a paper towel
   - Open vial(s) and ampoule(s)
   - Attach 21 gauge needle to appropriate-sized syringe
   - Draw up accurate dose of steroid
   - Draw up accurate dose of local anaesthetic if used
   - Discard drawing up needle in sharps box
   - Attach needle for injection of correct length firmly to the syringe
   - Take loaded syringe and fresh cotton wool ball to the patient

INJECTION TECHNIQUE FLOWCHART

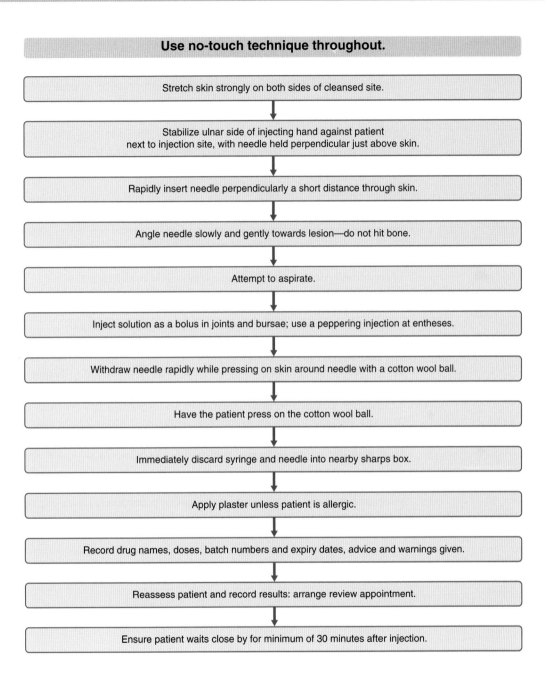

Use no-touch technique throughout.

Stretch skin strongly on both sides of cleansed site.

Stabilize ulnar side of injecting hand against patient
next to injection site, with needle held perpendicular just above skin.

Rapidly insert needle perpendicularly a short distance through skin.

Angle needle slowly and gently towards lesion—do not hit bone.

Attempt to aspirate.

Inject solution as a bolus in joints and bursae; use a peppering injection at entheses.

Withdraw needle rapidly while pressing on skin around needle with a cotton wool ball.

Have the patient press on the cotton wool ball.

Immediately discard syringe and needle into nearby sharps box.

Apply plaster unless patient is allergic.

Record drug names, doses, batch numbers and expiry dates, advice and warnings given.

Reassess patient and record results: arrange review appointment.

Ensure patient waits close by for minimum of 30 minutes after injection.

SECTION 2

REFERENCES

1. Longworth S. Chronic back and neck pain. In: Warburton Louise, ed. *Musculoskeletal Disorders In Primary Care – A Guide For GPs*. RCGP Curriculum Statement 15.9; 2011.
2. Price Z, Murphy D, Mackay K. Intra-articular injection and driving advice: a survey of UK rheumatologists' current practice. *Musculoskeletal Care*. 2011;9(4):188–193.
3. Jackson DW, Evans NA, Thomas BM. Accuracy of needle placement into the intra-articular space of the knee. *JBJS(A)*. 2002;84:1522–1527.
4. Chartered Society of Physiotherapy. Practice Guidance for Physiotherapist Supplementary and/or Independent Prescribers in the safe use of medicines. (3rd Edition) PD026 2016.
5. MHRA UK/H/4817/001/DC.
6. Zulian F, Martini G, Gobber D, et al. Triamcinolone acetonide and hexacetonide intra-articular treatment of symmetrical joints in juvenile idiopathic arthritis: a double-blind trial. *Rheumatology* (Oxford). 2004;43(10):1288–1291.
7. Lomonte AB, de Morais MG, de Carvalho LO, et al. Efficacy of triamcinolone hexacetonide versus methylprednisolone acetate intraarticular injections in knee osteoarthritis: a randomized, double-blinded, 24-week study. *J Rheumatol*. 2015;42(9):1677–1684.
8. British National Formulary No 72 (September 2016–March 2017) BMA/RPSGB, London.
9. WHO. WHO Guidelines on Hand Hygiene in Health Care (Advanced Draft), World Alliance for Patient Safety. 2006: p101WHO, Geneva.
10. Courtney P, Doherty M. Joint aspiration and injection and synovial fluid analysis. *Best Pract Res Clin Rheumatol*. 2009;23(2):161–192.
11. Griffith RJ, Jordan V, Herd D, et al. Vapocoolants (cold spray) for pain treatment during intravenous cannulation. *Cochrane Database Syst Rev*. 2016;(4):CD009484.
12. Azar FM, Lake JE, Grace SP, et al. Ethyl chloride improves antiseptic effect of betadine skin preparation for office procedures. *J Surg Orthop Adv*. 2012;21(2):84–87.

SECTION 3

UPPER LIMB INJECTIONS

EXAMINATION OF THE UPPER LIMB

The capsular pattern (CP) is a set pattern of loss of motion for each joint. It indicates that there is some degree of joint capsulitis caused by degeneration, inflammation or trauma. There may be a hard end feel in advanced capsulitis

Palpation of the shoulder is not usually particularly helpful, but is performed if required at the start of the examination of the elbow or hand, specifically for heat, swelling and synovial thickening, and at the end to localize the lesion; comparison with the other side clarifies if any tenderness felt is normal.

Additional tests can be performed if the diagnosis is in doubt; these include repeated movements, stability tests, individual joint play tests or neurological tests such as reflexes and skin sensation.

Objective tests, such as imaging and blood tests, should be undertaken only after careful consideration of the additional costs involved.

Abbreviations

Hx = History
OE = On examination
DD = Differential diagnoses
OA = Osteoarthritis
RA = Rheumatoid arthritis
LA = Local anaesthetic

Remember that all anatomical measurements are based on the patient's fingers, not the clinician's.

SECTION 3

THE SHOULDER

SHOULDER EXAMINATION

First eliminate the cervical spine by testing active movements in all directions.

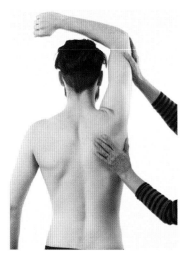

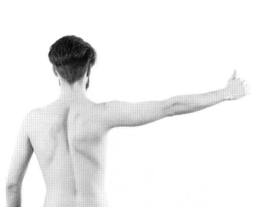

1 Active flexion, followed by passive flexion with overpressure

2 Active abduction to ear for painful arc

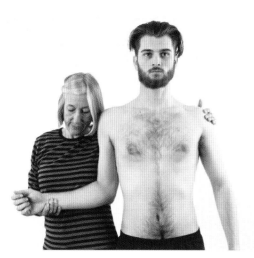

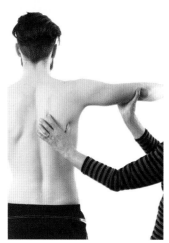

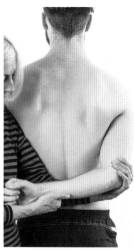

3 Passive lateral rotation

4 Passive abduction

5 Passive medial rotation

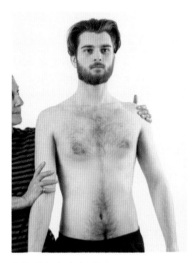

6 Resisted abduction

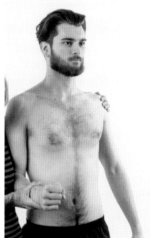

7 Resisted lateral rotation

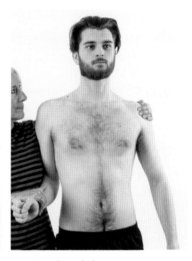

8 Resisted medial rotation

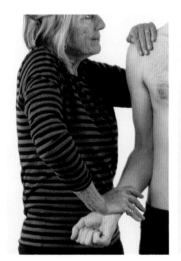

9 Resisted elbow flexion

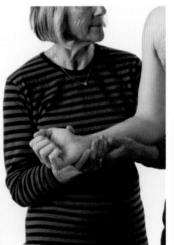

10 Resisted elbow extension

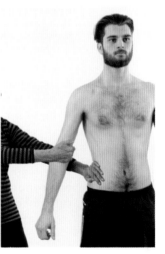

11 Resisted adduction

SECTION 3

Shoulder capsular pattern

- Most loss of lateral rotation, less of abduction, least of medial rotation

Additional shoulder tests if necessary

- Impingement, lag, stability, proprioception, scarf test for acromioclavicular joint (full passive horizontal adduction)

GLENOHUMERAL JOINT

Acute or chronic capsulitis – frozen shoulder

Hx – Trauma, RA or OA idiopathic, secondary to stroke, or neurological disease

OE – Pain in deltoid, radiating down to hand in severe cases, aggravated by arm movements and lying on shoulder; CP: most loss of lateral rotation, less of abduction, least of medial rotation

DD – Bursitis tendonitis; infection; referred from neck; psychological distress

Equipment

Syringe	Needle	Kenalog 40	Lidocaine	Total volume
5 ml	Green, 21 gauge 1.5–2 inches (40–50 mm)	40 mg	4 ml, 1%	5 ml

Anatomy

The shoulder joint is surrounded by a large capsule, and the easiest and least painful approach is posteriorly, where there are no major blood vessels or nerves. An imaginary oblique line running anteriorly from the posterior angle of the acromion to the coracoid process passes through the shoulder joint. The needle follows this line, passing through the deltoid, infraspinatus and posterior capsule. The end point should be the sticky feel of cartilage on the head of the humerus or the glenoid.

Technique

- Patient sits with arms folded, thus opening up posterior joint space
- Identify posterior angle of acromion with thumb and coracoid process with index finger
- Insert needle directly below posterior angle and pass anteriorly and obliquely towards coracoid process until needle gently touches intraarticular cartilage
- Inject solution as a bolus

Aftercare

Maintain mobility with pendular and stretching exercises within the pain-free range, progressing to greater stretching when pain reduces. Temporary sling support and oral analgesia can help in the acute stage. Strong passive stretching may commence when the pain abates. A strengthening and stabilizing rotator cuff programme is then started, together with postural correction.

Practice point

Frozen shoulder typically affects patients aged 40 to 60. In older patients, or those with obvious features of OA elsewhere, consider an x-ray for associated glenohumeral OA (looks normal in frozen shoulder). The less the radiation of pain and the earlier the joint is treated, the more dramatic may be the relief of symptoms. Usually one injection suffices in the early stages but more can safely be given at increasing intervals; in advanced capsulitis, 4 to 6 injections may be given over about 2 months. Warn the patient that a repeat dose might be needed if symptoms are severe.

   If there is resistance to the injection, the needle has probably been inserted too laterally and must be repositioned more medially. Rarely, the posterior approach is not effective, so an anterior approach is used; the arm is held in slight lateral rotation and the needle inserted anteriorly between the coracoid process and the lesser tuberosity of the humerus, aiming posteromedially towards the spine of the scapula with the same dose and volume are used. The disadvantages to this approach are that the patient can see the needle advancing, the flexor skin surfaces are more sensitive and there are more neurovascular structures on the anterior aspect of the shoulder.

40 mg of Adcortyl with 40 mg of 1% LA can be used in large shoulders where more volume is required. Smaller patients may require only 30 mg.

A number of conditions can coexist shoulder and neck and shoulder problems may interact, adding to potential diagnostic confusion. Reassessment after treating what appears to be the likeliest lesion may reveal another lesion. Judicious use of imaging may help. There is inconclusive evidence to support or refute the use of these injections.

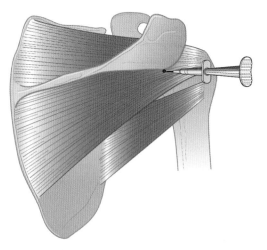

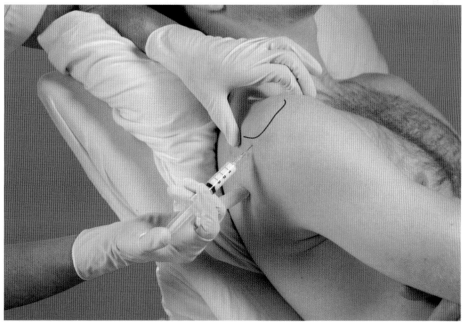

ACROMIO-CLAVICULAR JOINT

Acute or chronic capsulitis

Hx – Trauma or occasionally prolonged overuse in a degenerative shoulder

OE – Pain at point of shoulder; bump of bone or swelling may be seen; pain on all full passive movements at end range, especially full passive horizontal adduction (scarf test); occasional painful arc on active elevation

DD – Osteolysis of lateral clavicle (rare, visible on x-ray); referred from neck, gallbladder, diaphragm, postlaparoscopic abdominal surgery, lung tumour

Equipment

Syringe	Needle	Kenalog 40	Lidocaine	Total volume
1 ml	Orange, 25 gauge 0.5 inch (16 mm)	10 mg	0.75 ml, 2%	1 ml

Anatomy

The acromioclavicular joint line runs in the sagittal plane, about a thumb's width medial to the lateral edge of the acromion. The joint plane runs obliquely medially from superior to inferior and usually contains a small meniscus. Often, a small step can be palpated where the acromion abuts against the clavicle, or a slight V-shaped gap can be felt at the anterior joint margin. Passively gliding the acromion downwards on the clavicle may help in finding the joint line.

Technique

- Patient sits supported, with arm hanging by the side to slightly separate joint surfaces
- Identify lateral edge of acromion. Move palpating digit medially about a thumb's width and mark midpoint of joint line
- Insert needle, angling medially about 30 degrees from the vertical and pass through capsule
- Inject solution as a bolus

Aftercare

Begin gentle mobilizing exercises as soon as possible. Acutely inflamed joints are helped by the application of ice, taping across the joint to stabilize it and by oral analgesia.

Practice point

Occasionally, the joint is difficult to enter; it is normally a narrow space and degenerative changes may make it more so. Traction on the arm can open up the joint space. To avoid unnecessary pain, peppering of the capsule with the solution will anaesthetize it while feeling for the joint space with the needle.

The joint can also be injected anteriorly and horizontally at the V-shaped anterior gap if the superior approach is difficult. The unstable or repeatedly subluxing joint can be helped by sclerosing injections or possibly surgery.

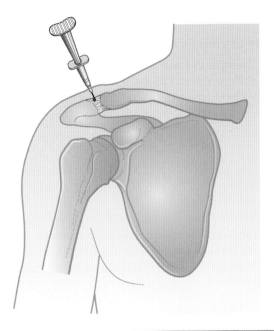

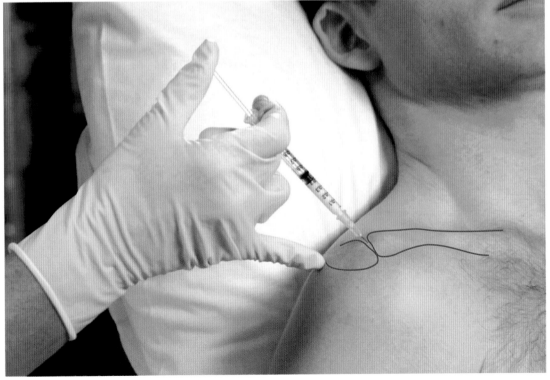

STERNO-CLAVICULAR JOINT

Acute or chronic capsulitis

Hx – Trauma, overuse in the degenerate shoulder or occasionally RA

OE – Pain over sternoclavicular joint; pain on shoulder retraction and protraction, full elevation, clicking and subluxation after trauma

DD – Sternocostal joints capsulitis; clavicle fracture; lung, oesophageal disease

Equipment

Syringe	Needle	Kenalog 40	Lidocaine	Total volume
1 ml	Orange, 25 gauge 0.5 inch (16 mm)	10 mg	0.5 ml, 2%	0.75 ml

Anatomy

The sternoclavicular joint contains a small meniscus that can sometimes be damaged and then elicit painful symptoms. The joint line runs obliquely laterally from superior to inferior and can be identified by palpating the joint medial to the end of the clavicle while the patient protracts and retracts the shoulder.

Technique

- Patient sits supported, with arm in slight lateral rotation
- Identify midpoint of joint line
- Insert needle perpendicularly through joint capsule
- Inject solution as a bolus

Aftercare

The patient should rest while pain is acute, followed by mobilization and a progressive postural and exercise regimen. Taping the joint helps stabilize it in the acute stage after trauma.

Practice point

Although not a common lesion, this usually responds well to one infiltration.

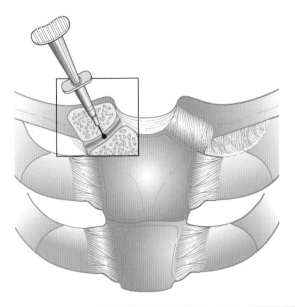

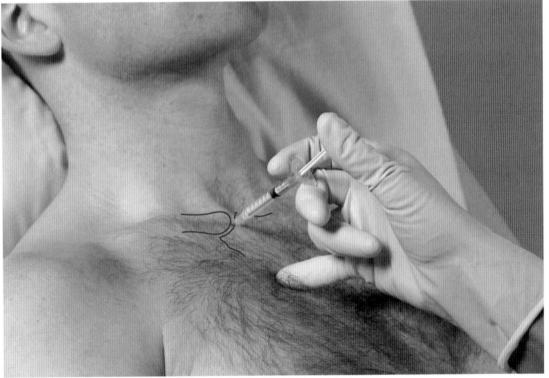

SUBACROMIAL BURSA

Chronic bursitis

Hx – Overuse or occasionally trauma

OE – Intermittent chronic pain in deltoid area, occasional referral down arm; passive elevation and medial rotation more than lateral rotation, resisted abduction and lateral rotation, especially on release of resistance, apparent weakness due to muscle inhibition; possible arc; often resisted tests less painful when joint is tested under distraction

DD – Shoulder capsulitis, rotator cuff tear, fracture; referred from neck

Equipment

Syringe	Needle	Kenalog 40	Lidocaine	Total volume
5 ml	Green, 21 gauge 1.5 inches (40 mm)	40 mg	4 ml, 1%	5 ml

Anatomy

The bursa lies mainly under the acromion but is very variable in size and can extend distally to the insertion of deltoid. Occasionally, a tender area can be palpated around the edge of the acromion. Sometimes the bursa communicates with the joint capsule, especially with a full-thickness rotator cuff tear.

Technique

- Patient sits with arm hanging to distract humerus from acromion
- Identify lateral edge of acromion
- Insert needle at midpoint of acromion and angle slightly upwards under acromion to its full length
- Slowly withdraw needle while simultaneously injecting as a bolus wherever there is no resistance

Aftercare

Maintain retraction and depression of the shoulders; avoid elevation of the arm above shoulder level for up to 2 weeks. Taping the shoulder in retraction and depression for a few days, with postural advice, is helpful. When pain free, the patient commences resisted lateral rotation and retraction exercises, followed by strengthening of abduction. Retraining of over-arm activities to avoid recurrence is essential, and sporting advice may be necessary.

Practice point

In our experience, this is the most common injectable lesion seen in musculoskeletal medicine (Appendix 5). Diagnosis can be difficult because the signs may be confusing. Results are usually excellent; relief of pain after one injection is not uncommon, but the rehabilitation programme must be scrupulously maintained. If, rarely, the symptoms persist after two injections, the shoulder should be scanned because a cuff tear might also be present. In thin patients, the fluid sometimes causes visible swelling around the edge of the acromion.

There is often loculation in long-standing bursitis. In this case, resistance is felt when injecting the solution, so the needle must be fanned around under the acromion to pepper separate pockets of the bursa – the sensation is that of injecting a sponge. Occasionally, calcification occurs within the bursa and hard resistance is felt, infiltration with a large-bore needle and local anaesthetic may help. Failing this, surgical clearance is recommended. If palpable tenderness is found either anterior or posterior to the acromion, the injection can be given at these sites.

Acute subacromial bursitis is much less common and presents with spontaneous, rapidly increasing severe pain over a few days, which may radiate down as far as the wrist. The patient is often unable to move the arm at all, and sleep is very disturbed. It can be injected in the same way but using a total volume of 2 ml.

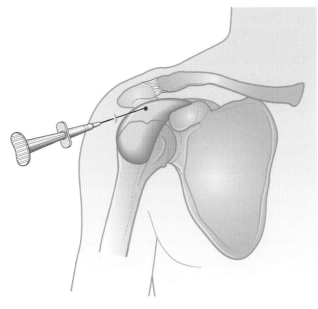

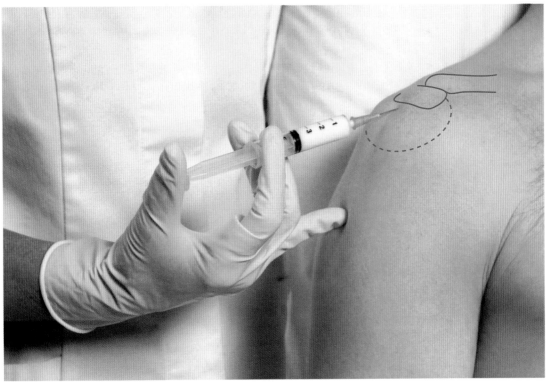

SUBSCAPULARIS BURSA AND TENDON

Acute or chronic tendinitis or bursitis

Hx – Overuse or trauma: haemorrhagic bursitis can follow a direct blow to the shoulder

OE – Pain in deltoid or anterior shoulder; resisted medial rotation, arc on active abduction, full passive horizontal adduction (scarf test)

DD – Shoulder capsullitis, bursa, pectoral muscle strain, fracture; referred from neck; lung disease

Equipment

Syringe	Needle	Kenalog 40	Lidocaine	Total volume
Bursa: 2 ml	Blue, 23 gauge	20 mg	1.5 ml, 2%	2 ml
Tendon: 1 ml	1.25 inches (30 mm)	10 mg	0.75 ml, 2%	1 ml

Anatomy

The subscapularis tendon inserts into the medial edge of the lesser tuberosity of the humerus. It is approximately two fingers wide at its teno-osseous insertion and is a thin fibrous structure that feels bony to palpation. The subscapularis bursa lies deep to the tendon in front of the neck of the scapula and usually communicates with the joint capsule of the shoulder. It is invariably extremely tender to palpation, even when not inflamed.

Technique

- Patient sits supported, with arm by the side and held in 45 degrees lateral rotation
- Identify coracoid process. Move laterally to feel small protuberance of lesser tuberosity while passively rotating the arm. Mark medial aspect of tuberosity
- Insert needle at this point, angling slightly laterally and touching bone at tendon insertion, or in the sagittal plane through tendon to enter bursa
- Pepper solution into tendon insertion or as a bolus deep to tendon into bursa

Aftercare

Relative rest for a week is advised, with a progressive stretching and rotator cuff strengthening programme when the patient is pain free. In sporting overuse injuries, the cause should also be addressed.

Practice point

Subscapularis bursitis and tendinitis are often difficult to differentiate. The bursa is implicated if there is more pain on the scarf test than on resisted medial rotation and if there is more than usual tenderness to palpation. If the bursa and tendon are inflamed together, they can both be infiltrated at the same time by peppering the tendon first and then going through it to infiltrate the bursa. The total dose is increased to 30 mg in a total volume of 3 ml.

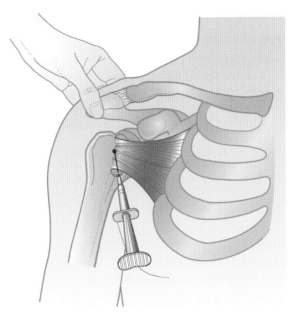

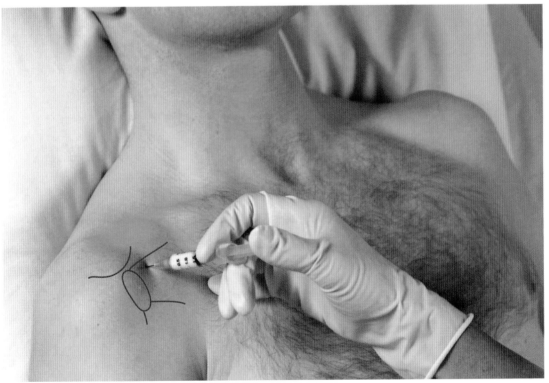

	BICEPS –	Chronic tendinitis

BICEPS – LONG HEAD

Chronic tendinitis

Hx – Overuse

OE – Pain at the anterior top end of the humerus; painful resisted elbow flexion with supination, passive shoulder extension, occasional arc on elevation

DD – Shoulder capsulitis, bursitis, subscapularis tendonitis; referred from neck

Equipment

Syringe	Needle	Kenalog 40	Lidocaine	Total volume
1 ml	Blue, 23 gauge 1–1.25 inches (25–30 mm)	10 mg	0.75 ml, 2%	1 ml

Anatomy

The long head of the biceps lies within a sheath in the bicipital groove between the greater and lesser tuberosities. It can be palpated by having the patient contract the muscle under the palpating finger in the groove.

Technique

- Patient sits with supported elbow held at a right angle
- Identify tender area of tendon
- Insert needle perpendicular to skin at the highest part of tenderness and then angle downwards parallel to tendon
- Inject solution as a bolus between tendon and sheath

Aftercare

Advise relative rest for about a week and then address the causes of the lesion and strengthening of the rotator cuff.

Practice point

There should be little or no resistance felt to the passage of the fluid. This lesion is commonly diagnosed but is, in our experience, quite rare. Palpation of what is normally a tender area can lead to a misdiagnosis of this tendinitis when it might be pain referred from the cervical spine, shoulder joint or rotator cuff lesion.

If there is a sudden onset of pain on flexing, a distinct bulge can appear midhumerus, indicating rupture of the long head of biceps. After the pain has subsided, the patient is usually able to function normally because the short head is sufficient to take over flexion activities.

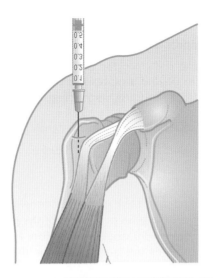

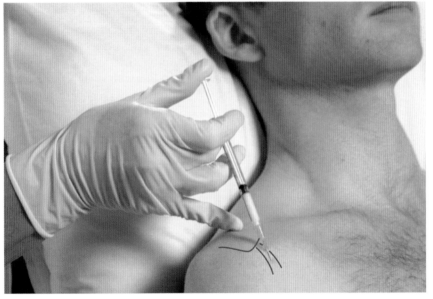

INFRASPINATUS TENDON

Chronic tendinitis

Hx – Overuse

OE – Pain in deltoid area; resisted lateral rotation, arc on active abduction

DD – Shoulder capsulitis, rotator cuff tear, fracture; referred from the neck

Equipment

Syringe	Needle	Kenalog 40	Lidocaine	Total volume
2 ml	Blue, 23 gauge 1.25 inches (30 mm)	20 mg	1.5 ml, 2%	2 ml

Anatomy

The infraspinatus and teres minor tendons insert together into the middle and lower facets on the posterior aspect of the greater tuberosity of the humerus. Placing the arm in 90 degrees of flexion, full adduction and lateral rotation brings the tendons out from under the thickest portion of the deltoid and puts them under tension. The tendons run obliquely upwards and laterally and are, together, approximately three fingers wide at the teno-osseous insertion.

Technique

- Patient sits or lies with supported arm flexed to a right angle and held in full adduction and lateral rotation
- Identify posterior angle of acromion. The tendon insertion now lies 45 degrees inferior and lateral in direct line with lateral epicondyle of the elbow
- Insert needle at midpoint of tendon at insertion. Pass through tendon and touch bone
- Withdraw slightly and pepper solution perpendicularly in two rows up and down into the teno-osseous junction. There will be some resistance to the passage of the fluid

Aftercare

Relative rest is advised for up to 2 weeks. A progressive rotator cuff exercise and postural correction regimen is begun when the patient is symptom free, and deep friction techniques can help.

Practice point

Usually a painful arc is present, which indicates that the lesion lies at the teno-osseous junction. If there is no arc, the lesion lies more in the body of the tendon. In this case, the needle is inserted more medially where there is often an area of tenderness. The same technique is applied.

This lesion might occur in conjunction with subacromial bursitis; if there is a possibility of a double lesion, inject the bursa first and the tendon later if symptoms persist.

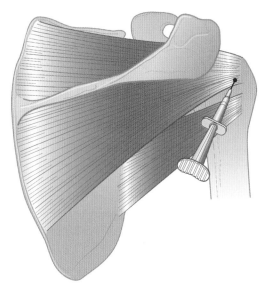

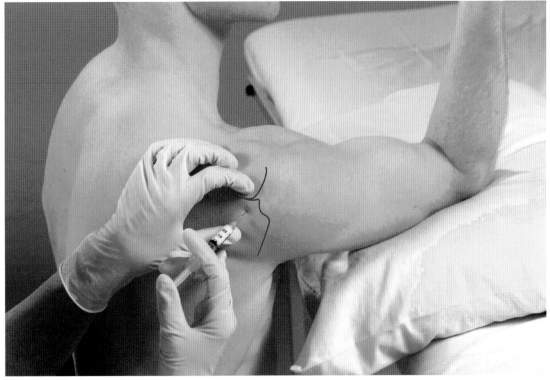

SUPRASPINATUS TENDON

Chronic tendinitis

Hx – Overuse
OE – Pain in deltoid area; painful resisted abduction, arc on active abduction
DD – Shoulder capsulitis, rotator cuff tear, fracture; referred from neck

Equipment

Syringe	Needle	Kenalog 40	Lidocaine	Total volume
1 ml	Orange, 25 gauge 0.5 inch (16 mm)	10 mg	0.75 ml, 2%	1 ml

Anatomy

The supraspinatus tendon inserts into the superior facet on the greater tuberosity of the humerus, which lies in a direct line with the lateral epicondyle of the elbow. A line joining the two points passes through the tendon, which is approximately the size of the middle finger at insertion.

Technique

- Patient sits supported at 45 degrees, with forearm medially rotated behind back, bringing tendon forward so it lies just anterior to edge of the acromion
- Identify rounded tendon in hollow between acromion and tuberosity, in direct line with lateral epicondyle
- Insert needle perpendicularly through tendon to touch bone
- Pepper solution perpendicularly into tendon

Aftercare

Relative rest is advised for up to 2 weeks. A progressive exercise for the rotator cuff muscles and postural control regimen is begun when the patient is symptom free.

Practice point

Supraspinatus tendinitis is another diagnosis commonly made in shoulder pain, but in our experience, it is more likely to be subacromial bursitis. If there is doubt about the existence of a double lesion, the bursa should be always injected first. If some pain then remains on resisted abduction, the tendon can be infiltrated 1 or 2 weeks later.

There is much controversy about injecting this tendon because of the possibility of rupture. If the patient is older, and the cause is traumatic, an ultrasound scan should be performed to determine if there is a tear in the tendon. Pain relief followed by deep friction and a muscle balancing regimen may then be the better treatment; surgery may be advised in some cases, although the results are variable.

Calcification can arise within the tendon and then a hard resistance to the needle would be found. It is worth attempting to break up the calcification with a large-bore needle and local anaesthetic, but if symptoms persist, a surgical opinion should be sought.

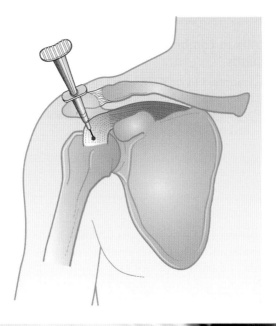

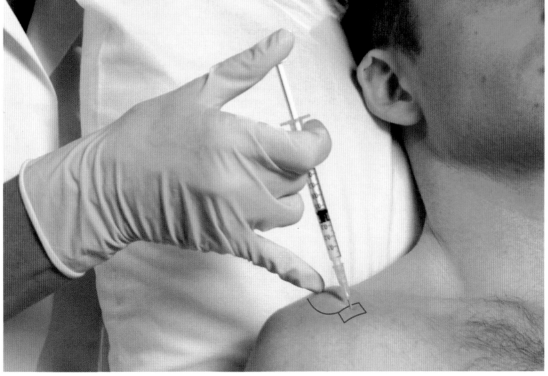

SUPRASCAPULAR NERVE

Neuritis in combination with acute or chronic glenohumeral capsulitis

Hx – Trauma, OA or RA causing frozen shoulder

OE – Pain in deltoid area possibly radiating down to the hand in severe cases; CP: most loss of lateral rotation, less of abduction, least of medial rotation

DD – Referred from the neck

Equipment

Syringe	Needle	Kenalog 40	Lidocaine	Total volume
1 ml	Green, 21 gauge 1.75 inches (40 mm)	20 mg	Nil	0.5 ml

Anatomy

The suprascapular nerve passes through the suprascapular notch into the supraspinous fossa, runs laterally to curl around the neck of the spine of the scapula and ends in the infraspinous fossa. It supplies the supraspinatus and infraspinatus and sends articular branches to the shoulder and acromioclavicular joints.

Technique

- Patient sits supported with arm in a neutral position
- Identify lateral end of spine of scapula, move one-third along medially and mark a spot one finger superiorly in suprascapular fossa
- Insert needle perpendicular to the fossa and touch bone
- Withdraw slightly and inject solution as a bolus

Aftercare

Mobility at the shoulder is maintained within the pain-free range. Stretching and mobilization of the joint are started when pain permits, together with strengthening and postural exercises.

Practice point

Symptoms of paraesthesia or burning when placing the needle indicate that it is within the nerve. It is worth trying an injection here when an intracapsular injection for shoulder capsulitis has not been successful. A small randomized trial has suggested that suprascapular nerve block is a safe and effective alternative treatment for frozen shoulder in primary care. Some clinicians advise the use of a longer lasting anaesthetic alone or with corticosteroid.

This injection might also be useful in patients with rotator cuff tears who are not fit for surgery. Should this happen, reposition the needle point and inject around the nerve – never inject corticosteroid directly into a nerve as this could permanently damage it.

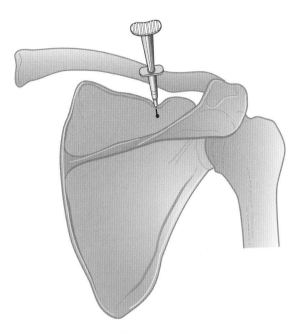

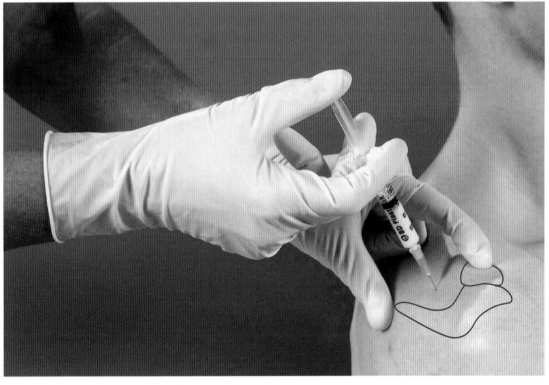

THE ELBOW

ELBOW EXAMINATION

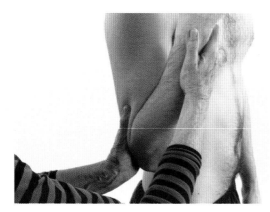

1 Passive flexion

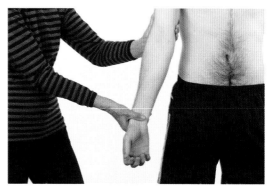

2 Passive extension

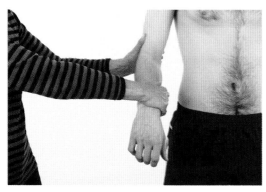

3 Passive pronation

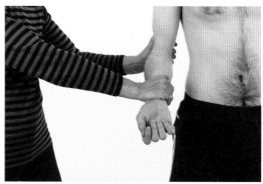

4 Passive supination

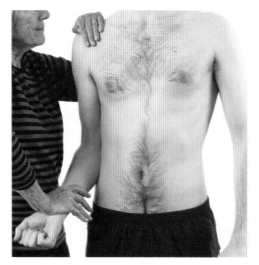

5 Resisted flexion

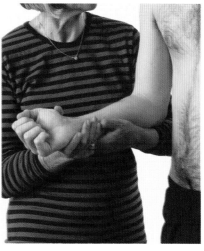

6 Resisted extension

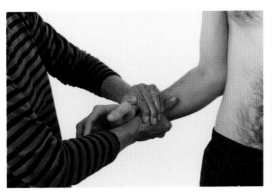

7 Resisted pronation

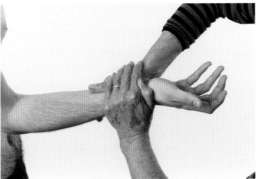

8 Resisted supination

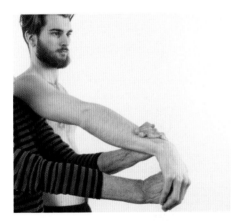

9 Resisted wrist flexion

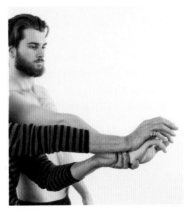

10 Resisted wrist extension

Elbow capsular pattern

● More loss of flexion than extension

Additional elbow tests if necessary

● Active bilateral flexion and extension of elbows with arms abducted horizontally

ELBOW JOINT   **Acute or chronic capsulitis**

Hx – Degenerative, inflammatory or traumatic arthropathies; occasionally overuse

OE – Pain in and around elbow joint; CP: more loss of flexion than extension, with hard end feel

DD – Tendinitis, bursitis, fracture; referred from the neck

Equipment

Syringe	Needle	Kenalog 40	Lidocaine	Total volume
2.5 ml	Blue, 23 gauge 1.25 inches (30 mm)	30 mg	1.75 ml, 2%	2.5 ml

Anatomy   The capsule of the elbow joint contains all three articulations – the radiohumeral, radioulnar and humeroulnar joints. The posterior approach into the small gap between the top of the head of the radius and the capitulum of the humerus is the safest and easiest.

Technique
- Patient sits with elbow supported in pronation at 45 degrees of flexion
- Identify gap of joint line above head of radius posteriorly by passively moving elbow into flexion and extension
- Insert needle at midpoint of joint line parallel to top of head of radius, and penetrate capsule
- Inject solution as a bolus

Aftercare   Begin early to increase the range of motion within the limits of pain using gentle stretching movements, especially into flexion. Passive mobilization techniques are effective in achieving full range but should be given with care so as not to traumatize the joint further.

Practice point

This is not a very common injection but may be useful after trauma or fracture of the radial head. If the cause of the symptoms is one or more loose bodies within the joint, the treatment is mobilization under strong traction. If the range is then improved by this but the pain persists, an injection may be considered.
Adolescents with loose bodies in the joint should be referred for advice on surgical removal.

If the joint is very degenerated, osteophytosis might be present around the joint margin, making entry with the needle more difficult. Deposition of a small amount of the solution into the capsule enables the clinician to pepper around the joint line, with minimal discomfort to the patient. Some clinicians favour the posterior approach to the joint, inserting the needle at the top of the olecranon and angling obliquely distally but this is slightly more difficult to perform.

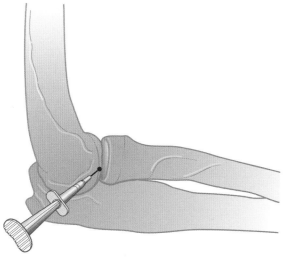

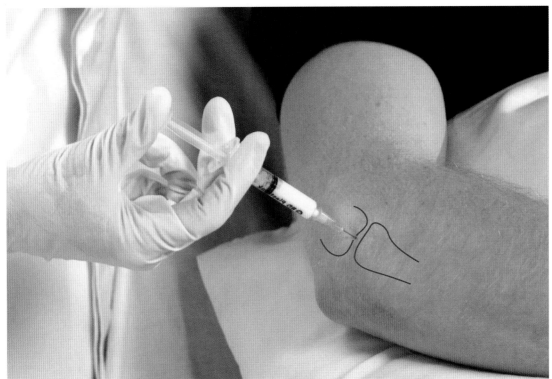

BICEPS BURSA AND TENDON INSERTION

Chronic tendinitis or bursitis

Hx – Overuse

OE – Pain at front of elbow: painful resisted flexion and supination for tendon, full passive flexion, extension and pronation for bursa

DD – Pronator teres tendinitis, tennis elbow; referred from neck

Equipment

Syringe	Needle	Kenalog 40	Lidocaine	Total volume
Tendon, 1 ml	Blue, 23 gauge 1 inch (25 mm)	Tendon, 10 mg	Tendon, 0.75 ml, 2%	Tendon, 1 ml
Bursa, 2 ml		Bursa, 20 mg	Bursa, 1.5 ml, 2%	Bursa, 2 ml

Anatomy

Although the biceps can be affected at any point along its length, the insertion into the radial tuberosity on the anteromedial aspect of the shaft of the radius is particularly vulnerable. A small bursa lies at this point and can be inflamed together with the tendon or on its own. The insertion of the biceps is identified by following the path of the tendon distal to the cubital crease while the patient resists elbow flexion. The patient then relaxes the muscle and the tuberosity can be palpated on the ulnar side of the radius while passively pronating and supinating the forearm. The site is always very tender to palpation, even in the normal elbow.

Technique

- Patient lies face down, with arm extended and palm flat. Fix humerus on the table and passively fully pronate forearm. This brings radial tuberosity around to face posteriorly
- Identify radial tuberosity at two fingers distal to radial head
- Insert needle perpendicularly to touch bone
- Pepper solution into tendon or as a bolus into bursa, or both, as necessary

Aftercare

The patient rests until pain free before beginning graded biceps strengthening and a stretching routine. The cause of the overuse should also be addressed.

Practice point

Differentiation between bursitis and tendinitis is often difficult. If there is more pain on passive flexion and pronation of the elbow than on resisted flexion, together with extreme sensitivity to palpation, the bursa is more likely to be the cause.

If a double lesion is suspected, infiltrate the bursa first and reassess a week later. The tendon can then be injected if necessary.

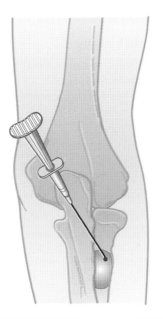

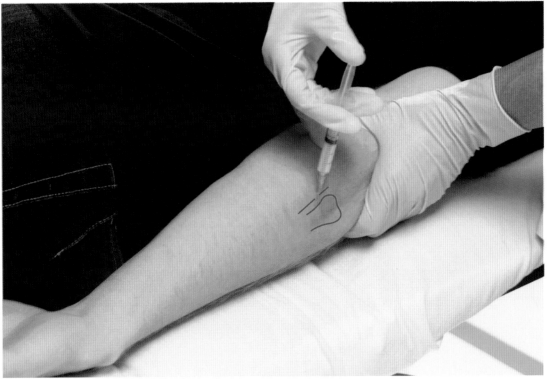

OLECRANON BURSA

Acute or chronic bursitis

Hx – Sustained compression or direct blow

OE – Pain at posterior aspect of elbow joint, often with obvious swelling; painful passive flexion and sometimes extension and resisted extension

DD – RA or gout; infection

Equipment

Syringe	Needle	Kenalog 40	Lidocaine	Total volume
2 ml	Blue, 23 gauge 1 inch (25 mm)	20 mg	1.5 ml, 2%	2 ml

Anatomy

The bursa lies subcutaneously at the posterior aspect of the elbow and is approximately the size of a golf ball.

Technique

- Patient sits with supported elbow at a right angle
- Identify centre of tender area of bursa
- Insert needle into this point
- Inject solution as a bolus

Aftercare

Advise relative rest for a week and then resumption of normal activities, avoiding leaning on the elbow.

Practice point

If swelling is present, always aspirate first. If suspicious fluid is withdrawn, infiltration should not be given until the aspirate has been investigated.

Occasionally a direct blow or fall can cause haemorrhagic bursitis. In these cases, the treatment should be immediate aspiration of all blood before infiltration.

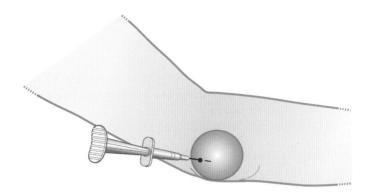

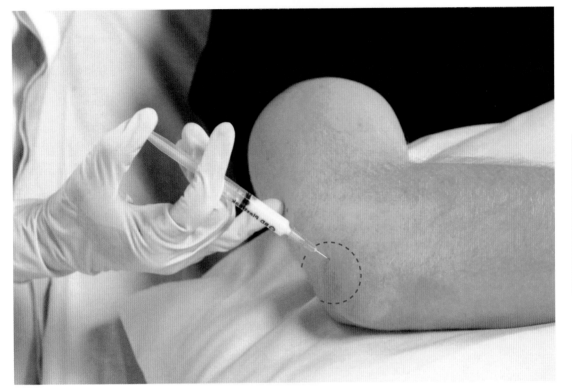

COMMON EXTENSOR TENDON

Chronic tendinitis – 'tennis elbow'

Hx – Overuse

OE – Pain at lateral aspect of elbow aggravated by gripping and twisting; painful resisted wrist extension with elbow extended, passive wrist flexion with ulnar deviation

DD – Radial bursitis, radial head fracture

Equipment

Syringe	Needle	Kenalog 40	Lidocaine	Total volume
1 ml	Orange, 25 gauge 0.5 inch (16 mm)	10 mg	0.75 ml, 2%	1 ml

Anatomy

Tennis elbow invariably occurs at the teno-osseous origin, or enthesis, of the common extensor tendon at the elbow. The tendon arises from the anterior flat facet of the lateral epicondyle, which is approximately the size of the little fingernail.

Technique

- Patient sits with supported elbow at a right angle and forearm supinated
- Identify lateral point of epicondyle, and then move anteriorly onto facet
- Insert needle in line with cubital crease, perpendicular to facet, to touch bone
- Pepper solution into tendon enthesis. Expect resistance to injecting fluid

Aftercare

Rest the elbow for at least 10 days. Any lifting must be done only with the palm facing upwards so that the flexors rather than the extensors are used; the causal activity must be avoided. When resisted extension is pain free, two or three sessions of deep friction massage with a strong extension manipulation (Mill's manipulation) may be given to prevent recurrence. Self-stretching of the extensors and a strengthening programme is then gradually introduced. If the cause was a racket sport, the weight, handle size and stringing of the racket should be checked, as should the technique and advice from a professional coach may be appropriate. Continuous static positions at work should be avoided.

Practice point

This is a very common injectable lesion, with a propensity for recurrence. Very often the reason for this is not that the injection has failed, but that, on relief of symptoms, the patient has returned too rapidly to their sport. Although the teno-osseous junction is the most usual site, the lesion can occur in other parts of the extensor complex. Ignore tender trigger points in the body of the tendon, present in everyone, and place the needle exactly at the very small site of the lesion. Repetitive strain injury can include true tennis elbow but neural stretching, relaxation techniques, cervical mobilization and postural advice might be effective if the tendon is clear. One injection usually suffices but, if symptoms recur, a second injection can be given followed by the above routine 10 days later. Ensure needle is very tightly attached to syringe to avoid spraying solution over both patient and clinician.

Sclerosant injection can be used, or tenotomy may be performed on recurrent tendinitis. Depigmentation and/or subcutaneous atrophy can occur in thin patients, especially those with dark skins, and they should be informed of this before giving consent. Hydrocortisone should be used if the patient is concerned about these possible side effects.

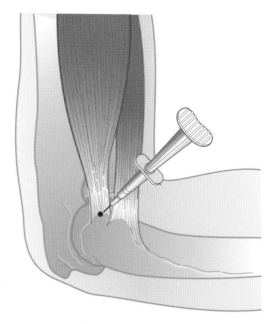

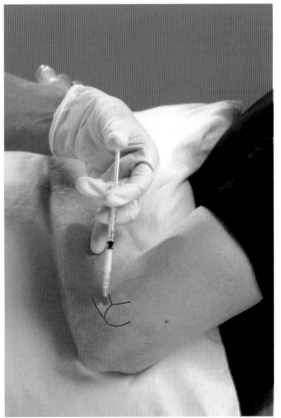

**COMMON
FLEXOR TENDON**

Chronic tendinitis – 'golfer's elbow'

Hx – Overuse

OE – Pain at medial aspect of elbow aggravated by gripping and lifting; painful resisted flexion of wrist, occasionally resisted pronation of forearm

DD – Pronator teres tendinitis; referred from neck

Equipment

Syringe	Needle	Kenalog 40	Lidocaine	Total volume
1 ml	Orange, 25 gauge 0.5 inch (16 mm)	10 mg	0.75 ml, 2%	1 ml

Anatomy

The common flexor tendon at the elbow arises from the anterior facet on the medial epicondyle. It is approximately the size of the little fingernail at its teno-osseous origin.

Technique

- Patient sits with supported arm extended
- Identify facet lying anteriorly on medial epicondyle
- Insert needle perpendicular to facet and touch bone
- Pepper solution into tendon. There will be some resistance

Aftercare

Advise relative rest for about 10 days, and then stretching and flexor and extensor strengthening exercises can be started. Deep transverse fiction massage may also be given.

Practice point

Occasionally, the lesion occurs at the musculotendinous junction, which is invariably a very tender point. Infiltration at this point might not be as effective but deep friction massage can be successful if the patient can tolerate it.

This lesion is not nearly as common as tennis elbow and is less prone to recurrence, so follow-up treatment of deep friction massage and manipulation do not seem to be necessary.

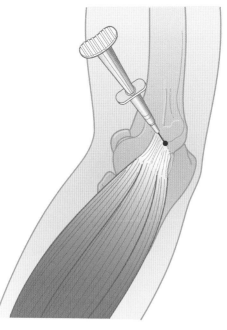

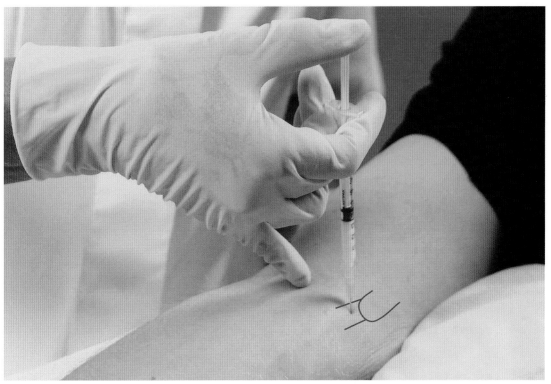

THE WRIST AND HAND

WRIST AND HAND EXAMINATION

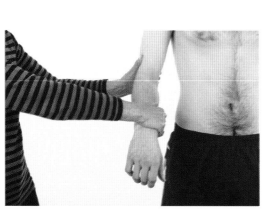

3 Passive extension

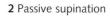

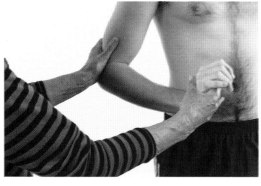

1 Passive pronation

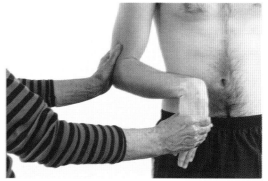

2 Passive supination

4 Passive flexion

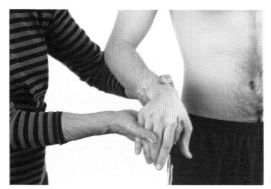

5 Passive ulnar deviation

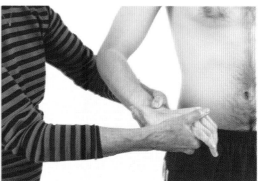

6 Passive radial deviation

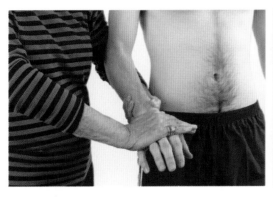

7 Resisted extension

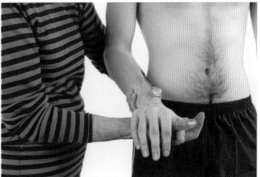

8 Resisted flexion

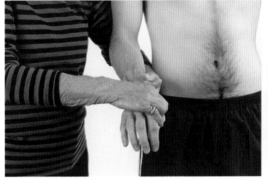

9 Resisted radial deviation

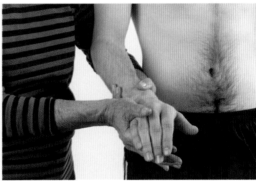

10 Resisted ulnar deviation

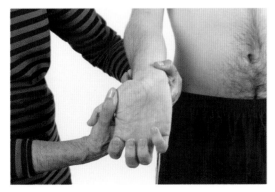

11 Passive thumb extension

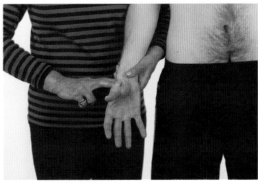

12 Resisted thumb abduction

SECTION 3

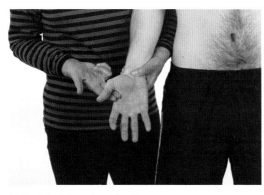

13 Resisted thumb adduction

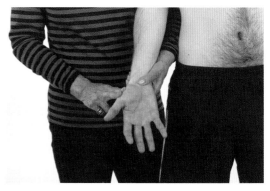

14 Resisted thumb extension

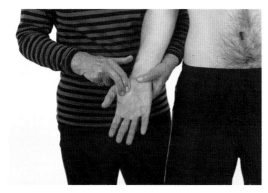

15 Resisted thumb flexion

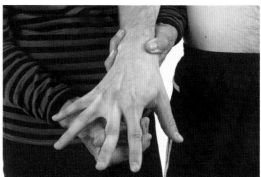

16 Resisted finger abduction

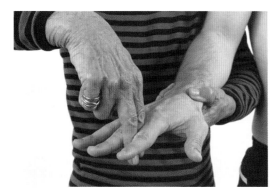

17 Resisted finger adduction

Wrist capsular pattern

- Equal loss of flexion and extension

Finger capsular patterns

Loss of:
- Thumb – extension and abduction
- Metacarpophalangeal joints – extension and radial deviation
- Interphalangeal joints – flexion
- Distal phalangeal joints – extension

Additional hand tests if necessary

- Finkelstein's test, skin sensation, pulses, pinch strength
- Paraesthesia with tapping the median nerve at wrist (Tinel's sign) or fully flexing wrist for 30 seconds and then releasing (Phalen's sign)

INFERIOR RADIOULNAR JOINT AND TRIANGULAR MENISCUS

Chronic capsulitis or acute tear of the meniscus

Hx – OA or RA trauma: fall on outstretched hand or strong traction of wrist

OE – Pain on ulnar side of wrist; painful and limited; CP: passive pronation and supination at end range

For meniscal tear: passive and resisted wrist flexion, resisted and passive ulnar deviation, plus scoop test (see below)

DD – Pisiform or ulnar fracture

Equipment

Syringe	Needle	Kenalog 40	Lidocaine	Total volume
2 ml	Orange, 25 gauge 0.5 inch (16 mm)	10 mg	1 ml, 2%	1.25 ml

Anatomy

The inferior radioulnar joint is an L-shaped joint about a finger's width in length and includes a triangular cartilage, which separates the ulna from the carpus. With the palm facing downwards, the joint line lies just medial to the bump of the end of the ulna, one-third across the wrist. The joint line is identified by gliding the ends of the radius and ulna against each other or by palpating the space between the styloid process of the ulna and the triquetral.

Technique

- Patient sits with hand palm down
- Identify styloid process of ulnar
- Insert needle just distal to styloid, aiming transversely towards radius and passing through ulnar collateral ligament to penetrate capsule
- Inject solution as a bolus

Aftercare

Advise rest for about a week, with avoidance of flexion and ulnar deviation activities. Mobilization with distraction can be effective in meniscal tears.

Practice point

Tears of the cartilage are relatively common, especially after trauma, such as falling on the outstretched hand, a traction injury or after Colles' fracture. The most pain-provoking test is the scoop test – compressing the supinated wrist into ulnar deviation and scooping it in a semicircular movement towards flexion. The patient often complains of painful clicking and occasionally the wrist locks.

Mobilization of the radioulnar joint can help relieve pain, but an injection, together with taping or splinting, may be given in the acute phase.

Often, an explanation of the condition and reassurance, together with advice on avoidance of impingement movements, such as turning a heavy steering wheel, doing handstands or a poor golf style, is sufficient.

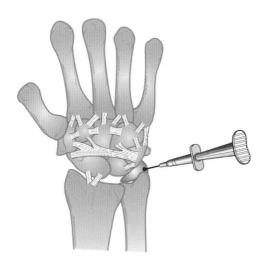

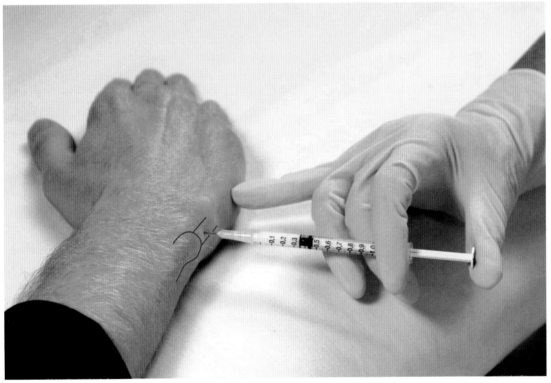

WRIST JOINT   ## Acute or chronic capsulitis

Hx – Overuse or trauma
OE – Pain in wrist joint, may be warm, with synovial thickening or swelling;
    painful and limited; CP: passive extension and flexion, with hard end feel
DD – RA or OA; fracture

Equipment

Syringe	Needle	Kenalog 40	Lidocaine	Total volume
2 ml	Blue, 23 gauge 1.25 inches (30 mm)	20 mg	1.5 ml, 2%	2 ml

Anatomy

The wrist joint capsule is not continuous and has septa dividing it into separate compartments. For this reason, it cannot be successfully injected at one spot but usually requires several areas of infiltration through one injection entry point.

Technique

- Patient places hand palm down in some degree of wrist flexion
- Identify midcarpus proximal to hollow dip of capitate
- Insert needle at midpoint of carpus
- Inject at different points across dorsum of the wrist, both into ligaments and also intracapsular, where possible

Aftercare

The patient rests in a splint until the pain subsides and then start gentle active and passive mobilizing exercises within the pain-free range. Simple wax baths can be most beneficial, and the wax can be used as an exercise ball after being peeled off the hands. Heavy hand work should be curtailed.

Practice point

This is a common area for injection in patients with rheumatoid arthritis. If the joint is badly affected and swollen, it might be necessary to use a longer needle to reach all around the area or to inject at several points.

Patients suffering from trauma, overuse or OA usually respond well to a short period of pain-relieving medication and rest in a splint. As in all cases of trauma, fracture, especially of the scaphoid, should be eliminated.

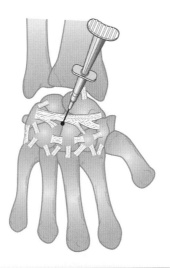

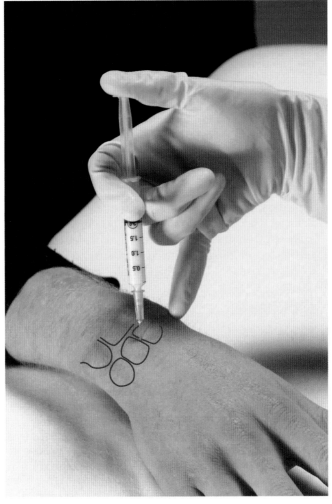

THUMB AND FINGER JOINTS

Acute or chronic capsulitis

Hx – Overuse or trauma
OE – Pain over joint line(s)
Thumb: CP: painful and limited extension and abduction;
Fingers: CP: painful and limited-distal finger joints extension, proximal finger joints flexion
DD – RA or OA; fracture

Equipment

Syringe	Needle	Kenalog 40	Lidocaine	Total volume
1 ml	Orange, 25 gauge 0.5 inch (16 mm)	Thumb, 10 mg Fingers, 10 mg	0.75 ml, 2% 0.5 ml, 2%	1 ml 0.75 ml

Anatomy

The first metacarpal articulates with the trapezium. The easiest entry site is at the apex of the snuffbox on the dorsum of the wrist. The joint line is found by passively flexing and extending the thumb while palpating for the joint space between the two bones. Mark the entry point slightly more proximally to allow for the rounded shape of the base of the metacarpal. Be aware that the radial artery lies at the base of the snuffbox. The distal thumb joint and all finger joints can best be infiltrated from the medial or lateral aspect at the joint line, with the digit in slight flexion.

Technique

- Patient rests hand in midposition, with thumb up, and applies traction of thumb with their other hand traction
- Identify gap of joint space at apex of snuffbox on dorsum of wrist
- Insert needle perpendicularly into gap
- Inject solution as a bolus

Aftercare

Tape the thumb using a spica technique, or tape two fingers together to splint them for a few days. The patient then begins gentle active and passive mobilizing exercise within the pain-free range and is advised against overuse of the thumb or fingers. Dipping the fingers into warm wax baths and using the wax ball as an exercise tool can be beneficial.

Practice point

Trapeziometacarpal joint capsulitis is a common lesion of older women, and the results of infiltration are uniformly excellent. Often, it is several years before a repeat injection is required, provided the patient does not grossly overuse the joint.

Infiltrating the thumb and finger joints can be difficult because osteophytosis will almost certainly be present. It is sometimes necessary to anaesthetize the capsule with some of the solution while trying to enter the joint. Gapping the side of the joint being entered also helps, and an even finer needle, such as a 30 gauge needle, can be used.

First carpometacarpal and scaphotrapezotrapezoidal (STT) OA of the thumb may coexist, with tenderness at the proximal joint line. If unsure of the main source of pain, inject the more distal joint first to avoid confusion from a possible anaesthetic block of surrounding cutaneous nerves.

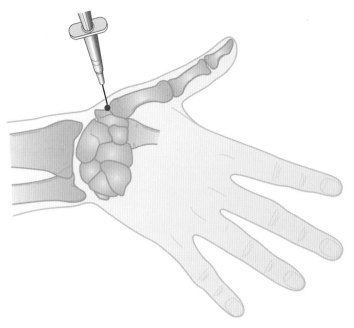

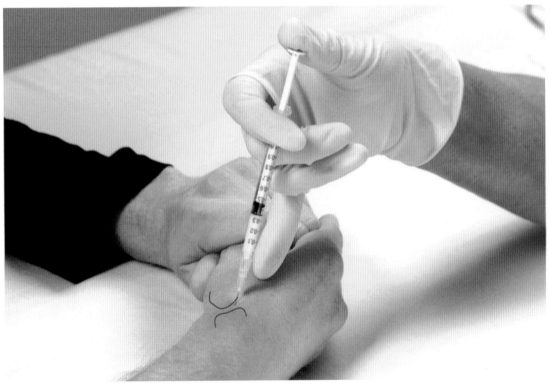

FLEXOR TENDON NODULE

Trigger finger or trigger thumb

Hx – Spontaneous onset

OE – Painful clicking and sometimes locking of finger or thumb, with inability to extend actively; a tender nodule can be palpated, usually at base of the digit

DD – RA or OA

Equipment

Syringe	Needle	Kenalog 40	Lidocaine	Total volume
1 ml	Orange, 25 gauge 0.5 inch (16 mm)	10 mg	0.25 ml, 2%	0.5 ml

Anatomy

Trigger finger is caused by enlargement of a nodule within the flexor tendon sheath, which then becomes inflamed and painful. It usually occurs at the joint lines where the tendon is tethered down by the ligaments and can occur in any digit, but more often is found in the thumb or index finger.

Technique

- Patient places hand palm up
- Identify and mark nodule
- Insert needle perpendicularly into nodule
- Deposit half of the solution in a bolus into nodule
- Angle needle distally into sheath
- Deposit remaining solution into sheath

Aftercare

No particular restriction is placed on the patient's activities except for relative rest for a few days.

Practice point

This injection is invariably effective. Although the nodule usually remains, it can continue to be asymptomatic indefinitely. Occasionally, a slight pop is felt as the needle penetrates the nodule. When the needle is in a tendon, a rubbery resistance is felt.

Some clinicians insert the needle alone first and then ask the patient to flex their finger; if the needle moves, this proves that the correct site has been reached and the syringe can then be attached, but this may involve delay and discomfort to the patient, Other clinicians like to bend the needle before inserting it into the tendon sheath, but there is a slight risk that the needle may snap.

The response rate to steroid injection is lower in patients with diabetes and rheumatoid arthritis, but up to 60% of diabetic patients are successfully treated with steroid injections. The success rate is lower if multiple digits are involved.

Modified from British Society for Surgery of the Hand. *Recommendations for Treatment of Trigger Digit in Adults.* 2014

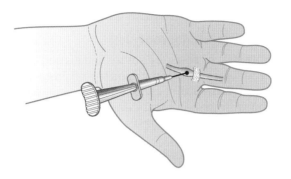

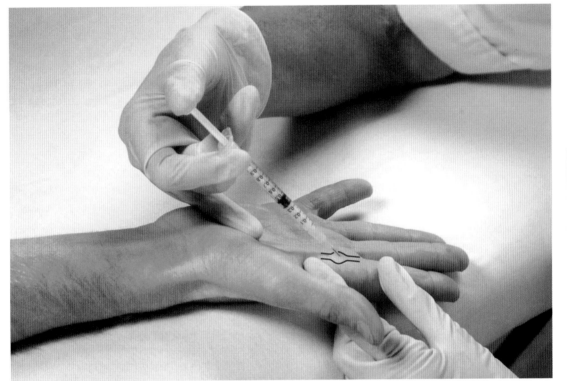

THUMB TENDONS

de Quervain's tenosynovitis

Hx – Overuse of abductor pollicis longus and extensor pollicis brevis

OE – Pain over base of thumb and styloid process of radius; occasional crepitus; painful resisted abduction, extension and passive flexion of thumb across palm with wrist in ulnar deviation (Finkelstein's test)

DD – Thumb joint capsulitis

Equipment

Syringe	Needle	Kenalog 40	Lidocaine	Total volume
1 ml	Orange, 25 gauge 0.5 inch (16 mm)	10 mg	0.75 ml, 2%	1 ml

Anatomy

The abductor pollicis longus and extensor pollicis brevis usually run together in a single sheath on the radial side of the wrist. The styloid process is always tender, so comparison should be made with the pain-free side. The two tendons can often be seen when the thumb is held in resisted extension or can be palpated at the base of the metacarpal. The aim is to slide the needle between the two tendons and deposit the solution within the sheath.

Technique

- Patient places hand vertically, with thumb held in slight flexion
- Identify gap between two tendons at base of first metacarpal
- Insert needle perpendicularly into gap, then slide proximally between tendons
- Inject solution as a bolus within tendon sheath

Aftercare

The patient should rest the hand, with taping of the tendons. This is followed by avoidance or curtailment of the provoking activity and a graded muscle-strengthening regimen, if necessary.

Practice point

Provided the wrist is not too swollen, a small sausage-shaped swelling can often be seen where the solution distends the tendon sheath. This is an area where depigmentation or subcutaneous fat atrophy can occur, especially noticeable in dark-skinned, thin females. Although recovery can take place, the results might be permanent. Patients should be warned of this possibility before giving their consent. The potential risk can be minimized by injecting with hydrocortisone.

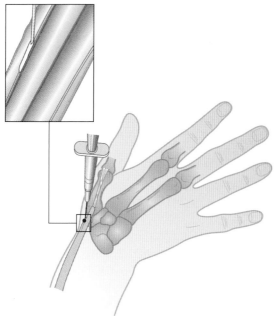

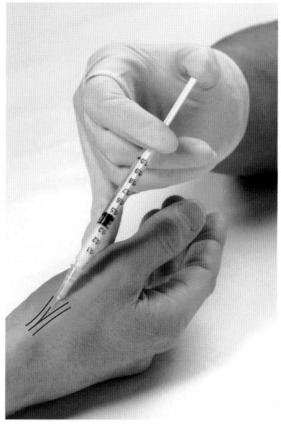

CARPAL TUNNEL   **Median nerve compression under flexor retinaculum**

Hx – Overuse or trauma, spontaneous

OE – Pins and needles in the distribution of the median nerve, especially at night; long-standing nerve compression may cause flattening of thenar eminence and weakness of thumb muscles

DD – Colles' fracture; referred from neck; pregnancy, hypothyroidism, acromegaly, rheumatoid or psoriatic arthropathy; idiopathic

Equipment

Syringe	Needle	Kenalog 40	Lidocaine	Total volume
1 ml	Blue, 23 gauge 1.25 inches (30 mm)	20 mg	Nil	0.5 ml

Anatomy

The flexor retinaculum of the wrist attaches to four sites – the pisiform, the scaphoid, the hook of hamate and the trapezium. It is approximately as wide as the thumb from proximal to distal, and the proximal edge lies at the distal wrist crease. The median nerve usually lies immediately under the palmaris longus tendon at the midpoint of the wrist and medial to the flexor carpi radialis tendon. If no palmaris longus is present, the patient presses the tip of the thumb onto the tip of the little finger; the crease seen at the midpoint of the palm points to where the median nerve should lie.

Technique

- Patient places hand palm up
- Identify point midway along proximal wrist crease, between flexor carpi radialis and median nerve
- Insert needle at this point and then angle it 45 degrees. Slide distally until needle end lies under the midpoint of retinaculum
- Inject solution as a bolus

Aftercare

The patient rests until symptoms abate and then resumes normal activities. A night splint helps in the early stages after the infiltration, and the patient is advised to avoid sleeping with the wrists held in full flexion – the dormouse position.

Practice point

No local anaesthetic is used here because the main symptom is paraesthesia, and more volume increases pressure within the tunnel. Avoid inserting the needle too vertically, when it will go into bone, or too horizontally, when it will enter the retinaculum. If the patient experiences paraesthesia, the needle is in the median nerve and must be withdrawn slightly and repositioned. The injection can be performed equally well by inserting the needle between the median nerve and the flexor tendons, using the same dose and volume. Although one injection is often successful, recurrences do occur. Further injections can be given, but if symptoms still recur, surgery may be required. If the patient has continuous numbness and/or thenar eminence wasting, refer promptly for decompressive surgery.

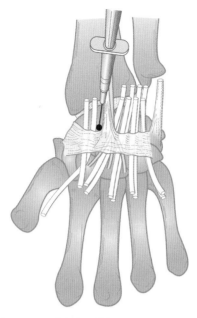

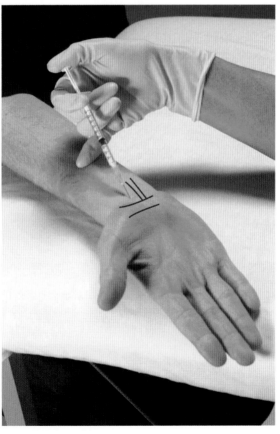

THE JAW

TEMPORO-MANDIBULAR JOINT

Acute or chronic capsulitis

Hx – OA, nocturnal teeth grinding, trauma, headaches, eating especially hard or large foods, clicking or locking

OE – Pain over joint line, poor jaw alignment; painful opening, deviation or protrusion of jaw with asymmetry of movement

DD – Dental or auditory causes; brain tumours; psychological distress

Equipment

Syringe	Needle	Kenalog 40	Lidocaine	Total volume
1 ml	Orange, 25 gauge 0.5 inch (16 mm)	10 mg	0.75 ml, 2%	1 ml

Anatomy

The temporomandibular joint space can be palpated just in front of the ear as the patient opens and closes the mouth. A meniscus lies within the joint, and the needle must be placed below this to enter the joint space. The joint can be infiltrated most easily when the jaw is held wide open. Occasionally the meniscus is torn during trauma.

Technique

- Patient lies on unaffected side, with head supported and mouth held open
- Identify and mark joint space
- Insert needle vertically into inferior compartment of joint space, below meniscus
- Inject solution as a bolus

Aftercare

Avoid excessive movement of the jaw, such as biting on a large apple or eating hard food. Gentle active movements and isometric exercises can be carried out. A mouth guard to prevent grinding the teeth at night and/or the advice of an orthodontist might be required.

Practice point

It might be necessary to manoeuvre the needle about to avoid the meniscus. If the meniscus is displaced, reduction by manipulation should be attempted about a week after giving the injection, when the inflammation has subsided. In resistant cases, surgery may be necessary.

Occasionally this condition arises in a patient suffering from severe tension; in this case an appropriate stress relieving approach is worth trying.

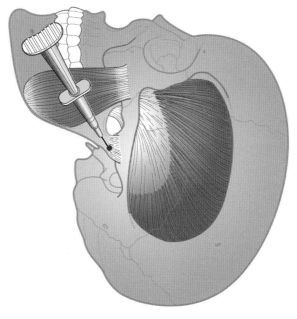

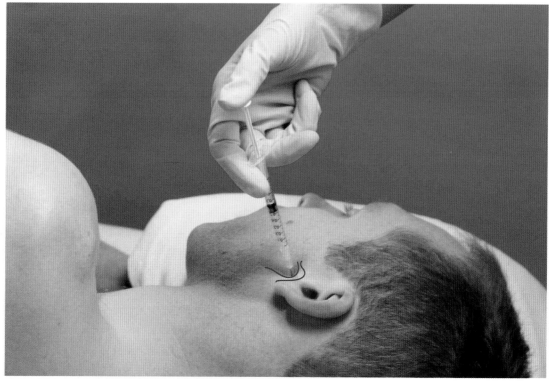

SUMMARY OF SUGGESTED UPPER LIMB DOSAGES

Area	Syringe (ml)	Needle (inches)	Kenalog 40 (mg)	Lidocaine	Total volume (ml)
Shoulder					
Glenohumeral joint	5	Green 1.5–2	40	4 ml 1%	5
Acromioclavicular joint	1	Orange 0.5	10	0.75 ml 2%	1
Sternoclavicular joint	1	Orange 0.5	10	0.75 ml 2%	1
Subacromial bursa	5	Green 1.25	40	4 ml 1%	5
Subscapularis bursa/tendon	2/1	Blue 1.5	20/10	1.5/0.75 ml 2%	2/1
Biceps long head	1	Blue 1–1.25	10	0.75 ml 2%	1
Infraspinatus tendon	2	Blue 1.25	20	1.5 ml 2%	2
Supraspinatus tendon	1	Orange 0.5	10	0.75 ml 2%	1
Suprascapular nerve	1	Green 1.75	20	–	0.5
Elbow					
Elbow joint	2.5	Blue 1.25	30	1.75 ml 2%	2.5
Biceps tendon/bursa	2	Blue 1.25	10/20	0.75/1.5 2%	1/2
Olecranon bursa	2	Blue 1.25	20	1.5 ml 2%	2
Common extensor tendon	1	Orange 0.5	10	0.75 ml 2%	1
Common flexor tendon	1	Orange 0.5	10	0.75 ml 2%	1
Biceps	2	Blue 1.25			
Hand					
Wrist joint	2	Blue 1.25	20	1.5 ml 2%	2
Inferior radioulnar joint/ meniscus	2	Orange 0.5	10	1 ml 2%	1.25
Thumb and finger joints	1	Orange 0.5	10	0.75/0.5	1/0.75
Flexor tendon nodule	1	Orange 0.5	10	0.25 ml 2%	0.5
Thumb tendons	1	Orange 0.5	10	0.75 ml 2%	1
Carpal tunnel	1	Blue 1.25	20	Nil	0.5
Jaw					
Temporomandibular joint	1	Orange 0.5	10	0.75 ml 2%	1

CLINICAL CASE HISTORIES

SELF-TESTING GUIDELINES

Each case history is taken from real patients encountered in our clinical practices. Most are common conditions frequently seen in musculoskeletal work. A few, however, are unusual presentations with rare diagnoses, which will hopefully challenge you more, as they did us. We hope you will find this a light-hearted way of considering the differential diagnoses possible in each case.

Summary of history

To simplify the exercise, the briefest history in each case contains only the relevant positive facts as given by the patient. We suggest you try to make a provisional diagnosis from the history first before moving onto the clinical findings.

Clinical findings

The information given here is what was found on examination using the routine as described in the text. Passive movements were tested for pain, limitation and end feel and resisted movements for pain and power. Additional confirming tests were performed if necessary.

Only the positive findings are listed. These are divided into which physical tests provoked pain, loss of power and/or limitation of range. Any test performed that produced none of these is not listed, so you can assume that they were negative.

On completion of each test, consider the most likely diagnosis and one possible alternative diagnosis. Also consider possible appropriate treatment, because not all cases require injection. (Answers are given in Appendix 1.)

THE SHOULDER

CASE HISTORY 1

A 22-year-old male skier falls at speed while jumping over a large mogul, and the end of his ski pole hits his right shoulder in the pectoral fold. The area becomes swollen within an hour. He presents a week later with severe bruising at the front of his shoulder, pain radiating down to the elbow and has difficulty in moving his arm. It is very painful to sleep on his shoulder at night, and painkillers relieve the pain only minimally. Pain ranges from 2/10 at rest to 8/10 on movement.

Painful – passive shoulder flexion, passive lateral rotation, passive medial rotation resisted medial rotation
Limited – flexion
Weak – flexion and medial rotation

CASE HISTORY 2

A 32-year-old male professional rugby player was tackled 2 weeks ago and landed on his right shoulder. He immediately felt pain at the point of his shoulder and has difficulty lying on it at night. There is some swelling and slight bruising over the shoulder. He has pain on movement at 6/10 and discomfort on lying on it in bed.

Painful – passive shoulder lateral rotation at end range, passive medial rotation, passive flexion, resisted adduction
Limited – passive flexion
Weak – abduction

CASE HISTORY 3   A 59-year-old woman gradually feels increasing pain in the deltoid area of her right dominant arm, which appeared to come on for no reason. Over the course of 2 months, the pain begins to move down the arm, and she visits you when it reaches the midforearm; she is unable to sleep on that shoulder at night or do up her bra. The pain is now constant and at a 6/10 to 7/10 level. Her past medical history includes a hysterectomy in 1987 for benign polyps.

Painful – passive shoulder lateral rotation (++), passive abduction, passive medial rotation, resisted medial rotation
Limited – mostly lateral rotation, less abduction and slight medial rotation
Weak – abduction

CASE HISTORY 4   A 27-year-old female physiotherapist enters a new job with heavy older patients and, at the same time, takes up squash. She complains of intermittent pain in the deltoid area of her dominant right arm on activities such as reaching up, lifting and reaching over to the back seat of the car. The symptoms have troubled her over a period of about 6 months.

Painful – end-range active shoulder flexion, arc on abduction, passive end range lateral, passive medial rotation, resisted abduction
Weak – resisted lateral rotation

CASE HISTORY 5   A 21-year-old doctoral student complains of dominant right shoulder pain on the anterior aspect over the joint line, travelling down the middle of the humerus, which began about 2 years ago. There is no history of injury but the pain is gradually getting worse. She swims competitively for university 100 m freestyle, and the pain is now affecting her swim training because she finds that her shoulder aches for about 2 hours after swimming.

Painful – end-range active shoulder elevation, passive lateral rotation
Weak – lateral rotation, elbow flexion

CASE HISTORY 6   A 64-year-old builder has developed gradual pain at the point of his dominant right shoulder over 2 months. He thinks it might have been caused by lifting a very heavy beam. Now the pain radiates up the right side of his neck, across the right scapular, into the deltoid and down to the elbow. He had previously had angina in the left arm but his recent cardiac workup was normal. The pain is now constant at 2/10 but increases to 6/10 on dressing, elevation, lying on the shoulder and reaching behind the back. Ibuprofen does not relieve the pain.

Limited: all cervical movements
Painful – passive shoulder lateral rotation (++), passive flexion, medial rotation and abduction
Weak – shoulder abduction, lateral rotation

THE ELBOW

CASE HISTORY 7   A 53-year-old woman complains of pain on the lateral aspect of her dominant right elbow spreading about 5 cm into her forearm after carrying heavy shopping bags one month previously. Pain is aggravated to 9/10 by any gripping or squeezing action, is worse at night and her elbow is stiff in the morning. The joint occasionally clicks on certain movements.

Painful – passive elbow extension, passive wrist flexion, resisted wrist extension, resisted supination
Weak – wrist extension

CASE HISTORY 8   A 64-year-old retired male groundskeeper has gradually developed pain on the medial aspect of his dominant right elbow. He had to stop tennis because of a quadruple bypass but wishes to get back to the sport. He gets twinges of pain at 7/10 on certain awkward activities such as pulling off a jumper or using a heavy mowing machine. The elbow occasionally locks and makes noises. His past medical history includes a quadruple bypass 1 year ago.

Painful – passive elbow extension, passive wrist extension, resisted wrist flexion, resisted pronation
Weak – wrist flexion

CASE HISTORY 9   A 52-year-old labourer presents with a 12-year history of intermittent pain in his dominant right elbow. Recently he had felt that the nature of the pain had changed from an intermittent dull ache to frequent sharp twinges of pain, and he is having difficulty trying to lift anything above head height. Occasionally the joint appears to temporally lock.

Painful – end range elbow passive flexion with hard end feel, passive supination
Limited – extension with a springy end feel

CASE HISTORY 10   A 35-year-old single mother decides she needs to get fit and plays a strenuous game of tennis with a friend. She swings wildly in an attempt to smash a backhand shot, misses the ball and feels an instant sharp pain at the back of her dominant right elbow. Within 2 hours she is unable to fully flex or extend

SECTION 3

her elbow. She consults you the next day and you observe that her elbow joint feels warm to the touch.

Painful – passive elbow flexion, passive extension
Limited – elbow flexion, 70 degrees; extension, 50 degrees

CASE HISTORY 11   A 40-year-old secretary slips and falls onto her left buttock and elbow at Piccadilly Station in the rush hour. Apart from feeling embarrassed, she is fine and able to continue to work. The next day, she wakes unable to flex or extend her left elbow fully. The pain is all around and in her elbow, particularly on the lateral aspect. Her sleep is disturbed, and the pain continues to increase. She consults you 3 days after the incident in some pain, 8/10.

Painful – passive elbow flexion, passive extension, passive supination, resisted extension, resisted wrist extension
Limited – flexion, 50 degrees; extension, 40 degrees
Palpation – warm and slightly swollen

CASE HISTORY 12   A 55-year-old pub landlord presents with gradual onset over several months of left (nondominant) elbow pain of 4/10 in the front of his elbow. This is made worse by pulling pints and lifting kegs of beer. Rest relieves the pain, but he needs to continue working.

Painful – end-range passive elbow flexion, passive elbow extension, passive pronation, resisted flexion, resisted supination

THE WRIST AND HAND

CASE HISTORY 13   A young man comes to see you on a Monday morning after a weekend of kayaking. He complains of severe pain (8/10) and crepitus on the dorsal aspect, midpoint of his dominant right forearm, which is aggravated by any wrist activity. There is some swelling present over the painful area and the skin is warm to the touch.

Painful – passive flexion, passive pronation, resisted extension, resisted radial deviation
Weak – extension, supination

CASE HISTORY 14   Eric, aged 70 years, has been doing a lot of gardening recently and using secateurs to prune his rose trees. He has subsequently developed pain at the base of the thumb in his dominant hand and now finds difficulty in gripping and lifting. The joint aches at night, is stiff in the morning and he complains of a weak and painful grip. His past medical history includes a transient ischemic cardiac attack 3 years ago.

Painful – passive thumb extension and abduction
Limited – thumb extension and abduction
Weak – thumb adduction and flexion, wrist extension and flexion

CASE HISTORY 15   A 42-year-old woman fell backwards onto her outstretched hand one month previously and complains of pain over the dorsum of her wrist. It is painful for her to lift heavy objects and she feels it will give way when she puts weight on it. It aches at night and is stiff in the morning. An x-ray taken at the time of the injury showed no bony abnormality.

Painful – passive wrist extension, passive wrist flexion
Limited – wrist extension

CASE HISTORY 16   A 76-year-old female artist has gradually developed pain over the radial side of her dominant right wrist and thumb, which spread up into the forearm while painting her new studio with a heavy paintbrush. Anti-inflammatories, splints and an injection have not helped. She has pain at 5/10 on all activities using her thumb and wrist. There is slight swelling over the lower forearm.

Painful – passive ulnar deviation of the wrist, resisted radial deviation, resisted thumb abduction and extension

CASE HISTORY 17   A 37-year-old teacher presents with 3 months of unilateral paraesthesia and aching in her dominant right hand. The symptoms occur at night and disturb her sleep. She is not sure, but thinks that the main symptoms are concentrated on the lateral side of her hand and digits. The whole hand feels swollen and tender.

Weak – thumb pinch grip
Paraesthesia – passive wrist flexion
Anaesthesia – palmar aspect of right thumb

CASE HISTORY 18   A 30-year-old physiotherapist feels a sharp pain on the ulnar side of her dominant right wrist when applying strong manual traction to a footballer's large neck. The pain gradually settles with rest and pain killers but now, 2 years later, she gets occasional twinges of pain on certain movements, such as twisting her wrist or turning the wheel of her large Range Rover, and the wrist often clicks. She is unable to treat the local football team effectively nor pursue her sport of martial arts, necessary for her own self-defence.

Painful – passive wrist supination, passive flexion, passive ulnar deviation, resisted flexion, resisted ulnar deviation

SECTION 3

KEY REFERENCES

General Accuracy

Daley EL, Bajaj S, Bison LJ, et al. Improving injection accuracy of the elbow, knee, and shoulder: does injection site and imaging make a difference? A systematic review. *Am J Sports Med*. 2011;39(3):656–662.

Glenohumeral Joint: Adhesive Capsulitis

American Academy of Orthopaedic Surgeons. The treatment of glenohumeral joint osteoarthritis: guideline and evidence report; December 4, 2009, recommendation 3. www.aaos.org/research/guidelines/gloguideline.pdf.

Buchbinder R, Green S, Youd JM, et al. Arthrographic distension for adhesive capsulitis (frozen shoulder). *Cochrane Database Syst Rev*. 2008;(1):CD007005.

Lee HJ, Lim KB, Kim DY, et al. Randomized controlled trial for efficacy of intra-articular injection for adhesive capsulitis: ultrasonography-guided versus blind technique. *Arch Phys Med Rehabil*. 2009;90(12):1997–2002.

Maund E, Craig D, Suekarran S, et al. Management of frozen shoulder: a systematic review and cost-effectiveness analysis. *Health Technol Assess*. 2012;16(11):1–264.

Murphy RJ, Carr AJ. Shoulder pain: intra-articular corticosteroid injections. *BMJ Best Pract*. 2012;16(11):1–264.

Uppal HS, Evans JP, Smith C. Frozen shoulder: a systematic review of therapeutic options. *World J Orthop*. 2015;6(2):263–268.

Acromioclavicular Joint

Wasserman BR, Pettrone S, Jazrawi LM, et al. Accuracy of acromioclavicular joint injections. *Am J Sports Med*. 2013;41(1):149–152.

Subacromial Bursa

Bloom JE, Rischin A, Johnston RV, et al. Image-guided versus blind glucocorticoid injection for shoulder pain. *Cochrane Database Syst Rev*. 2012;(8):CD009147.

Coghlan JA, Buchbinder R, Green S, et al. Surgery for rotator cuff disease. *Cochrane Database Syst Rev*. 2008;(1):CD005619.

Suprascapular Nerve

Pehora C, Pearson AME, Kaushal A, et al. Dexamethasone as an adjuvant to peripheral nerve block. *Cochrane Database Syst Rev*. 2017;(11):CD011770.

Common Extensor Tendon

Buchbinder R, Johnston RV, Barnsley L, et al. Surgery for lateral elbow pain. *Cochrane Database Syst Rev*. 2011;(3):CD003525.

Coombs BK, Connelly L, Bisset L, et al. Economic evaluation favours physiotherapy but not corticosteroid injection as a first-line intervention for chronic lateral epicondylalgia: evidence from a randomised clinical trial. *Br J Sports Med*. 2016;50:1400–1405.

Dong W, Goost H, Lin XB, et al. Injection therapies for lateral epicondylalgia: a systematic review and Bayesian network meta-analysis. *Br J Sports Med*. 2016;50:900–908.

Wrist Joint

Burke FD, Melikyan EY, Bradley MJ, et al. Primary care referral protocol for wrist ganglia. *Postgrad Med J*. 2003;79:329–331.

Thumb and Finger Joints

Wolf JM, Delaronde S. Current trends in nonoperative and operative treatment of trapeziometacarpal osteoarthritis: a survey of US hand surgeons. *J Hand Surg Am*. 2012;37(1):77–82.

Flexor Tendon Nodule

Amirfeyz R, McNinch R, Watts A, et al. Evidence-based management of adult trigger digits. *J Hand Surg Eur Vol*. 2017;42(5):473–480.

de Quervain's Tenosynovitis

Mirzanli C, Ozturk K, Esenyel CZ, et al. Accuracy of intrasheath injection techniques for de Quervain's disease: a cadaveric study. *J Hand Surg Eur Vol*. 2012;37(2):155–160.

Peters-Veluthamaningal C, van der Windt DA, Winters JC, et al. Corticosteroid injection for de Quervain's tenosynovitis. *Cochrane Database Syst Rev*. 2009;(3):CD005616.

Richie CA 3rd, Briner WW Jr. Corticosteroid injection for treatment of de Quervain's tenosynovitis: a pooled quantitative literature evaluation. *J Am Board Fam Pract*. 2003;16(2):102–106.

Carpal Tunnel

American Academy of Orthopaedic Surgeons. *Clinical Practice Guideline on Treatment of Carpal Tunnel Syndrome*. Rosemont, IL: American Academy of Orthopaedic Surgeons; 2008.

Huisstede BM, Hoogvliet P, Randsdorp MS. Carpal tunnel syndrome. Part I: effectiveness of nonsurgical treatments – a systematic review. *Arch Phys Med Rehabil*. 2010;91(7):981–1004.

Marshall SC, Tardif G, Ashworth NL. Local corticosteroid injection for carpal tunnel syndrome. *Cochrane Database Syst Rev*. 2007;(2):CD001554.

Van Dijk MAJ, Reitsma JB, Fischer JC, et al. Indications for requesting laboratory tests for concurrent diseases in patients with carpal tunnel syndrome. *Clin Chem*. 2003;49(9):1437–1444.

Verdugo RJ, Salinas RA, Castillo JL, et al. Surgical versus non-surgical treatment for carpal tunnel syndrome. *Cochrane Database Syst Rev*. 2008;(4):CD001552,

Temperomandibular Joint

de Souza RF, Lovato da Silva CH, Nasser M, et al. Interventions for the management of temporomandibular joint osteoarthritis. *Cochrane Database Syst Rev*. 2012;(4):CD007261.

SECTION 3

SECTION 4

LOWER LIMB INJECTIONS

EXAMINATION OF THE LOWER LIMB

The capsular pattern (CP) is a set pattern of loss of motion for each joint. It indicates that there is some degree of joint capsulitis caused by degeneration, inflammation or trauma. There may be a hard end feel in advanced capsulitis.

Palpation is performed at the start of the examination of the knee or foot, specifically for heat, swelling and synovial thickening, and at the end for tenderness to localize the lesion; comparison with the other side clarifies if any tenderness felt is normal.

Additional tests can be performed if the diagnosis is in doubt or to confirm a provisional diagnosis. These include repeated movements, stability tests, individual joint play tests and neurological tests such as tests for reflexes and skin sensation.

Objective tests, such as imaging and blood tests, should be undertaken only after careful consideration of the additional costs involved or if possible red flags occur.

All lower limb examinations begin with watching the patient walk in and performing active lumbar extension to eliminate the lumbar spine as a cause of the symptoms.

Abbreviations

Hx = History
OE = On examination
DD = Differential diagnoses
CP = Capsular pattern
OA = Osteoarthritis
RA = Rheumatoid arthritis
LA = Local anaesthetic
ACL = Anterior cruciate ligament
PLC = Posterior cruciate ligament

THE HIP

**HIP
EXAMINATION
(IN SUPINE)**

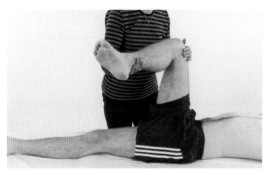

1 Passive lateral rotation

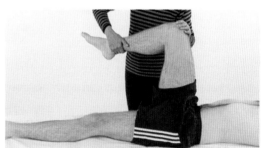

2 Passive medial rotation

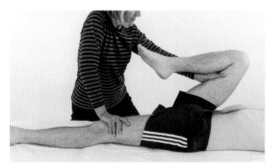

3 Passive flexion

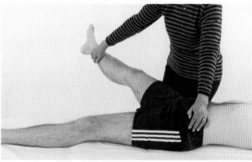

4 Passive abduction

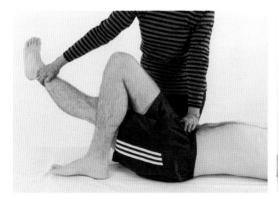

5 Passive adduction

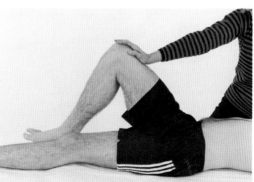

6 Resisted flexion

SECTION 4

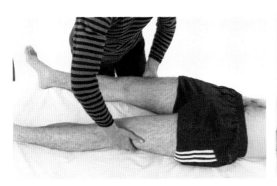

7 Resisted abduction

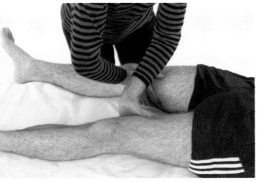

8 Resisted adduction

HIP
EXAMINATION
(IN PRONE)

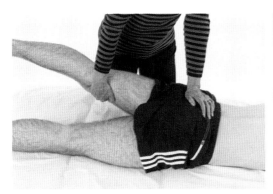

1 Passive extension

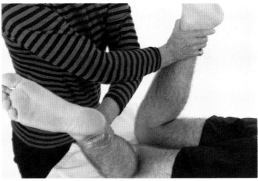

2 Resisted lateral rotation

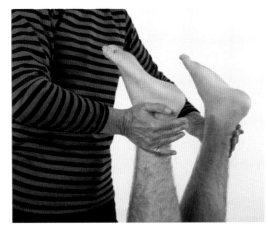

3 Resisted medial rotation

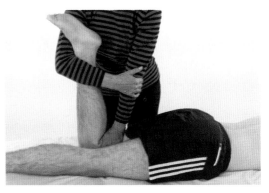

4 Resisted knee extension

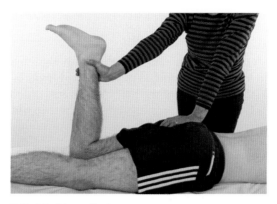

5 Resisted knee flexion

Hip capsular pattern

- Most loss of medial rotation, less of flexion and abduction and least of extension

Additional hip tests if necessary

- Trendelenburg test – one leg standing
- Psoas compression test – full passive hip flexion, with scoop into adduction

SECTION 4

HIP JOINT   **Acute or chronic capsulitis**

Hx – OA, RA or traumatic capsulitis with night pain and severe radiating pain no longer responding to physiotherapy; pain in groin and/or anterior thigh

OE – CP: most loss of medial rotation, less of flexion, least of extension

DD – Fracture in femur, rarely stress fracture in osteoporotic postnatal woman; aseptic necrosis, bony metastases, groin strain; L3 referred, visceral; rarely, psychological distress in females

Equipment

Syringe	Needle	Kenalog 40	Lidocaine	Total volume
5 ml	Spinal, 22 gauge 3.5 inches (90 mm)	40 mg	4 ml, 1%	5 ml

Anatomy   The hip joint capsule attaches to the base of the surgical neck of the femur, so if the needle is touching the neck, the solution will be deposited within the capsule. The greater trochanter is a triangular bone with a sharp angulation of the apex overhanging the neck. This part is difficult to palpate, especially on large patients, so allow at least a thumb's width proximal to the most prominent part of the trochanter. The safest and easiest approach is from the lateral aspect.

Technique
- Patient lies on pain-free side, with lower leg flexed and upper leg straight, resting horizontally on a pillow
- Palpate the triangular greater trochanter with thumb and middle finger of caudal hand, placed on either side of base, and identify dip at apex of bone with index finger
- Place index finger of cephalic hand here while passively abducting leg
- Insert needle perpendicularly about a thumb's width proximal to the apex until it touches hard neck of femur
- Inject solution as a bolus

Aftercare   Gradually increase pain activity, maintaining the range with a stretching routine, but with limitation of weight-bearing exercise. During the early stages of the degenerative process, when the pain is localized with minimal night pain, elastic end feels and reasonably good function, physiotherapy can be effective.

Practice point

The lateral approach to the hip joint is simple, safe and is not painful; there is usually no sensation of penetrating the capsule and it is not essential to perform the technique under fluoroscopy. This injection is usually given to patients awaiting hip replacement, but should not be used in the run-up to surgery because this might increase the risk of postoperative infection; discuss with the surgeon before proceeding. It usually gives temporary pain relief and can, if necessary, be repeated at intervals of no less than 3 months if the patient is still awaiting or is unsuitable for surgery. An annual x-ray monitors degenerative changes.

For large patients, the total injection volume can be increased to 8 ml to 10 ml. Adcortyl (40 mg in a volume of 4 ml) might be preferred here, and a longer spinal needle may be required.

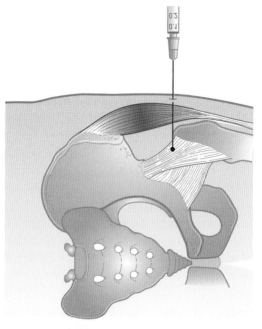

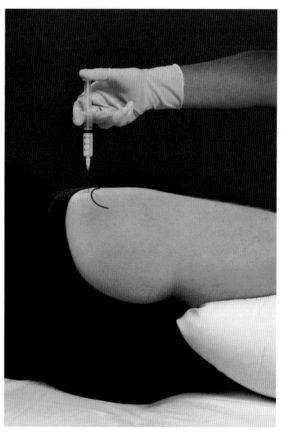

GLUTEAL BURSA **Chronic bursitis**

Hx – Overuse or fall onto buttock

OE – Pain and tenderness over the upper lateral quadrant of the buttock; painful passive flexion, abduction adduction; resisted abduction and extension

DD – Sacroiliac joint strain; referred from L4-5

Equipment

Syringe	Needle	Kenalog 40	Lidocaine	Total volume
5 ml	Spinal, 22 gauge 3.5 inches (90 mm)	40 mg	4 ml, 1%	5 ml

Anatomy

Gluteal bursae are variable in number, size and shape. They can lie deep to the gluteal muscles on the blade of the ilium and also between the layers of the three muscles. Palpation for the centre of the painful site guides the placement of the needle, but comparison between the two sides is essential because this area is always tender.

Technique

- Patient lies on unaffected side, with lower leg extended and upper leg flexed
- Identify and mark centre of tender area in upper outer quadrant of buttock
- Insert needle perpendicular to skin until it touches bone of ilium
- Inject solution in areas of no resistance while moving the needle in a circular manner, out towards surface; imagine needle point walking up a spiral staircase

Practice point

There are no major blood vessels or nerves in the area of the bursae, so the injection is straightforward. Feeling for a loss of resistance beneath and within the glutei guides the clinician in depositing the fluid. Pain referred from the lumbar spine or sacroiliac joint may be mistaken for gluteal bursitis. The mere presence of tenderness midbuttock, which is normal in most individuals, should not be considered diagnostic of an inflamed bursa.

For large individuals, a longer spinal needle might be required.

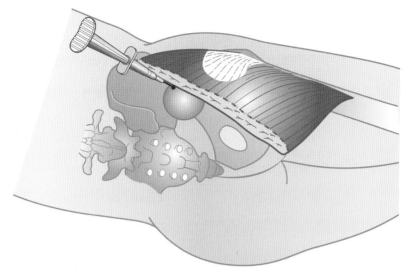

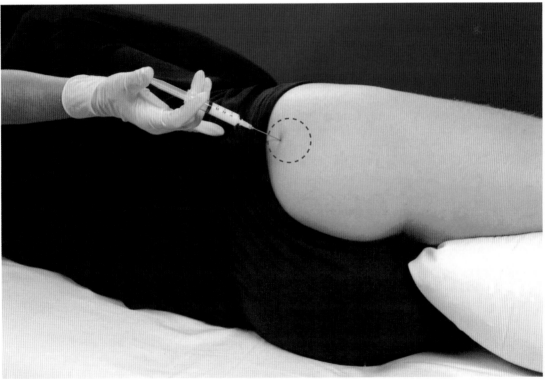

PSOAS BURSA Chronic bursitis

Hx – Overuse – especially activities involving repeated hip flexion, such as running, hurdling

OE – Pain in groin; painful passive flexion, adduction, abduction, extension; resisted flexion and adduction; scoop test – passive circular compression of femur from full flexion into adduction

DD – Hip joint OA, fracture, bony metastases, adductor strain, pubic symphysitis, hernia, abdominal muscles strain, cutaneous nerve; referred from L3, sacroiliac joint, genitourinary organs

Equipment

Syringe	Needle	Kenalog 40	Lidocaine	Total volume
2.5 ml	Spinal, 22 gauge 3.5 inches (90 mm)	20 mg	2 ml, 2%	2.5 ml

Anatomy

The psoas bursa lies between the iliopsoas tendon and the anterior aspect of the capsule over the neck of the femur. It is situated deep to three major structures in the groin – the femoral vein, artery and nerve, lying at the level of the inguinal ligament. For this reason, careful placement of the needle is essential. The following technique aims to pass the needle obliquely upwards and medially beneath the neurovascular bundle

Technique

- Patient lies supine
- Identify femoral pulse at midpoint of inguinal ligament. Mark a point three fingers distally and three fingers laterally, in line with the anterior superior iliac spine on medial edge of sartorius
- Insert needle at this point and aim 45 degrees cephalad and 45 degrees medially. Visualize needle sliding under the three major vessels through the psoas tendon until point touches bone on the hard anterior aspect of neck of femur
- Withdraw slightly and inject as a bolus deep to tendon

Aftercare

Avoidance of the activities that irritated the bursa must be maintained until symptom free, and then stretching of the hip extensors and a muscle-balancing programme can be initiated.

Practice point

Although this injection might appear intimidating at the first attempt, in our experience the approach outlined above is safe and effective. Occasionally, it is possible to catch a lateral branch of the femoral nerve and cause temporary loss of power in the quadriceps. If the patient complains of a tingling or burning pain during the process, either reposition the needle before depositing solution or abandon the procedure and reschedule.

In view of the many differential diagnoses outlined above, a high index of suspicion should be maintained until the clinician is satisfied with the diagnosis. If in doubt, a diagnostic injection of local anaesthetic alone is an option. For large patients, a longer spinal needle might be required.

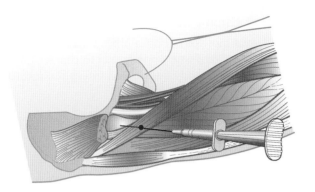

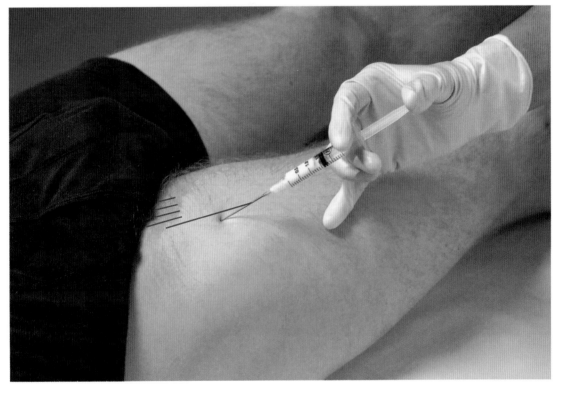

TROCHANTERIC BURSA

Acute or chronic bursitis

Hx – Direct blow or fall onto hip; spontaneous, overuse

OE – Pain and tenderness over greater trochanter; painful passive hip abduction, adduction, possibly flexion and extension; resisted abduction

DD – Fracture; referred from L2-3

Equipment

Syringe	Needle	Kenalog 40	Lidocaine	Total volume
2 ml	Blue, 23 gauge 1.25 inches (30 mm)	20 mg	1.5 ml, 2%	2 ml

Anatomy

The trochanteric bursa lies over the greater trochanter of the femur. It is approximately the size of a golf ball and is usually tender to palpation.

Technique

- Patient lies on unaffected side, with lower leg flexed and upper leg extended
- Identify and mark centre of the tender area over greater trochanter
- Insert needle perpendicularly at this point and advance to touch bone
- Inject by feeling for area of no resistance, and introduce fluid as a bolus

Aftercare

The patient should avoid overuse until they are pain free, with gradual return to normal activity. In the thin, older patient, lying on the same side every night on a hard mattress may be the cause; the trochanter can be padded with a large ring of sticky felt, and a change of lying position is encouraged. The mattress might also need to be replaced. Stretching of the iliotibial band may help.

Practice point

A fall or direct blow onto the trochanter may cause a haemorrhagic bursitis. This calls for immediate aspiration.

Severe pain over the trochanter with rapid onset and exquisite tenderness to palpation may be caused by acute calcific bursitis, similar to that seen in the shoulder. This may be visible on x-ray and often responds extremely well to injection therapy.

In resistant or recurrent cases, consider imaging to exclude tears in the short rotator muscles of the hip.

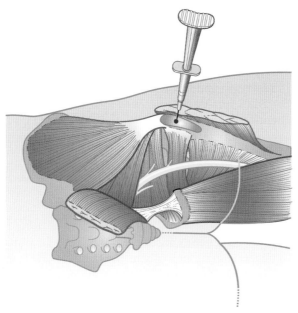

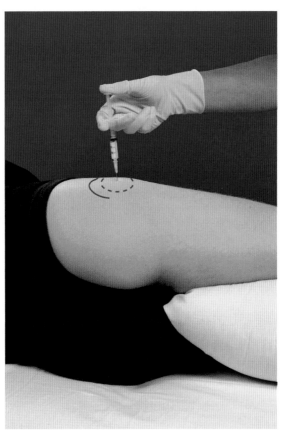

ADDUCTOR TENDONS

Chronic tendinitis

Hx – Overuse or trauma

OE – Pain in groin at origin from pubis or mid tendon; painful resisted adduction and passive abduction

DD – Hip joint OA, fracture, bony metastases, psoas bursitis, pubic symphysitis, hernia, inguinal disruption (previously called *sportsman's groin*), cutaneous nerve; referred from L3, sacroiliac joint, genitourinary organs

Equipment

Syringe	Needle	Kenalog 40	Lidocaine	Total volume
2 ml	Blue, 23 gauge 1.25 inches (30 mm)	20 mg	1.5 ml, 2%	2 ml

Anatomy

The adductor tendons arise commonly from the pubis and are approximately two fingers wide at their origin. The lesion can lie at the teno-osseous junction or in the body of the tendon. The technique described is for the more common site at the teno-osseous junction.

Technique

- Patient lies supine, with leg slightly abducted and laterally rotated
- Identify and mark origin of the tendons
- Insert needle into this spot, angle towards pubis, and touch bone
- Pepper solution into teno-osseous junction

Aftercare

The patient should rest until symptom free, and then start a graduated stretching and strengthening programme. Deep friction massage may also be used.

Practice point

For the less common site in the body of the tendon, physical therapy (including deep friction massage and stretching) may be more effective.

There are many alternative causes of pain in the groin and these may coexist, making this region one of the most diagnostically challenging in musculoskeletal medicine.

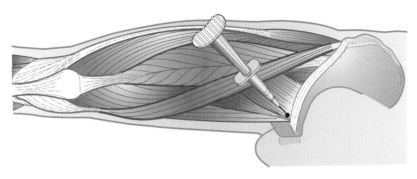

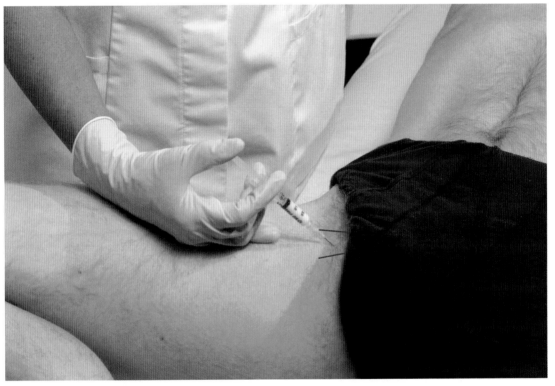

HAMSTRING TENDON AND ISCHIAL BURSA

Acute or chronic tendinitis or ischial bursitis

Hx – Friction overuse, such as prolonged cycling; trauma, such as a fall onto buttock

OE – Pain in buttock over tuberosity; painful resisted extension, passive straight leg raise

DD – Pelvic disease or fracture; referred from L4-5, S1

Equipment

Syringe	Needle	Kenalog 40	Lidocaine	Total volume
2 ml	Green, 21 gauge 2 inches (50 mm)	20 mg	1.5 ml, 2%	2 ml

Anatomy

The hamstring tendons have a common origin arising from the ischial tuberosity and are approximately three fingers wide at this point. The ischial bursa lies between the gluteus maximus and the bone of the ischial tuberosity, just deep to the tendon.

Technique

- Patient lies on unaffected side, with lower leg straight and upper leg flexed
- Identify ischial tuberosity and mark tendon origin lying immediately distal
- Insert needle into midpoint of tendon, and angle up towards tuberosity to touch bone
- Pepper solution into teno-osseous junction of tendon, or inject as a bolus into bursa

Aftercare

Avoid precipitating activities such as continually sitting on hard surfaces or prolonged running until pain eases, and then a graduated stretching and strengthening programme can be started.

Practice point

Tendinitis and bursitis can occur together at this site, in which case a larger volume is drawn up and both lesions are infiltrated. It may be difficult to differentiate between the two lesions, but if there is extreme tenderness at the tuberosity and history of a fall onto buttocks, bursitis is suspected.

Occasionally, haemorrhagic bursitis can occur as a result of a hard fall. Aspiration of the blood is then performed before infiltration.

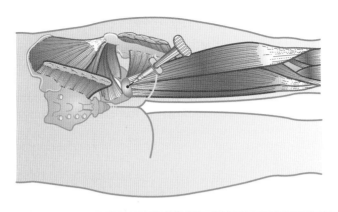

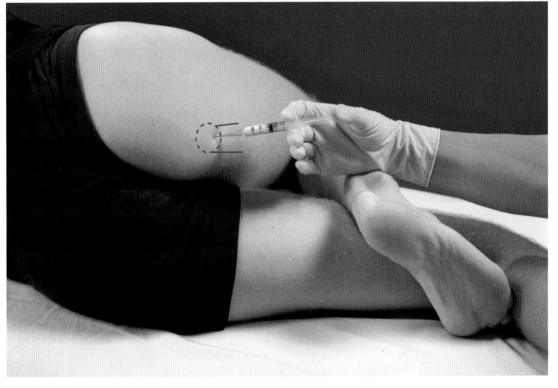

LATERAL CUTANEOUS NERVE OF THIGH

Meralgia paraesthetica

Hx – Spontaneous onset of anaesthesia, burning pain, paraesthesia on front of the thigh

OE – Clearly defined oval area of numbness over the anterolateral thigh; tender at inguinal ligament or where the lateral cutaneous nerve emerges through the fascia on the lateral thigh

DD – Referred from L3, sacroiliac joint; arterial claudication

Equipment

Syringe	Needle	Kenalog 40	Lidocaine	Total volume
1 ml	Green, 21 gauge 2 inches (50 mm)	20 mg	Nil	0.5 ml

Anatomy

The lateral cutaneous nerve of the thigh arises from the outer border of the psoas and crosses over the iliacus. It passes under or through the inguinal ligament, through the femoral fascia, and emerges superficially about a hand's width distal and in line with the anterior superior iliac spine.

Technique

- Patient lies supine
- Identify tender area at the inguinal ligament or at a distal point in the thigh
- Inject as a bolus around the compressed nerve, avoiding nerve itself

Aftercare

This entrapment neuropathy can be caused by compression of the lateral cutaneous nerve from obesity, tight underwear, prolonged sitting with a flexed posture (so-called *crane driver's thigh*) or pregnancy. Removing the cause is therefore of prime importance, such as losing weight, avoiding tight clothing, or correcting sitting posture. If the patient is pregnant, the compression might be from the growing foetus, and symptoms will normally abate after delivery.

Practice point

As with other nerve compression injections, the nerve itself must not be injected. If the patient reports increased tingling or burning pain during the procedure, the needle should be moved before the steroid is injected around, not into, the nerve.

This lesion often resolves spontaneously. Advice on avoidance of compression and reassurance as to the nature and normal outcome of the condition might be all that is required.

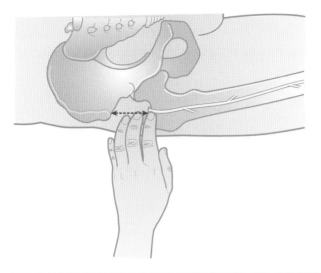

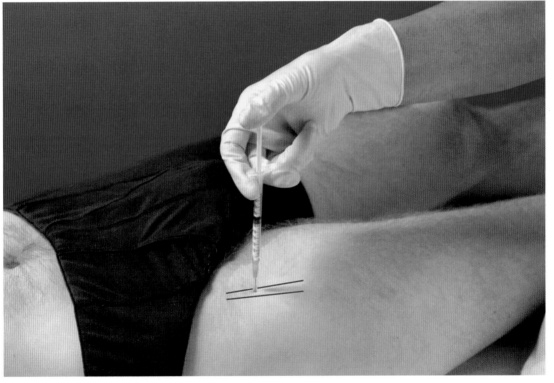

THE KNEE

KNEE EXAMINATION

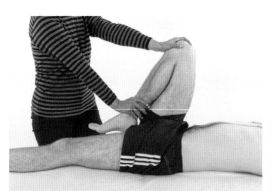

1 Passive flexion

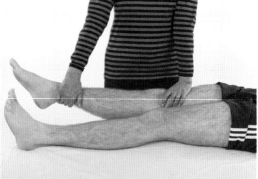

2 Passive extension

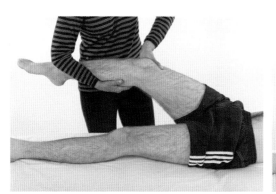

3 Passive valgus

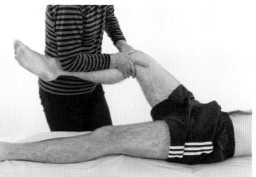

4 Passive varus

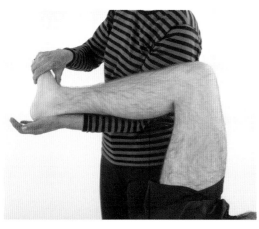

5 Passive lateral rotation

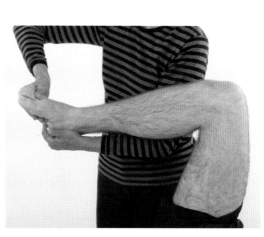

6 Passive medial rotation

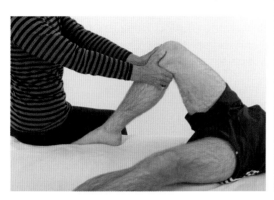

7 Draw test. Anterior and posterior draw test for anterior cruciate ligament/posterior cruciate ligament

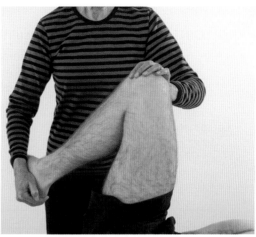

8 Meniscal tests. Four meniscal tests in full flexion into combined medial rotation + varus-valgus, lateral rotation + varus-valgus

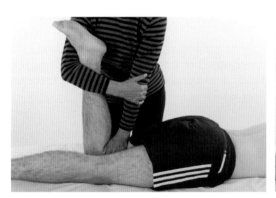

9 Resisted extension

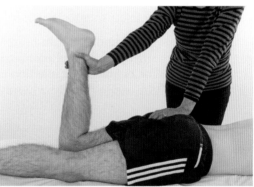

10 Resisted flexion

Additional knee tests if necessary
- Proprioception, squat, Lachman's or Ober's
- Popliteus test – resisted combined knee flexion with medial rotation of tibia

KNEE JOINT **Acute or chronic capsulitis**

Hx – OA, RA, gout or trauma

OE – Pain in knee joint, possible warmth, effusion, crepitus; CP: more passive flexion than extension, hard end feel on flexion

DD – Soft tissues around knee, menisci; referred from L3

Equipment

Syringe	Needle	Adcortyl	Lidocaine	Total volume
10 ml	Green, 21 gauge 1.5 inches (40 mm)	40 mg Adcortyl	5 ml, 1%	9 ml

Anatomy
The knee joint has a potential capacity of approximately 120 ml or more in the average-sized adult. The capsule is lined with synovium, which is convoluted and thus has a large surface area; in the larger knee, therefore, more volume will be required to bathe all the target area. Plicae, which are bands of synovium, might exist within the joint and can also become inflamed. The suprapatellar pouch is a continuum of the synovial capsule. and there are many bursae around the joint.

Technique
- Patient sits with knee supported in slight flexion
- Identify and mark medial edge of patella
- Insert needle and angle laterally and slightly upwards under patella
- Inject solution as bolus, and/or aspirate if required

Aftercare
Avoid undue weight-bearing activity until symptoms abate, and then start strengthening and mobilizing exercises. One study found that total bed rest for 24 hours after injection in rheumatoid knees shows better results; however, the bed rest involved hospital stay, which is not cost-effective.

Practice point

In obese patients using a longer needle and a larger volume of 40 mg of Adcortyl, enables more of the joint surface to be bathed. Hyaluronans may be injected but are more expensive than corticosteroids and do not appear to have longer lasting benefits.

The injection provides a variable length of pain relief, but if the knee is not overused this may be prolonged. Repeat injections can be given at intervals of not less than 3 months, with an annual x-ray to monitor joint degeneration. If the patient is awaiting surgery, discuss with the surgeon before proceeding.

There are several ways to enter the knee joint; one study showed more successful placement using the supralateral approach than through the eyes of the knee, but did not compare the lateral with this medial approach. The advantage here is that there is plenty of space to insert the needle between the medial condyle and the patella, where even small amounts of serous fluid or blood can be aspirated with a large (19 gauge) needle. Sometimes an obvious effusion is difficult to aspirate; in this case, moving the needle point around within the joint may be more successful.

Only one RCT looked at whether LA should be injected into the aspiration site first to make the procedure more comfortable; it made no difference to patient comfort.

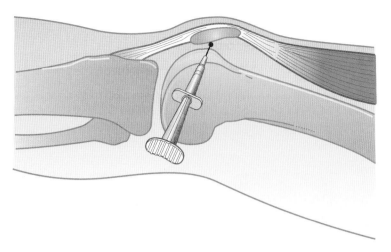

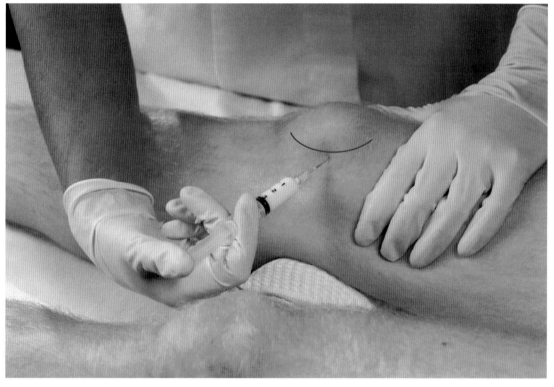

SUPERIOR TIBIOFIBULAR JOINT

Acute or chronic capsulitis

Hx – Usually trauma, such as a fall with forced medial rotation and varus on the flexed knee

OE – Pain over the lateral side of the knee; painful resisted flexion, and full passive medial rotation of knee

DD – Lateral collateral ligament strain, lateral meniscus tear; referred from L4-5

Equipment

Syringe	Needle	Kenalog 40	Lidocaine	Total volume
2 ml	Orange, 25 gauge 0.5 inch (13 mm)	20 mg	1 ml, 2%	1.5 ml

Anatomy
The superior tibiofibular joint runs medially under the lateral slope of the tibia, from superior to inferior. The anterior approach is safer because the peroneal nerve lies immediately posterior to the joint.

Technique
- Patient sits with knee at a right angle
- Identify head of fibula and mark joint line medial to it
- Insert needle at midpoint of joint line and aim obliquely and laterally to penetrate capsule
- Deposit solution as a bolus

Aftercare
Advise relative rest until symptom free, and then resume normal activities. Strengthening of the biceps femoris might be necessary.

Practice point

This is an uncommon injection. Occasionally the joint is subluxed and has to be manipulated before infiltration. The condition may occur after a severe ankle sprain.

The unstable joint could be treated with sclerotherapy and taping.

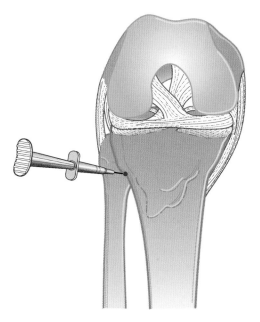

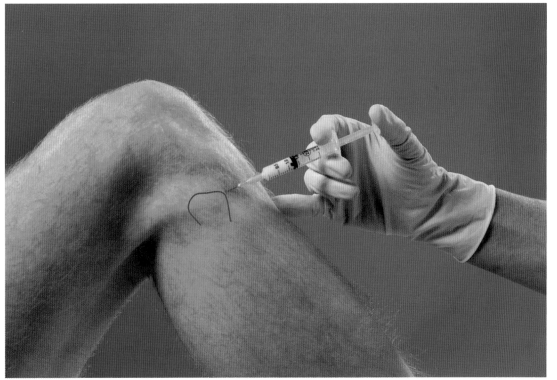

**BAKER'S CYST
ASPIRATION**

Baker's cyst aspiration

Hx – Spontaneous, insidious onset, usually in an osteoarthritic joint
OE – Obvious swelling in the popliteal fossa, often quite large; limited active
    and passive knee flexion
DD – Ruptured Baker's cyst may mimic deep vein thrombosis of the calf

Equipment

Syringe	Needle	Kenalog 40	Lidocaine	Total volume
10 ml	White, 19 gauge 1.5 inches (40 mm)	Nil	Nil	

Anatomy

A Baker's cyst is an enlarged sac of synovial fluid caused by seepage through a defect in the posterior wall of the capsule of the knee joint or by effusion within the semimembranosus bursa. The popliteal artery and vein and posterior tibial nerve pass centrally in the popliteal fossa and must be avoided when injecting.

Technique

- Patient lies prone
- Mark spot two fingers medial to midline of fossa and two fingers below popliteal crease
- Insert needle at marked spot and angle laterally at a 45 degree angle
- Aspirate excess fluid

Aftercare

A firm compression bandage can be applied for 1 or 2 days.

Practice point

If anything other than clear synovial fluid is removed, a specimen should be sent for culture and the appropriate treatment instigated. The swelling frequently returns at some point but can be reaspirated if the patient wishes.

A Baker's cyst is often found in association with a knee effusion and disappears on aspirating the knee, implying that they communicate.

Refrain from putting a needle into a pulsatile Baker's cyst; this is almost certainly a popliteal artery aneurysm.

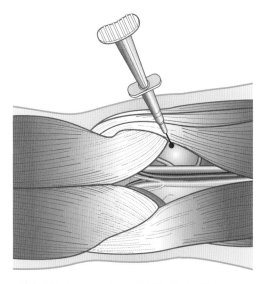

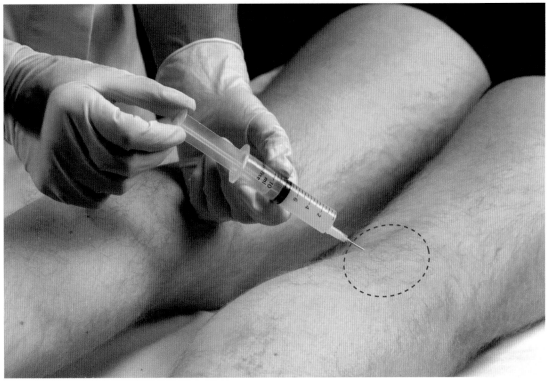

ILIOTIBIAL BAND BURSA

Chronic bursitis

Hx – Overuse, especially long distance runners

OE – Pain on the outer side of the knee above the lateral femoral condyle; painful resisted abduction and passive adduction of leg, painful Ober's test

DD – Iliotibial band bursitis; referred from L4-5

Equipment

Syringe	Needle	Kenalog 40	Lidocaine	Total volume
2 ml	Blue, 23 gauge 1.25 inches (30 mm)	20 mg	1.5 ml, 2%	2 ml

Anatomy

The bursa lies deep to the iliotibial band, just above the lateral condyle of the femur, and is approximately the size of a golf ball.

Technique

- Patient sits with knee supported
- Identify and mark tender area on lateral side of femur
- Insert needle into bursa, passing through tendon to touch bone
- Deposit solution as a bolus

Aftercare

Absolute rest should be maintained for about 10 days and then a stretching and strengthening programme initiated. Footwear and running technique should be assessed and corrected if necessary.

Practice point

The lower end of the iliotibial tract itself can be irritated, but invariably the bursa is also at fault. If both lesions are suspected, infiltration of both at the same time can be performed by peppering a small amount into the tendinous insertion and injecting a bolus of remaining fluid into the bursa beneath.

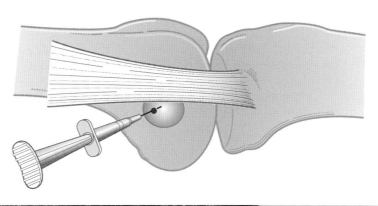

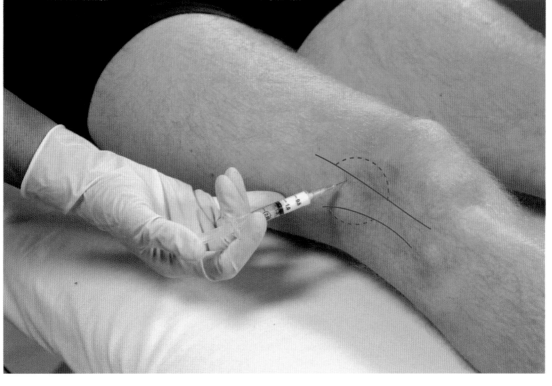

INFRAPATELLAR BURSA

Acute or chronic bursitis

Hx – Overuse – prolonged running or kneeling; trauma – direct blow

OE – Anterior knee pain distal to the lower pole of the patella; painful resisted extension of knee, full passive flexion of knee, tenderness midtendon

DD – Infrapatellar tendinitis, patella fracture, meniscal tear; Osgood-Schlatter's disease

Equipment

Syringe	Needle	Kenalog 40	Lidocaine	Total volume
2 ml	Blue, 23 gauge 1.25 inches (30 mm)	20 mg	1.5 ml, 2%	2 ml

Anatomy

There are two infrapatellar bursae; one lies superficial to and one deep to the tendon. In a small study, it was found that the deep bursa consistently lay posterior to the distal third of the tendon and was slightly wider. A fat pad apron extends from the retropatellar fat pad to compartmentalize the bursa partially. The technique described is for the deep bursa, which is more commonly affected.

Technique

- Patient sits with leg extended and knee supported
- Identify and mark tender area at midpoint of tendon
- Insert needle horizontally at lateral edge of tendon, just proximal to tibial tubercle; ensure that needle enters deep to posterior surface of tendon. There should be no resistance to fluid flow
- Deposit solution as a bolus

Aftercare

Avoid overuse of the knee until pain free, when correction of footwear, running style and quadriceps and hamstring strengthening exercises may be necessary. When the cause is occupational, such as in carpet layers, a pad with a hole in it to relieve pressure on the bursa can be used.

Practice point

It is tempting to believe that pain found at the midpoint of the patellar tendon is caused by tendinitis, but in our experience, this is extremely rare at this site. Infrapatellar tendinitis is found consistently at the proximal teno-osseous junction on the patella or, rarely, at insertion into the tibial tubercle. Pain here in an active adolescent should be considered to be Osgood-Schlatter's disease and should not be injected because of its proximity to the growing end plate; taping and rest may relieve the symptoms.

For the superficial infrapatellar bursa and the prepatellar bursa, palpate for the centre of the tender area and, using the same equipment, inject just deep to the skin and superior to the bone. Free flow of the fluid confirms the correct placement within the structure. Consider using hydrocortisone for thin, dark-skinned individuals to avoid skin depigmentation or fat atrophy.

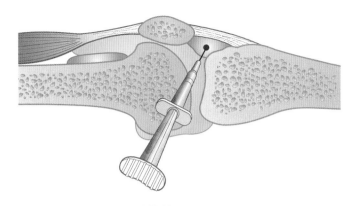

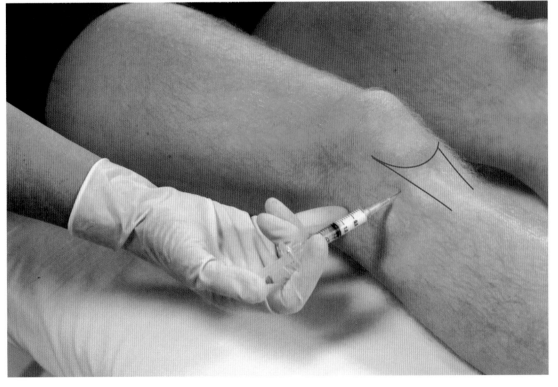

PES ANSERINE BURSA	## Chronic bursitis

Hx – Overuse, especially dancers or runners

OE – Pain, localized tenderness and possible visible or palpable swelling just proximal to insertion of medial flexors of knee; painful resisted knee flexion

DD – Individual sartorius, gracilis or semitendinosis tendon lesions

Equipment

Syringe	Needle	Kenalog 40	Lidocaine	Total volume
2 ml	Blue, 23 gauge 1.25 inches (30 mm)	20 mg	1.5 ml, 2%	2 ml

Anatomy   The pes anserine, or so-called *goose's foot,* is the combined tendon of insertion of the sartorius, gracilis and semitendinosis. It attaches on the medial side of the tibia, just below the knee joint line. The bursa lies immediately under the tendon, just posterior to its insertion into the tibia, and is normally very tender to palpation.

Technique
- Patient sits with knee supported
- Identify pes anserine tendon by flexing knee against resistance. Follow easily palpated flexor tendons distally to where they disappear at insertion into tibia. Mark tender area slightly proximal to insertion
- Insert needle into centre of this area, through tendon to touch bone
- Deposit solution as a bolus

Aftercare   Avoid overuse activities until pain free. A change in the causal activity and possible footwear correction or advice from a podiatrist may need to be considered.

Practice point

Remember that the bursa is extremely tender to palpation in everyone, so always compare palpation with the other knee.

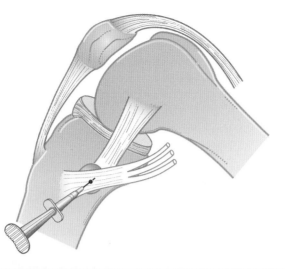

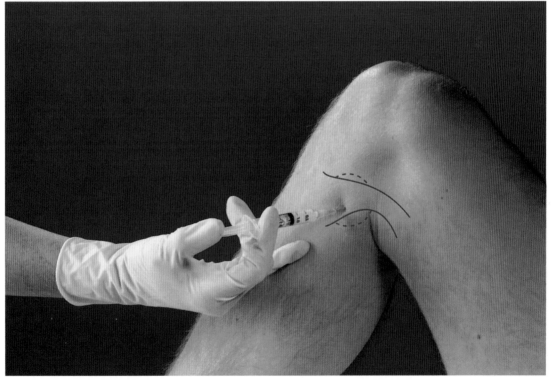

CORONARY LIGAMENTS

Ligamentous sprain

Hx – Trauma – strong forced rotation of the knee with or without meniscal tear, postmeniscectomy or constant running on the same side of the road

OE – Pain usually at medial joint line painful – passive lateral rotation; possibly meniscal grind tests

DD – Meniscal tear

Equipment

Syringe	Needle	Kenalog 40	Lidocaine	Total volume
1 ml	Orange, 25 gauge 0.5 inch (13 mm)	10 mg	0.75 ml, 2%	1 ml

Anatomy

The coronary ligaments are small, thin, fibrous bands attaching the menisci to the tibial plateau. The medial coronary ligament is much more usually affected. It can be found by flexing the knee to a right angle and turning the planted foot into lateral rotation. This brings the medial tibial plateau into prominence, and the tender area is found by pressing in and down onto the plateau.

Technique

- Patient sits with knee at a right angle and planted foot laterally rotated
- Identify and mark tender area on tibial plateau
- Insert needle vertically down onto plateau
- Pepper all along tender area; strong resistance will be felt

Aftercare

Early mobilizing exercises to full range of motion without pain are started immediately. Advice on athletic choices may be needed.

Practice point

This lesion is commonly missed; apparent meniscal tears, anterior cruciate sprain or patellofemoral joint lesions might be simple coronary ligament sprains. It is always worth checking the ligament after a meniscal tear or surgery, as often both structures are damaged concurrently.

The classic history is of the so-called *cinema seat syndrome*; sitting for a prolonged period in a cramped position causes pain when getting up. Often there are no objective tests, and the only sign is pain on palpation along the joint line when compared with the other knee.

These ligaments usually respond extremely well to deep friction massage; it is not uncommon to cure the symptoms in one session. The injection therefore should be reserved for when the friction treatment is not available or the pain is too intense to allow the pressure of the finger. This is a fairly common knee lesion, but is usually nonrecurrent with appropriate avoidance of aggravating activities and possible use of orthotics.

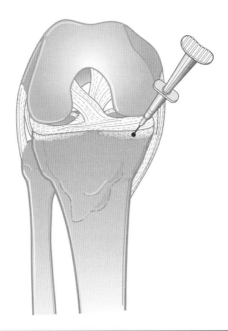

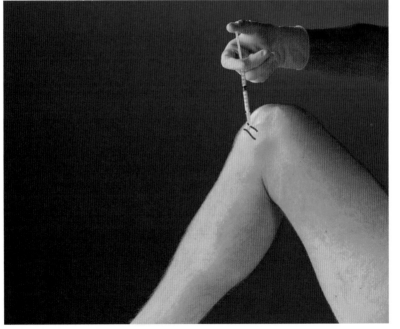

MEDIAL COLLATERAL LIGAMENT

Chronic sprain

Hx – Trauma – typically flexion, valgus and lateral rotation of the knee, such as a fall while skiing

OE – Pain along the medial knee joint line; painful passive valgus and lateral rotation of the knee

DD – Medial meniscal tear, anterior cruciate ligament sprain

Equipment

Syringe	Needle	Kenalog 40	Lidocaine	Total volume
2 ml	Blue, 23 gauge 1.25 inches (30 mm)	20 mg	1 ml, 2%	1.5 ml

Anatomy

The medial collateral ligament of the knee passes distally from the medial condyle of the femur to the medial aspect of the shaft of the tibia and is approximately a hand's width long and three fingers wide at the joint line. It is difficult to palpate the ligament because it is so thin and is intimately connected to the joint capsule. It is usually sprained at the joint line.

Technique

- Patient lies with knee supported and slightly flexed
- Identify and mark medial joint line and tender area of ligament
- Insert needle at midpoint of tender area. Do not penetrate into joint capsule
- Pepper solution along the width of ligament in two rows

Aftercare

In the acute phase, ice knee supports, oral analgesia and early instruction on normal gait, using stairs and placing a pillow under the knee at night are very helpful. Gentle passive and active movement within the pain-free range is started immediately.

Practice point

Sprain of this ligament rarely needs to be injected because early physiotherapeutic treatment with ice, massage and mobilization is very effective. The injection approach could be used when this treatment is not available or the patient is in a great deal of pain.

Occasionally, the distal or proximal end of the ligament is affected, so the solution can be deposited there.

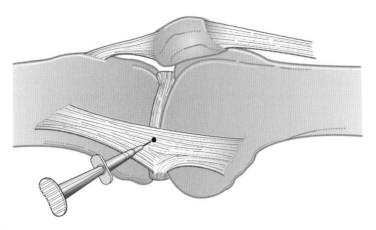

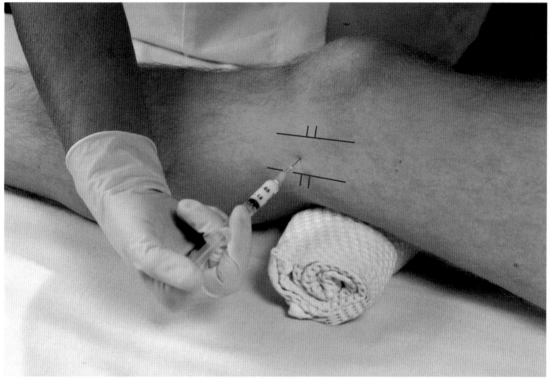

INFRAPATELLAR TENDON

Chronic tendinitis

Hx – Overuse, jumpers and runners

OE – Pain at inferior pole of patella; painful resisted extension of the knee

DD – Infrapatellar bursitis; Osgood-Schlatter's disease; referred from hip or L3

Equipment

Syringe	Needle	Kenalog 40	Lidocaine	Total volume
2 ml	Blue, 23 gauge 1.25 inches (30 mm)	20 mg	1.5 ml, 2%	2 ml

Anatomy

The infrapatellar tendon arises from the inferior pole of the patella, and it is here that it is usually affected. The tendon is at least two fingers wide at its origin. It is an absolute contraindication to inject corticosteroid into the body of the tendon because it is a large, weight-bearing and relatively avascular structure. Tenderness at the midpoint of the tendon is usually related to infrapatellar bursitis.

Technique

- Patient sits with knee supported and extended
- Place web of the cephalic hand on superior pole of patella and tilt inferior pole up. Mark tender area at the origin of tendon on distal end of patella
- Insert needle at midpoint of tendon origin at an angle of 45 degrees
- Pepper solution along tendon origin in two rows. Resistance to flow of the drug ensures that needle is not intraarticular

Aftercare

Absolute rest from strong exercise is recommended, and when symptoms are relieved, a stretching and strengthening programme is initiated. Retraining should be undertaken gradually.

Practice point

In an older patient with a chronic tendinopathy, scanning is recommended before considering injection to ensure that there are no significant degenerative changes in the substance of the tendon.

In the case of the committed athlete, or if scanning shows changes as above, a conservative physiotherapeutic approach should be used. This might include an eccentric exercise programme, a glyceryl trinitrate patch, taping, deep friction and/or electrotherapy together with running and orthotic advice.

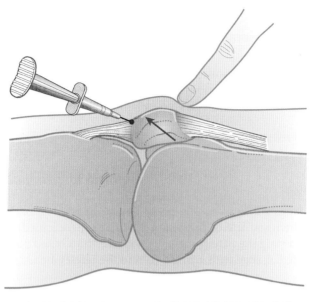

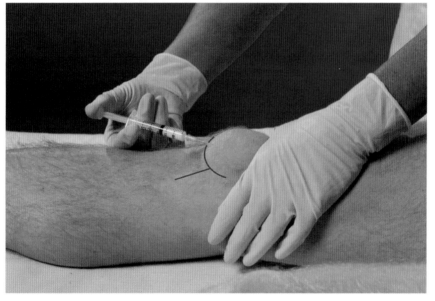

QUADRICEPS
EXPANSION

Muscle sprain

Hx – Overuse

OE – Pain usually on superomedial side of patella on going downstairs or cycling; painful resisted extension of the knee

DD – Patellofemoral joint inflammation, medial collateral ligament sprain

Equipment

Syringe	Needle	Kenalog 40	Lidocaine	Total volume
2 ml	Orange, 25 gauge 0.5 inch (13 mm)	10 mg	1.75 ml, 2%	2 ml

Anatomy

The quadriceps muscle inserts as an expansion around the edges of the patella. The usual site of the lesion is at the superior medial pole. This is found by pushing the patella medially with the thumb and palpating up and under the medial edge with a finger to find the tender area.

Technique

- Patient half-lies with knee relaxed
- Identify and mark tender area, usually on medial edge of superior pole of patella
- Insert needle and angle horizontally to touch bone of patella
- Pepper solution along line of insertion. Some resistance will be felt

Aftercare

Avoid overusing the knee until pain free, when a progressive strengthening and stretching programme may be started.

Practice point

This is an uncommon injection; in our experience, this lesion usually responds very well to two or three sessions of strong deep friction massage. The injection might be used therefore when friction is not available or the area is too tender or to reduce pain in the expansion prior to friction a week later, in a combination approach.

The same dose and technique may be used to inject inflamed plicae around the patella rim.

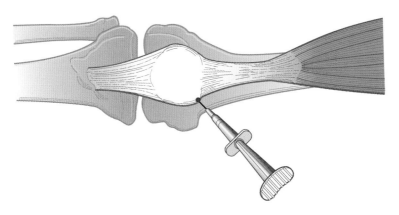

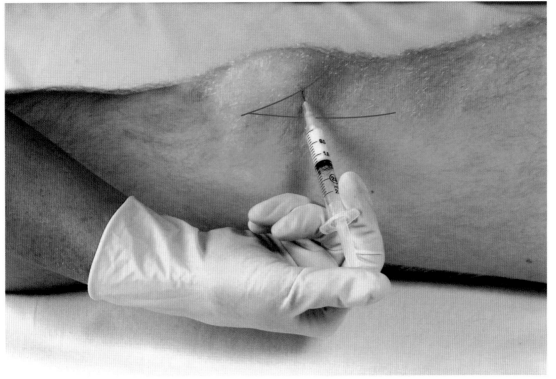

THE ANKLE AND FOOT

ANKLE
EXAMINATION

Ankle and foot tests
Palpate for heat, swelling and synovial thickening

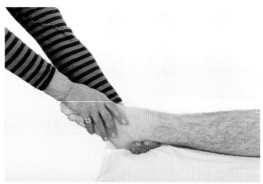

1 Ankle passive dorsiflexion

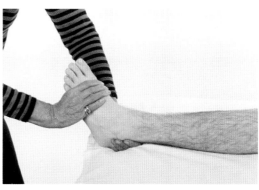

2 Ankle passive plantarflexion

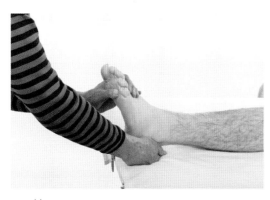

3 Ankle passive eversion

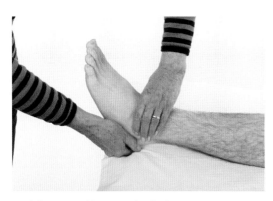

4 Ankle passive inversion

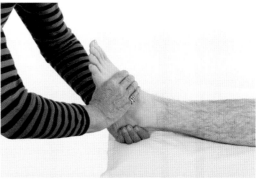

5 Abduction-adduction of subtalar joint

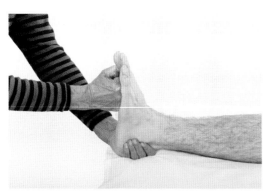

6 Midtarsal joint testing – passive flexion, extension, eversion and inversion

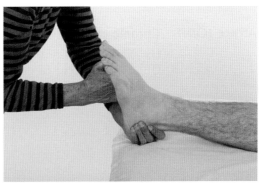

7 Resisted dorsiflexion

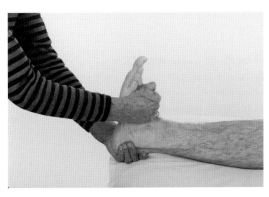

8 Resisted plantarflexion

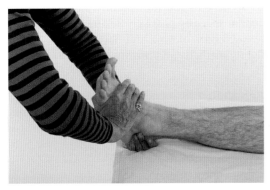

9 Resisted eversion

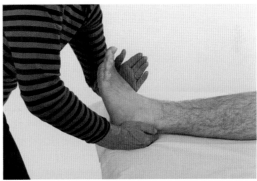

10 Resisted inversion

Ankle and foot capsular patterns

- Ankle – more loss of plantarflexion than dorsiflexion
- Subtalar joint – more loss of adduction
- Forefoot – loss of adduction, dorsiflexion and supination
- Big toe – more loss of extension than flexion
- Toes – more loss of flexion than extension
- Palpate to localize lesion

Additional foot tests

- Proprioception
- Individual ligament tests
- Draw test for ankle instability – fix planted foot with other hand, grip fibular base between thumb base and fingers of other hand and glide bone anterior and posterior. Compare sides

SECTION 4

ANKLE JOINT   Chronic capsulitis

Hx – Post trauma or fracture, sometimes many years later

OE – Pain at front of or within the ankle; CP: more passive plantarflexion than dorsiflexion with hard end feel

DD – Tendinitis of dorsiflexors; fracture; referred from L3, 4, 5

Equipment

Syringe	Needle	Kenalog 40	Lidocaine	Total volume
2.5 ml	Blue, 23 gauge 1.25 inches (30 mm)	30 mg	1.75 ml, 2%	2.5 ml

Anatomy   The easiest and safest entry point to the ankle joint is at the junction of the tibia and fibula, just above the talus. A small triangular space can be palpated here.

Technique
- Patient lies with knee bent to 90 degrees and foot slightly plantarflexed
- Identify and mark small triangular space by passively flexing and extending ankle while palpating gap between base of tibia and fibula
- Insert needle here, angling slightly medially and proximally into joint space
- Deposit solution as a bolus

Aftercare   Excessive weight-bearing activities should be avoided until symptoms ease. Advise the patient that heavy overuse will cause a recurrence of symptoms, and therefore long distance running should be curtailed. Weight control is also advised, and footwear should be assessed to ensure correct support; appropriate insoles often help maintain pain-free walking.

Initiate passive joint mobilization and strengthening of the dorsiflexors and evertors, and assess muscle balance around the ankle because this is often a contributing factor.

Practice point

The ankle joint rarely causes problems except after severe trauma or fracture, and then often many years later.

In our experience the injection is often successful in giving reasonably prolonged pain relief, provided excessive weight bearing is avoided. This can be repeated if necessary at intervals of at least 3 months with an annual x-ray to monitor degenerative changes.

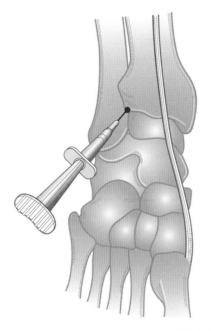

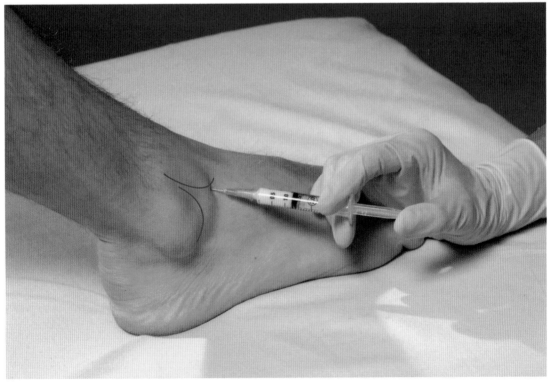

SUBTALAR JOINT   **Chronic capsulitis**

Hx – Trauma after fracture or severe impaction injury, often years later. RA overuse in older obese patient

OE – Pain deep in medial and lateral sides of heel; CP: passive adduction of the calcaneus

DD – Deltoid or lateral ligaments; gout

Equipment

Syringe	Needle	Kenalog 40	Lidocaine	Total volume
2 ml	Blue, 23 gauge 1.25 inches (30 mm)	30 mg	1.25 ml, 2%	2 ml

Anatomy

The subtalar joint is divided by an oblique septum into anterior and posterior portions. It is slightly easier to enter the joint just above the sustentaculum tali, which projects a thumb's width directly below the medial malleolus.

Technique

- Patient lies on side with foot supported so that medial aspect of heel faces upwards
- Identify bump of sustentaculum tali
- Insert needle perpendicularly immediately above and slightly posterior to sustentaculum tali
- Deposit half solution here
- Withdraw needle slightly, angle obliquely anteriorly through septum into anterior compartment of joint space and deposit remaining solution here

Aftercare

Avoid excessive weight-bearing activities until pain free. Orthotics and weight control are helpful in preventing recurrence.

Practice point

This is a difficult injection to perform because of the anatomical shape of the joint. If the needle does not enter the joint immediately, deposit a small amount of the mixed solution into the area. This will allow more comfortable further attempts to place the needle intraarticularly. It may be repeated at infrequent intervals if necessary.

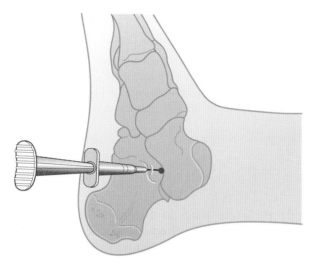

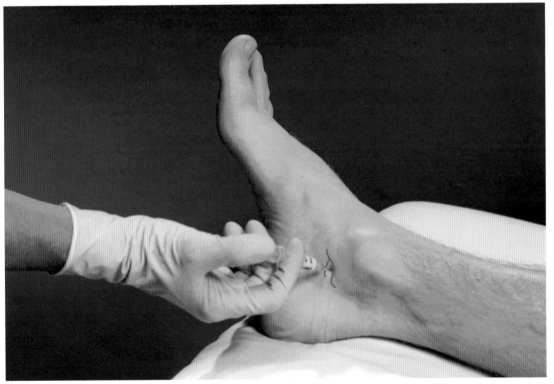

MIDTARSAL JOINTS

Acute or chronic capsulitis

Hx – Overuse or trauma, such as dancers who overpoint

OE – Pain on dorsum of foot, often at third metatarsocuneiform joint line; CP: adduction and inversion of midtarsal joints

DD – Tendinitis of dorsiflexors metatarsal stress fracture; gout

Equipment

Syringe	Needle	Kenalog 40	Lidocaine	Total volume
2 ml	Blue, 23 gauge 1 inch (25 mm)	20 mg	1.5 ml, 2%	2 ml

Anatomy

There are several joints in the midtarsus, each with its own capsule. Gross passive testing in all six directions followed by local joint gliding and palpation should identify the joint or joints involved.

Technique

- Patient lies with foot supported in a neutral position
- Identify and mark tender joint line
- Insert needle down into joint space
- Pepper some solution into capsule and remainder as a bolus into joint cavity

Aftercare

Avoid excessive weight-bearing activities until the pain is eased. Mobilizing and strengthening exercises and retraining of causal activities follow. Orthotics and weight control, if necessary, are useful additions.

Practice point

A successful outcome is more likely if sensible attention is paid to aftercare. For example, it is very difficult for an adult female ballet dancer to stop overpointing, so different dance methods should be discussed tactfully.

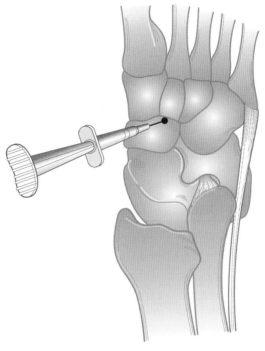

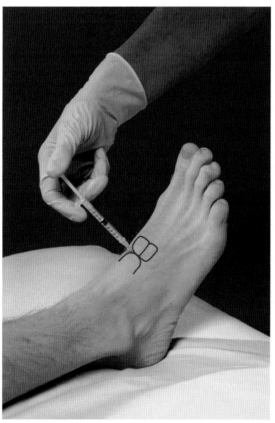

TOE JOINTS   **Acute or chronic capsulitis**

Hx – Overuse or trauma; hallux valgus or hammer toe may be present

OE – Pain locally in toe joint(s); CP: extension of big toe, flexion of other toes

DD – Hallux valgus or rigidus; infected toenail, sesamoid stress fracture

Equipment

Syringe	Needle	Kenalog 40	Lidocaine	Total volume
1–2 ml	Orange, 25 gauge 0.5 inch (13 mm)	10–20 mg	0.5–1 ml, 2%	0.75–1 ml

Anatomy   The first metatarsophalangeal joint line is found by palpating the space produced at the base of the metatarsal on the dorsal aspect while passively flexing and extending the toe. Palpation of the collateral ligaments at the joint line on the sides of the other toes will help identify the affected joint.

Technique
- Patient lies with foot supported
- Distract affected toe with one hand
- Identify and mark joint line
- Insert needle perpendicularly into joint space, avoiding extensor tendons
- Deposit the solution as a bolus

Aftercare   Avoid excessive weight-bearing activities until comfortable, together with taping of the joint and a toe pad between the toes. Care in choice of footwear and orthotic advice will usually be necessary.

Practice point

This treatment may be long-lasting in early degenerative disease of the first metatarsophalangeal joint but less so in advanced cases. The other toe joints are usually more easily injected from the medial or lateral aspect while under traction using a smaller dose and volume, such as 10 mg Kenalog plus 0.5 ml lidocaine (0.75 ml total volume).

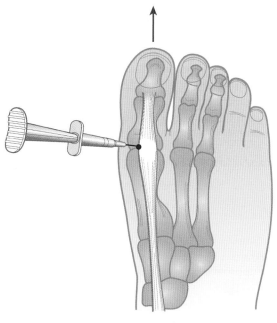

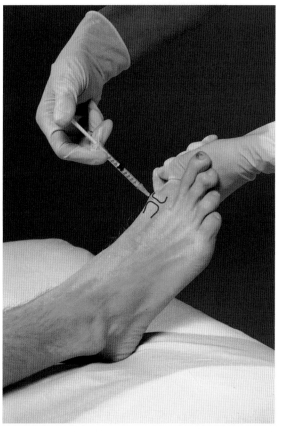

ACHILLES BURSA   ## Chronic bursitis

Hx – Overuse, often runners and dancers

OE – Pain posterior to tibia and anterior to the body of Achilles tendon; painful resisted plantarflexion, especially at end range; full passive plantarflexion

DD – Achilles tendinitis, referred from S1, early sign of ankylosing spondylitis, gout, calcaneal stress fracture

Equipment

Syringe	Needle	Kenalog 40	Lidocaine	Total volume
2 ml	Blue, 23 gauge 1.25 inches (30 mm)	20 mg	1.5 ml, 2%	2 ml

Anatomy
The Achilles bursa lies in the triangular space anterior to the tendon and posterior to the base of the tibia and the upper part of the calcaneus. The safest approach is from the lateral side to avoid the posterior tibial artery and nerve.

Technique
- Patient lies prone. with foot held in dorsiflexion
- Identify and mark tender hollow on lateral side of tendon
- Insert needle into bursa anterior to tendon; avoid piercing tendon
- Deposit solution as a bolus

Aftercare
Avoid overuse activities until pain free, and then start a stretching and eccentric exercise programme.

Practice point

It is important to differentiate between tendinitis and bursitis here because both are caused by overuse. In bursitis, there is usually more pain on full passive plantarflexion when the heel is pressed up against the back of the tibia, thereby squeezing the bursa. Also, palpation of the bursa is very sensitive, and the pain is usually felt more at the end of rising on tiptoe rather than during the movement. Female ballet dancers need to avoid overplantarflexing the ankle when on point.

Avoid penetrating the Achilles tendon and depositing the solution there. Any resistance to the needle requires immediate withdrawal and repositioning well anterior to the tendon.

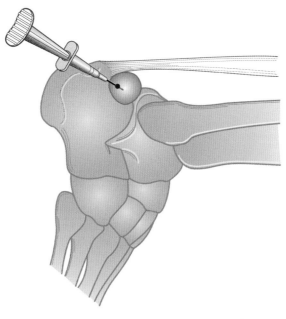

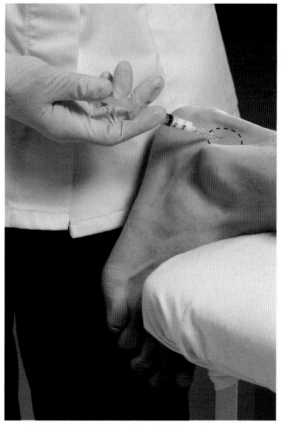

DELTOID LIGAMENT

Chronic sprain

Hx – Trauma, overuse or obesity, sometimes after severe lateral ligament sprain

OE – Pain over medial side of heel below the medial malleolus, overpronated foot; painful passive eversion of ankle in plantarflexion

DD – Flexor tendinitis, calcaneus fracture; referred from L4

Equipment

Syringe	Needle	Kenalog 40	Lidocaine	Total volume
1 ml	Orange, 25 gauge 0.5 inch (13 mm)	10 mg	0.75 ml, 2%	1 ml

Anatomy

The deltoid ligament is a strong cuboid structure with two layers. It runs from the medial malleolus to the sustentaculum tali on the calcaneus and to the tubercle on the navicular. The inflamed part is usually at the origin on the malleolus.

Technique

- Patient sits with medial side of foot accessible
- Identify lower border of medial malleolus and mark midpoint of ligament
- Insert needle and angle upwards to touch bone at midpoint of ligament
- Pepper solution along ligamentous attachment to bone. There should be resistance here

Aftercare

Activity should be limited until the patient is symptom free. To prevent recurrence, the biomechanics of the foot must be carefully checked. Orthotics are almost always necessary and, where appropriate, advice on weight loss muscle building and proprioception retraining may also help.

Practice point

This is an uncommon injection. Sprains here are not as common as at the lateral ligament, but because they do not seem to respond well to deep friction and mobilization, injection is worth trying.

When this problem follows a severe sprain of the lateral ligament, the patient often is not aware of the medial pain until sometime later. The presumed cause in this case is bruising of the calcaneus as it impinges on the sustentaculum tali.

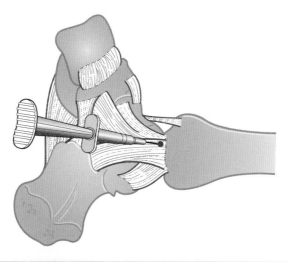

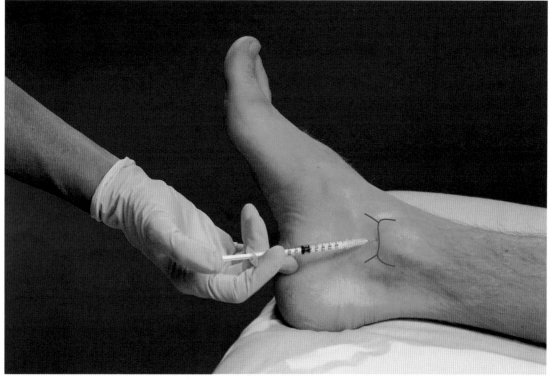

LATERAL LIGAMENT

Chronic sprain

Hx – Inversion injury
OE – Pain at lateral side of ankle; painful passive inversion of ankle
DD – Peroneal tendinitis, fibular or ankle fracture, lateral ligament rupture

Equipment

Syringe	Needle	Kenalog 40	Lidocaine	Total volume
1 ml	Orange, 25 gauge 0.5 inch (13 mm)	10 mg	0.75 ml, 2%	1 ml

Anatomy

Three ligaments make up the lateral ligament complex, of which the anterior talofibular ligament is most commonly sprained. It runs distally and medially from the anterior inferior edge of the lateral malleolus to attach to the talus and is a thin structure, approximately the width of the little finger. The bifurcate calcaneocuboid ligament runs from the calcaneus to the cuboid and is often also involved in ankle sprains. Both ligaments run parallel to the sole of the foot. The calcaneofibular runs obliquely distally and posteriorly from the posterior edge of the lateral malleolus to the calcaneum and is approximately two fingers' width in length. It is rounder, so it is more easily palpated than the other two ligaments and less commonly injured. The technique below is for the anterior talofibular ligament.

Technique

- Patient lies supported
- Identify and mark anterior inferior edge of lateral malleolus
- Insert needle to touch bone
- Pepper half of the solution around origin of ligament
- Turn needle and pepper remainder into insertion on talus

Aftercare

This lesion usually responds very well in the acute stage to an immediate regimen of ice, elevation and gentle massage. Taping, together with a pressure pad behind the malleolus, helps control swelling. The patient keeps the ankle constantly moving within the pain-free range while elevated, and active and passive mobilization with balance training and instruction on normal heel-toe gait should be administered. A hairline fracture of the fibula should be suspected if pain is worse on weight bearing. If the above regimen has not been followed, and the lesion is in the chronic stage, physiotherapeutic treatment with deep massage, manipulation, exercises to strengthen the peronei and proprioception techniques is probably the best approach.

Practice point

This is not a common injection because the treatment of choice is early physiotherapy, but is an option when conservative treatment has failed in the chronic stage or the ligament is too painful. The automatic use of crutches in the acute stage should be avoided if at all possible because this tends to reinforce limping and delays normal healing.

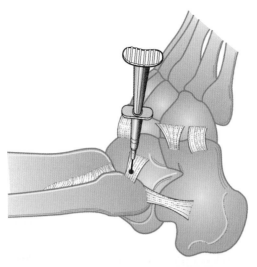

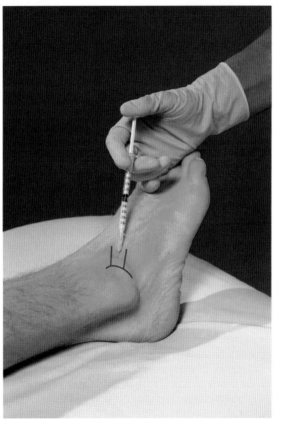

ACHILLES TENDON

Chronic tendinitis

Hx – Overuse especially in maturing person

OE – Pain at posterior aspect of ankle on both sides of tendon; painful resisted plantarflexion standing on one foot or from full dorsiflexion

DD – Achilles bursitis, referred from S1; early sign of ankylosing spondylitis; gout

Equipment

Syringe	Needle	Kenalog 40	Lidocaine	Total volume
2 ml	Blue, 23 gauge 1.25 inches (30 mm)	20 mg	1.5 ml, 2%	2 ml

Anatomy

The Achilles tendon lies at the end of the gastrocnemius as it inserts into the posterior surface of the calcaneus. It is a large dense tendon and is affected usually at the midpoint.

Technique

- Patient lies prone, with foot held in dorsiflexion over end of the bed. This keeps tendon under tension to facilitate procedure
- Identify and mark tender area of tendon, usually midpoint along the sides
- Insert needle on medial side and angle parallel to tendon. Slide needle along side of tendon, taking care not to enter into tendon itself
- Deposit half of the solution while slowly withdrawing needle
- Insert needle on lateral side and repeat procedure with remaining solution

Aftercare

Absolute avoidance of any overuse is essential until pain free. In the case of the committed athlete, or if scanning shows significant degenerative changes, a conservative physiotherapeutic approach should be used. This might include an eccentric exercise programme, a glyceryl trinitrate patch, taping, orthotics, deep friction and/or electrotherapy. Retraining in the causal activity is usually necessary.

Practice point

It is absolutely contraindicated to infiltrate the body of the tendon because this is a large, weight-bearing, relatively avascular tendon, with a known propensity to rupture.

Although there have been reports of tendon rupture after injection here, this has usually occurred as a result of repeated bolus injections of large doses and volumes into the body of a degenerated tendon, followed by excessive exercise postinjection. Because of this recognized risk, we recommend always scanning the tendon before injecting to ascertain the extent of any degeneration (see Section 1, Chapter 6). Tears and degenerative changes within the substance of the tendon would be an absolute contraindication to injection. This challenging disorder can frustrate both patients and clinicians.

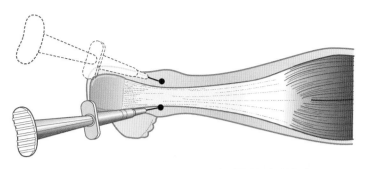

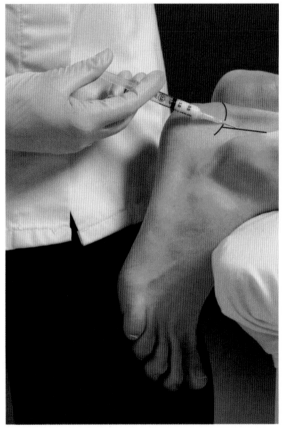

PERONEAL TENDONS

Acute or chronic tendinitis

Hx – Overuse

OE – Pain above, behind or below the lateral malleolus; painful resisted eversion of the foot; passive inversion

DD – Lateral ligaments sprain, fibular stress fracture; referred from S1

Equipment

Syringe	Needle	Kenalog 40	Lidocaine	Total volume
1 ml	Orange, 25 gauge 0.5 inch (13 mm)	10 mg	0.75 ml, 2%	1 ml

Anatomy

The peroneus longus and brevis run together in a synovial sheath behind the lateral malleolus. The longus then divides to pass under the arch of the foot to insert at the base of the big toe, and the brevis inserts into the base of the fifth metatarsal. The division of the two tendons is the entry point for the needle to slide inside the sheath; it can be found by having the patient hold the foot in strong eversion and palpating for the V-shaped fork of the tendons.

Technique

- Patient sits with foot supported in some medial rotation
- Identify and mark division of two tendons
- Insert needle perpendicularly at this point; turn and slide horizontally within the sheath proximaly towards malleolus
- Deposit solution into combined tendon sheath. There should be minimal resistance, and often a sausage-shaped bulge is observed

Aftercare

Avoid any overuse until symptom free. A few sessions of deep transverse massage may help in the chronic stage. Resolution of symptoms should then lead to consideration of change in footwear, orthotics and strengthening of the evertors; usually, proprioception retraining is necessary.

Practice point

This lesion often occurs together with acutely sprained lateral ligaments of the ankle. Examination of the joint should ascertain if one or more ligaments are also affected, and all should be treated if necessary. Obtain a scan first if there is any doubt that there is a tendon tear.

Occasionally, the tendinitis occurs at the insertion of the peroneus brevis. The same amount of solution is then peppered into the teno-osseous junction by inserting the needle parallel to the skin to touch the base of the fifth metatarsal.

Less common is a sprain of the flexor tendons on the medial side of the foot; the signs there will be pain on resisted flexion and inversion. The same dose and volume as above is recommended.

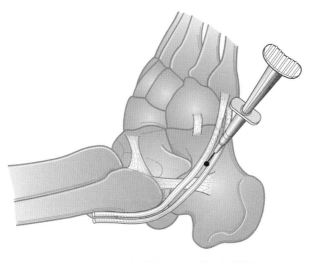

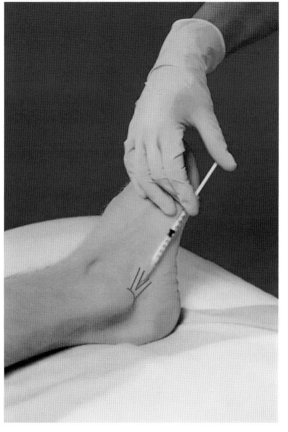

PLANTAR FASCIA   Acute fasciitis

Hx – Idiopathic, overuse, obesity or poor footwear

OE – Pain on medial aspect of heel pad, especially on weight bearing first thing in the morning; tender area over medial edge of the origin of fascia from the calcaneus

DD – Heel spur; referred from S1; early sign of ankylosing spondylitis

Equipment

Syringe	Needle	Kenalog 40	Lidocaine	Total volume
2 ml	Green, 21 gauge 2 inches (50 mm)	20 mg	1.5 ml, 2%	2 ml

Anatomy   The plantar fascia, or long plantar ligament, arises from the medial and lateral tubercles on the inferior surface of the calcaneus. The lesion is invariably found at the medial head, and significant localized tenderness of this area can be elicited by deep pressure with the thumb.

Technique
- Patient lies prone, with foot held in strong dorsiflexion
- Identify tender area on medial side of heel
- Insert needle perpendicularly into medial side of soft part of sole, just distal to heel pad. Advance at 45 degrees towards calcaneus until touching bone
- Pepper solution in two rows into fascia at its medial bony origin

Aftercare   Advise gel heel raises in both ankle boots for men or low-heeled shoes in women after the injection, followed by intrinsic muscle exercise and daily active stretching of the fascia. Rolling the foot on a golf ball or dense squash ball to apply deep friction can be helpful, and orthotics or taping can be applied.

Practice point

The classic history of pain under the heel when putting the foot to the floor on arising from bed in the morning is usually diagnostic.

Although this would appear to be an extremely painful injection, this approach is much kinder than inserting the needle straight through the heel pad. Patients usually tolerate it surprisingly well, and depositing a few drops of the solution as the needle passes through the tissue will give an anaesthetic result.

Heel spurs are often seen on x-rays of this area and may be an incidental finding. If this is the cause, the patient complains of pain more on static weight bearing. The use of a pad with a hole in the middle can relieve the symptoms, but a surgical solution might be considered.

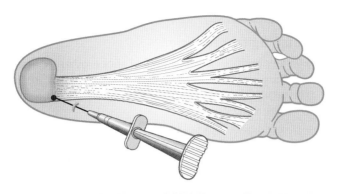

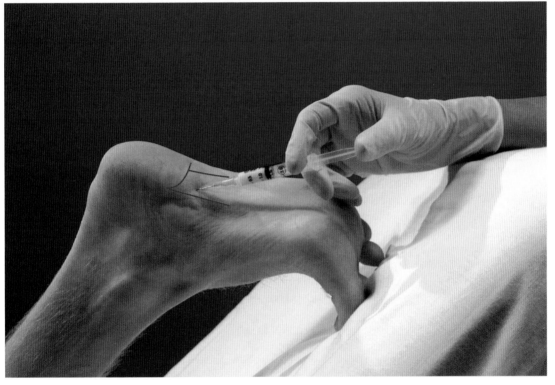

MORTON'S NEUROMA

Plantar digital neuritis

Hx – Very high heels or thin-soled shoes, overpronated foot, abnormal gait
OE – Burning pain or paraesthesia in the first or second interspace between metatarsal heads; painful squeezing metatarsal heads or pressure at site
DD – Neurological disease

Equipment

Syringe	Needle	Kenalog 40	Lidocaine	Total volume
1 ml	Blue, 23 gauge 1.5 inches (30 mm)	20 mg	Nil	0.5 ml

Anatomy A painful fusiform swelling develops in the common digital nerve below the transverse intermetatarsal ligament, usually in the first or second interspace between or slightly distal to the metatarsal heads. The history of burning pain, especially at night, and squeezing of the heads or stretching the nerve by hyperextending the toes is usually indicative of this lesion.

Technique
- Patient sits supported, with foot placed flat
- Identify and mark tender area between metatarsal heads
- Insert needle perpendicularly at this point
- If a sharp burning sensation is reported, slightly withdraw needle tip
- Deposit solution around inflamed neuroma

Aftercare This injection is often successful in relieving symptoms, but these may recur unless the patient is prepared to forego wearing thin-soled, very high heels or other inappropriate footwear. Placing a small pad just proximal to the metatarsal head to lift the bone and reduce the compression for the first weeks postinjection is helpful.

Recurrence of symptoms usually indicates that the patient should discuss operative options with a foot surgeon.

Practice point

As with all injections around neural tissue, care must be taken to approach the nerve slowly because the sudden sharp pain induced if the nerve is entered may make the patient jump. The drug is deposited around the neuroma, not into the substance of the nerve, which might permanently damage it.

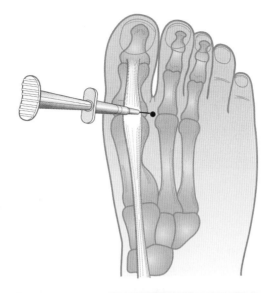

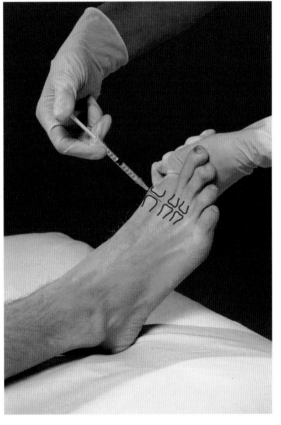

SUMMARY OF SUGGESTED LOWER LIMB DOSAGES

Area	Syringe (ml)	Needle (Inches)	Kenalog 40 (mg)	Lidocaine	Total volume (ml)
Hip					
Hip joint	5	Spinal 3.5	40	4 ml 1%	5
Gluteal bursa	5	Spinal 3.5	40	4 ml 1%	5
Psoas bursa	2.5	Spinal 3.5	20	2 ml 2%	2.5
Trochanteric bursa	2	Blue 1.25	20	1.5 ml 2%	2
Adductor tendon	2	Blue 1.25	20	1.5 ml 2%	2
Hamstring tendon	2	Green 2	20	1.5 ml 2%	2
Ischial bursa	2	Green 2	20	1.5 ml 2%	2
Lateral cutaneous nerve	1	Green 2	20	Nil	0.5
Knee					
Knee joint	10	Green 1.5	40 Adcortyl	5 ml 1%	9
Superior tibiofibular joint	2	Orange 0.5	20	1 ml 2%	1.5
Iliotibial bursa	2	Blue 1.25	20	1.5 ml 2%	2
Infrapatellar bursa	2	Blue 1.25	20	1.5 ml 2%	2
Pes anserine bursa	2	Blue 1.25	20	1.5 ml 2%	2
Coronary ligament	1	Orange 0.5	10	0.75 ml 2%	1
Medial collateral ligament	2	Blue 1.25	20	1 ml 2%	1.5
Infrapatellar tendon	2	Blue 1.25	20	1.5 ml 2%	2
Quadriceps expansion	2	Orange 0.5	10	1.75 ml 2%	2
Foot					
Ankle joint	2.5	Blue 1.25	30	1.75 ml 2%	2.5
Subtalar joint	2.5	Blue 1.25	30	1.75 ml 2%	2.5
Midtarsal joints	2	Blue 1	20	1.5 ml 2%	2
Toe joints	1-2	Orange 0.5	10-20	0.5–1 ml 2%	0.75–1
Deltoid ligament	1	Orange 0.5	10	0.75 ml 2%	1
Lateral ligament	1	Orange 0.5	10	0.75 ml 2%	1
Achilles bursa	2	Blue 1.25	20	1.5 ml 2%	2
Achilles tendon	2	Blue 1.25	20	1.5 ml 2%	2
Peroneal tendons	1	Orange 0.5	10	0.75 ml 2%	1
Plantar fascia	2	Green 2	20	1.5 ml 2%	2
Morton's neuroma	1	Blue 1	20	Nil	0.5

CLINICAL CASE HISTORIES

SELF-TESTING
GUIDELINES

Each case history is taken from real patients encountered in our clinical practices. Most are common conditions frequently seen in musculoskeletal work. A few, however, are unusual presentations with rare diagnoses, which will hopefully challenge you more, as they did us. We hope you will find this a light-hearted way of considering the differential diagnoses possible in each case.

Summary of history

To simplify the exercise, the briefest history in each case contains only the relevant positive facts as given by the patient. We suggest you try to make a provisional diagnosis from the history first before moving onto the clinical findings.

Clinical findings

The information given here is what was found on examination using the routine as described in the text. Passive movements were tested for pain, limitation and end feel and resisted movements for pain and power. Additional confirming tests were performed if necessary.

Only the positive findings are listed. These are divided into which physical tests provoked pain, loss of power and/or limitation of range. Any test performed that produced none of these is not listed, so you can assume that they were negative.

On completion of each test, consider the most likely diagnosis and one possible alternative diagnosis. Also consider possible appropriate treatment, because not all cases require injection. (Answers are given in Appendix 1.)

THE HIP

CASE HISTORY 19

A 60-year-old male company director, whose passion is downhill skiing, fell onto his left hip while trying to impress his young son on a steep hill. He has had 4 months of manipulation for his lumbar spine, with no relief. He now complains of constant ache around his left greater trochanter, aggravated by lying on it, walking and sitting for long periods. He is often stiff first thing in the morning.

Painful – passive hip flexion, passive hip medial rotation, passive hip lateral rotation, passive adduction, resisted hip abduction

CASE HISTORY 20

A 66-year-old retired chauffeur has gradually developed pain in his right buttock over a 5-year period, and 6 months ago he had sudden pain in his right groin while doing abduction exercises in the gym. Since then, he has had severe pain on getting up from sitting, the hip occasionally locks and it seems as if it is about to give way. Heat and exercises have not helped. Anti-inflammatory medication helps relieve the pain slightly.

SECTION 4

Painful – passive hip flexion, passive medial rotation, passive lateral rotation, passive abduction

Limited – medial rotation (++), flexion, abduction

CASE HISTORY 21 A 39-year-old fit policeman decides to show off to his admiring family while on holiday in Turkey. He takes off at great speed on water skis behind the hotel motor boat, immediately does the splits and feels a searing pain on the inner side of his right groin. The pain is severe, and the next few days produce spectacular bruising. Painkillers and ice help a little. He limps in to see you a week later with his multicoloured right groin and inner thigh

Painful – standing lumbar extension, passive hip extension and abduction, resisted hip adduction and flexion

Weak – hip adduction and flexion (++)

CASE HISTORY 22 A 31-year-old secretary consults you because she is finding it more difficult to ride her rather large horse. She has suffered pain in both buttocks and groins from the age of 14, with no history of trauma. Over the past few years, the pain has occasionally spread down the front of both thighs, right (R) more than left (L), and the riding aggravates this. Her x-rays show degenerative changes in both hips, R more than L.

Painful – passive flexion, medial rotation (++), abduction and extension

Limited – medial rotation, R, 0 degrees, L, 5 degrees; flexion, R, 80 degrees, L, 90 degrees; abduction, R, 20 degrees, L, 30 degrees; extension, R, 5 degrees, L, 10 degrees

---

CASE HISTORY 23 A 20-year-old male trainee army officer presents with a gradual onset of severe groin pain while competing in an ultramarathon competition in the Sahara 4 weeks ago. Pain began after 20 miles and was relieved by high doses of oral anti-inflammatory medication, enabling the patient to complete the competition. He is now complaining of low-level constant groin pain, 4/10, which radiates down the anterior aspect of the thigh when trying to run. There is no swelling or bruising.

Painful – passive flexion (++), passive medial rotation, resisted hip flexion

Limited – medial rotation

CASE HISTORY 24 A 91-year-old woman tells you she has had increasing severe pain in her right groin for about one month. The onset was gradual, with no history of trauma. It is worse on walking and has become so bad that she is unable to lie down in bed at night, so has to sleep sitting up. She grades her pain as 8/10, but also says she "doesn't want to make a fuss."

Past medical history (PMH) – mild congestive heart failure, controlled by medication

Painful – passive hip medial rotation (+++), passive hip flexion (++)

Limited – passive hip medial rotation, passive hip flexion

THE KNEE

CASE HISTORY 25   A 63-year-old farmer has a 3-month history of right medial knee pain after jumping down from his tractor and twisting the joint. He has pain on squatting and turning his body to the left, and occasionally it feels as if the leg is about to give way. It sometimes swells slightly when the pain is pronounced, and the joint temporally locks occasionally. It is worse after prolonged driving of his Fiat 500.

Painful – passive knee flexion, passive valgus, passive lateral rotation, combined compression in lateral rotation and valgus
Limited – passive knee flexion

CASE HISTORY 26   A 27-year-old man complains of several months of pain over the medial aspect of his right knee after increasing his road running training on the right-hand side of the road (he lives in the United Kingdom). His knee is stiff in the morning and aches if he sits still for a long time. He has pronated feet.

PMH – skiing injury to same knee 7 years ago
Painful – passive knee flexion, passive valgus, passive lateral rotation

CASE HISTORY 27   A 22-year-old woman falls downstairs and hurts her right knee on the lateral aspect and also twists her right ankle. There was some paraesthesia around the lateral ankle initially. Some months later, she still has pain on twisting and squatting and the knee occasionally feels unstable.

Painful – passive medial rotation of the tibia, resisted flexion of the knee, passive plantarflexion and inversion of the ankle

CASE HISTORY 28   A 28-year-old homemaker goes on a cycling tour of Scotland and, after 3 days is unable to continue cycling because of severe bilateral pain around both her patellae. She limps slightly and is unable to climb stairs without pain. All investigations are normal and painkillers help temporally, but an exercise treatment programme has aggravated the condition. She is on the waiting list for surgery.

Painful – resisted extension of both knees, squatting, full passive knee flexion

CASE HISTORY 29   A 22-year-old male student presents with severe pain in his left knee after a forward fall on his skis 5 days previously. He felt a sharp pain at the time of the fall, was taken down the mountain on the blood wagon and the knee was swollen when examined an hour later. His leg was splinted. and he was flown home with advice to rest and ice the joint and take nonsteroidal anti-inflammatory drugs (NSAIDs). His knee is very swollen and warm, and he has constant pain of 8/10, rising to 10/10 on any movement.

SECTION 4

Painful – passive knee flexion and extension (++), passive valgus, passive knee lateral rotation

Limited – flexion (++), extension

CASE HISTORY 30   A 25-year-old computer programmer presents with a history of being kicked in the front of his left thigh just above the knee joint during a fierce football game 6 months ago. There was severe bruising shortly afterwards, and he limped for a while. He is now able to resume normal activities but the front of his thigh is still tender to pressure, and he is unable to flex his knee fully while standing.

Weak – knee extension

Limited – 45 degrees knee flexion lying prone, normal when supine

THE ANKLE AND FOOT

CASE HISTORY 31   A young footballer presents with a history of a sliding tackle on hard ground, producing a severe pain on the front of his left ankle, which was under him at the time. The ankle was swollen the next day, he was limping and 3 weeks later he finds it painful in the morning and is unable to play his sport without pain.

Painful – passive ankle plantarflexion, passive dorsiflexion, passive inversion

Limited – ankle flexion more than extension

CASE HISTORY 32   A 28-year-old runner puts her right foot down a rabbit hole and feels a sharp pain on the lateral side of her ankle and foot. After six treatments of electrotherapy and exercise, she is still complaining of pain on the later side of her ankle, which is slightly swollen, but also on the medial side. She is unable to run without pain.

Painful – passive inversion of ankle, passive supination of the forefoot, passive adduction of the talus

CASE HISTORY 33   Roger is a very keen 65-year-old walker, but has noticed increasing pain and stiffness under the ball of his left big toe. This has lasted for longer than 1 year, and he is worried that he may have to stop walking. He has also noticed an ache recently in the front of his left shin and dorsum of his ankle.

Painful – passive extension of big toe (+), passive flexion, passive abduction

Limited – extension of the big toe

CASE HISTORY 34   Lesley, 53 years old, has a chronically pronated foot and, over the past 12 months, has gradually developed pain and swelling behind and below the medial malleolus. It is usually much worse after prolonged walking. Because she cannot exercise, she has been putting on extra weight, and the symptoms are increasing.

Painful – passive plantar flexion, passive eversion
Limited – adduction of talus

CASE HISTORY 35 A 65-year-old female civil servant has noticed a gradual increase of a burning pain on the dorsum of her right foot, between her second and third metatarsals. She is distressed because she has had to give up wearing high heels, and the foot now aches most of the time, but is worse on weight bearing. She has also noticed her foot swelling at the end of the day.

Painful – passive flexion and extension of toes, passive compression of the metatarsal heads

CASE HISTORY 36 A fit 44-year-old male pharmacist presents with an 18-year history of bilateral pain at the back of both heels, L more than R, which occurs every rugby season. Every year, he promises himself he will give up the sport next year. The pain now comes on earlier in the season and lasts longer. He is getting fed up with the problem.

Painful – passive dorsiflexion of ankles with knees extended, more passive dorsiflexion with knees flexed, resisted ankle plantarflexion
Weak – rising on tiptoes at end range
Limited – hamstring length and gastrocnemius length

SECTION 4

KEY REFERENCES

General Accuracy

Daley EL, Bajaj S, Bison LJ, et al. Improving injection accuracy of the elbow, knee, and shoulder: does injection site and imaging make a difference? A systematic review. *Am J Sports Med.* 2011;39(3):656–662.

Hip Joint

Hoeber S, Aly AR, Ashworth N, et al. Ultrasound guided hip joint injections are more accurate than landmark-guided injections: a systematic review and meta-analysis. *Br J Sports Med.* 2016;50:392–396.

Trochanteric Bursa

Brinks A, van Rijn RM, Willemsen SP, et al. corticosteroid injections for greater trochanteric pain syndrome: a randomized controlled trial in primary care. *Ann Fam Med.* 2011;9(3):226–234.

Lievense A, Bierma-Zeinstra S, Schouten B, et al. Prognosis of trochanteric pain in primary care. *Br J Gen Pract.* 2005;55(512):199–204.

Lateral Cutaneous Nerve

Khalil N, Nicotra A, Rakowicz W. Treatment for meralgia paraesthetica. *Cochrane Database System Rev.* 2012;(12):CD004159.

Knee Joint

Hermans J, Bierma-Zeinstra SM, Bos PK, et al. The most accurate approach for intra-articular needle placement in the knee joint: a systematic review. *Semin Arthritis Rheum.* 2011;41(2):106–115.

Jackson DW, Evans NA, Thomas BM. Accuracy of needle placement into the intra-articular space of the knee. *J Bone Joint Surg Am.* 2002;84:1522–1527.

Jüni P, Hari R, Rutjes AWS, et al. Intra-articular corticosteroid for knee osteoarthritis. *Cochrane Database System Rev.* 2015;(10):CD005328.

Kirwan JR, Haskard DO, Higgens CS. The use of sequential analysis to assess patient preference for local skin anaesthesia during knee aspiration. *Br J Rheumatol.* 1984;23:210–213.

Foot and Ankle Joint

Ward ST, Williams PL, Purkayastha S. Intra-articular corticosteroid injections in the foot and ankle: a prospective 1-year follow-up investigation. *J Foot Ankle Surg.* 2008;47:138–144.

Achilles Tendon

Kearney RS, Parsons N, Metcalfe D, et al. Injection therapies for Achilles tendinopathy. *Cochrane Database System Rev.* 2015;(5):CD010960.

Plantar Fascia

Tsikopoulos K, Vasiliadis HS, Mavridis D. Injection therapies for plantar fasciopathy ('plantar fasciitis'): a systematic review and network meta-analysis of 22 randomised controlled trial. *Br J Sports Med.* 2016;50:1367–1375.

Morton's Neuroma

Thomson CE, Gibson JA, Martin D. Interventions for the treatment of Morton's neuroma. *Cochrane Database System Rev.* 2004;(3):CD003118.

SECTION 5

SPINAL INJECTIONS

SPINAL INJECTION GUIDELINES

We strongly recommend that clinicians wishing to give spinal injections attend reputable training courses and undergo a period of supervised practice with an experienced colleague before attempting them on their own.

OVERVIEW

Low back pain, with or without lower extremity pain, is the most common problem among chronic pain disorders with significant economic, societal and health impact. Epidural injections are one of the most commonly performed interventions.[1] A study of back pain prevalence in US adults found that about 25% reported low back pain over a 3-month period,[2] but pathoanatomical causes could be established in only 15% of all cases.[3]

There have been many treatments to relieve this affliction, including spinal injections, which has engendered much controversy in the literature. Opinions about efficacy, safety and relevance have differed greatly since their inception in the 1920s, with many studies considered to be of poor quality.[4-10]

Although epidural injections are one of the most commonly used invasive interventions in the treatment of low back pain, with or without radicular pain, there is currently little consensus about this technique and wide variation in practice.[11] There is also no agreement on the most effective approach for lumbar epidural injection, whether to use steroid, local anaesthetic or saline (or a combination) and the exact volume required. Depot steroids are not licensed for spinal use, but orthopaedic and pain specialists, rheumatologists and others use these injections extensively.[12] One randomized controlled trial (RCT) evaluating the benefits of cortisone versus saline reported improvement during the follow-up period in both the methylprednisolone and saline groups. The combination of methylprednisolone and bupivacaine appeared to have a short-term effect but, at 3 and 6 months, the steroid group seemed to experience a rebound phenomenon.[13]

Almost every study recommends that more studies are needed and that future studies should include more placebo-controlled trials. These would conclusively define the role of lumbar injections, although current studies support their use in the treatment of lumbosacral radicular pain.

INDICATIONS FOR SPINAL INJECTION

The techniques described here include caudal epidural, nerve root, facet joint, sacroiliac joint (SIJ) and sacrococcygeal joint injections. The choice between giving a caudal or nerve root injection can be aided by the site of pain; if this is clearly unilateral in the lumbar area, or radiating down one leg, a nerve root injection may be effective. If the pain is bilateral or central in the lumbar spine, a caudal epidural may be a better choice; however, this guide is not an absolute.

The following are the main indications for caudal and nerve root injections:

- Acute back and/or leg pain, for which pain makes manipulation impossible to perform
- Chronic back and/or leg pain, for which conservative treatment has failed
- Before considering surgery

SECTION 5

Older patients with chronic back pain and stiffness increased on active extension may benefit from facet joint injections. A retrospective study of patients with spinal stenosis has found that 35% of patients had at least 50% improvement; those with spondylolisthesis, single-level stenosis and aged older than 73 years had better outcomes.[14] Less commonly, injections for coccydynia or SIJ pain can be attempted in cases of acute traumatic or postnatal pain and, in our experience, can be helpful.

SAFETY

All the contraindications clearly listed in Section 2 apply. We do not use, or recommend using, local anaesthetic in caudal, nerve root and facet joint injections due to the risk of intrathecal deposition. The temporary benefit of analgesic and diagnostic outcomes is outweighed by the greater risks. Our advice to 'listen to the needle' here is invaluable; appreciating the difference between the hard endfeel of bone, the sticky endfeel of cartilage and the leathery endfeel of ligament not only helps ensure correct placement, but also installs confidence in the operator.

The incidence of intravascular uptake during lumbar spinal injection procedures is approximately 8.5%; it is greater in patients older than 50 years and, if the caudal route is used, rises to 11%. Absence of flashback of blood on preinjection aspiration does not predict extravascular needle placement.[3] An epidural steroid injection is safe in patients receiving aspirin-like antiplatelet medications, with no excess risk of serious haemorrhagic complications, such as spinal haematoma. Increased age, large needle gauge, needle approach, insertion at multiple interspaces, number of needle passes, large volume of injectant and accidental dural puncture are all relative risk factors for minor haemorrhagic complications.[15]

Safety precautions and strict aseptic techniques are the same as for all injections. An additional hazard is the rare possibility of an intrathecal injection of local anaesthetic, which can be avoided by using corticosteroid alone. The rationale is that the benefit of the brief relief of pain and the diagnostic information obtained from using an anaesthetic does not outweigh the potential risks. Normal saline can be added, or Adcortyl can be used instead of Kenalog if additional volume is required.

New neurological symptoms or worsening of preexisting complaints that persist for more than 24 hours (median duration of symptoms, 3 days; range, 1–20 days) might occur after epidural injection,[15] but in our experience this is rare.

The British Society for Rheumatology and the Royal College of Anaesthetists have recommended guidelines for the use of epidural injections. We suggest their use to all practitioners who give these injections. They can be found at www.rheumatology.org.uk and www.rcoa.ac.uk.

A study recording the complications and side effects of cervical and lumbosacral selective nerve root injections stated that there were no major complications, such as death, paralysis, spinal nerve injury, infection or allergic reaction during the study; 91% of subjects had no side effects during the procedure. A positive response on interview was reported by 39.4% of the study subjects immediately after the procedure. The only significant lumbosacral side effect was increased pain at the injection site (17.1%).[16]

ACCURACY Performing spinal injections under imaging can ensure correct placement but requires specialized training and is much more expensive to perform, especially if done in theatre. Many clinicians undertake these techniques using their advanced knowledge of spinal anatomy (so-called 'blind' injecting) and obtain satisfactory results.

The accuracy of 'blind' caudal epidural injections compared with targeted placement has been assessed in a few studies. In one study, successful placement on the first attempt occurred in three of four subjects. Results were improved when anatomical landmarks were identified easily (88%), and no air was palpable subcutaneously over the sacrum when injected through the needle (83%). The combination of these two signs predicted a successful injection in 91% of attempts. In another study, blind injections were correctly placed in only two of three attempts, even when the operator was confident of accurate placement. When the operator was less certain, the success rate was less than half and, if the patient was obese, the success rate was reduced even further. In a third prospective randomized, double-blind trial, the results showed no advantage of spinal endoscopic placement compared with the more traditional caudal approach.[14,17,18]

EFFICACY ## Lumber epidurals

There is a paucity of well-designed, randomized controlled studies and a lack of quality evidence with statistically significant results in the existing literature and contemporary interventional pain management practices. This means that a solid foundation for the effectiveness of spinal injection therapy is lacking.[4,19] The UK National Institute for Health and Clinical Excellence (NICE), has recommended that patients with persistent, nonspecific, low back pain should not be offered injections of therapeutic substances,[20] but what impact this has had on clinical practice is uncertain.

A Cochrane Review has found minor side effects such as headache, dizziness, transient local pain, tingling, numbness and nausea reported in a small number of patients in only 50% of the trials reviewed. The report concluded that there is no strong evidence for or against the use of any type of injection therapy for individuals with subacute or chronic low back pain.[12]

A comprehensive review with systematic analysis of the published data has stated that in a substantial number of patients with lumbar radicular pain from disc herniation, corticosteroid injection was effective in reducing pain, restoring function, avoiding surgery and decreasing referrals for other health care. The evidence was found to be much more compelling than it would have been if the literature review had been of the limited scope of a traditional systematic review of RCTs only.[21] A randomized, double-blind, controlled trial has concluded that lumbar interlaminar epidural of local anaesthetic with steroid is effective in 86% of patients and, without steroid, in 74%.[3]

A systematic review has indicated positive evidence (level II2) for short-term relief of pain from disc herniation or radiculitis using blind interlaminar epidural steroid injections. However, there was weaker evidence for long-term pain relief for these conditions and for the short-term and long-term relief of pain from spinal stenosis and discogenic pain without radiculitis or disc herniation.[18]

SECTION 5

Another review of both caudal and lumbar epidurals has also concluded that the best studies showed inconsistent results, and benefits were of short duration only.[7] Yet another showed strong evidence for epidurals in the management of nerve root pain caused by disc prolapse, but limited evidence in spinal stenosis.[22] A multicentre RCT of epidurals for sciatica has reported significant relief at 3 weeks but no long-term benefit.[23]

There is fair evidence supporting transforaminal epidural steroid injections (TFESIs) as superior to placebo for treating radicular symptoms. There is good evidence that TFESIs should be used as a surgery-sparing intervention and that TFESIs are superior to interlaminar ESIs (ILESIs) and caudal ESIs for radicular pain. In patients with subacute or chronic radicular symptoms, there is good evidence that a single TFESI has similar efficacy as a single transforaminal injection of bupivacaine or saline. In the past, large volumes were injected into the epidural space; however, a total injection volume of 8 ml appears to be sufficient for a caudal epidural injection to reach the L4–5 level.

Selective guided nerve root injections of corticosteroids

These are significantly more effective than those of bupivacaine alone in obviating the need for operative decompression for 13 to 28 months following the injections in operative candidates. This finding suggests that patients who have lumbar radicular pain at one or two levels should be considered for treatment with selective nerve root injections of corticosteroids before operative intervention. A significantly greater proportion of patients treated with a transforaminal injection of steroid achieve relief of pain compared with those treated by transforaminal injection of local anaesthetic, saline or intramuscular steroids.[24] When symptoms have been present for more than 12 months, local anaesthetic alone may be just as effective as steroid and local anaesthetic together.

When conservative measures fail, nerve root injections are effective in reducing radicular pain in patients with osteoporotic vertebral fractures and no evidence of nerve root palsy. These patients may be considered for this treatment before percutaneous vertebroplasty or operative intervention is attempted.[20]

Injection of the sacroiliac joints

This has been rarely discussed in recent literature, but using this treatment for very painful sacroiliitis appears to be safe and effective. It can be considered in patients with contraindications or complications with nonsteroidal anti-inflammatory drugs (NSAIDs), or if other medical treatment is ineffective, although manipulative techniques can often obviate the need for an injection. However, accurate placement of the drug without the use of fluoroscopy is estimated to be successful in only 12% of patients.[25]

SUMMARY There is a wide variation of opinion about the efficacy of spinal injections for back pain. Adverse effects are generally minor, and it cannot be ruled out that specific subgroups of patients may respond to a specific type of injection therapy. A cost-effective intervention that may be performed safely as an outpatient procedure and rapidly relieve pain, even in the short term, is worth considering for carefully selected patients with both acute and chronic low back pain.[26,27]

As with all injection techniques, resuscitation facilities must be easily available and the guidelines on aseptic technique strictly followed.

EXAMINATION OF LUMBAR SPINE AND SACROILIAC JOINT

The capsular pattern (CP) is a set pattern of loss of motion for each joint. It indicates that there is some degree of joint capsulitis caused by degeneration, systemic disease or trauma. There may be a hard end feel in advanced capsulitis.

Additional spinal tests can be performed if the diagnosis is in doubt or to confirm a provisional diagnosis. Objective tests, such as imaging and blood tests, should be undertaken only after careful consideration of the additional costs involved, but be aware of the possible presence of red flags.

LUMBAR SPINE EXAMINATION

Observe patient from front, sides and back – a full length mirror in front of the patient while examiner stands behind is useful.

Check whether there is any pain at rest before commencing examination.

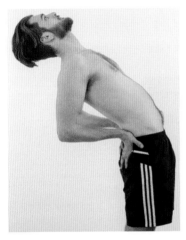

1 Active extension

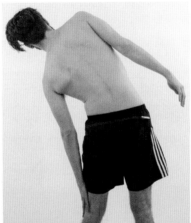

2 Active left side flexion

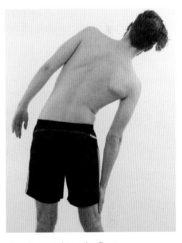

3 Active right side flexion

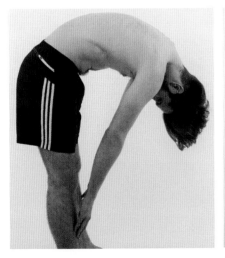

4 Active flexion

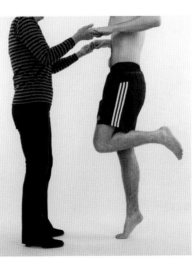

5 Resisted plantar flexion, S1-2

SECTION 5

Eliminate sacroiliac joint as source of pain

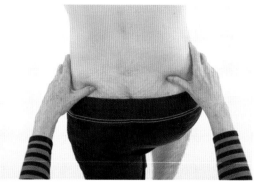

6 'Walk' test – slowly lifting one leg to right angle while palpating posterior sacroiliac spines – checks for asymmetry of sacroiliac joint movement

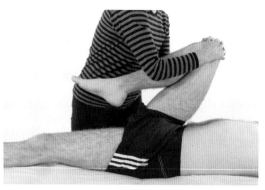

7 Posterior sacroiliac ligaments: passive flexion with overpressure

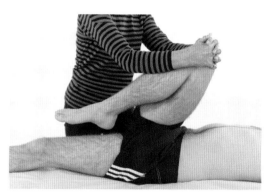

8 Posterior sacroiliac ligaments: passive oblique flexion with overpressure

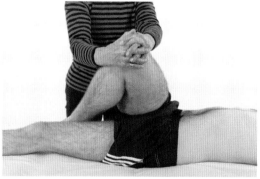

9 Posterior sacroiliac ligaments: passive transverse flexion with overpressure

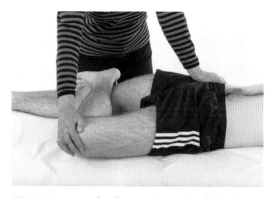

10 Anterior sacroiliac ligaments: passive lateral rotation with overpressure – '4 test'

Eliminate hip joint as source of pain

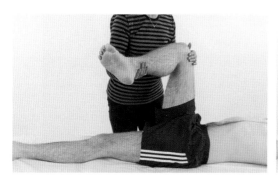

11 Hip: passive lateral rotation

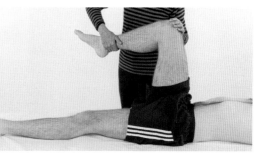

12 Hip: passive medial rotation

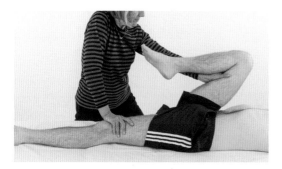

13 Hip: passive flexion

Lumbar spine neurological tests for nerve root mobility and muscle power

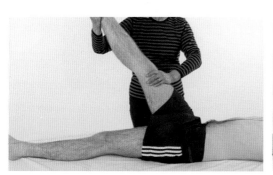

14 Straight leg raise L4-5, S1-2

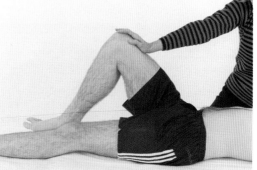

15 Resited hip flexion, L2-3

SECTION 5

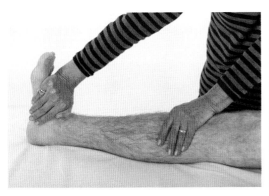

16 Resisted foot dorsiflexion, L4

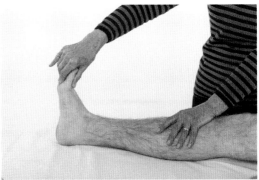

17 Resisted toe extension, L4 5

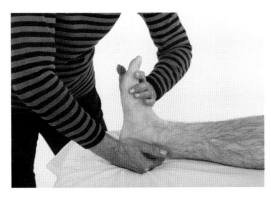

18 Resisted foot eversion L5 S1

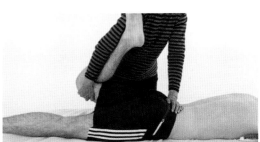

19 L3 stretch

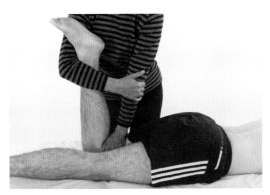

20 Resisted knee extension, L3

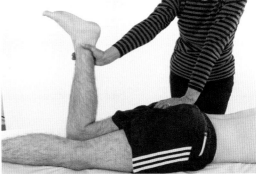

21 Resisted knee flexion S1 2

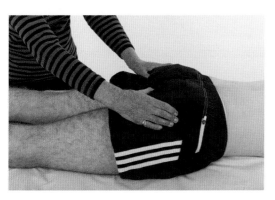

22 Clench gluteal muscles for tone S1

Reflexes

Knee L3
Ankle L5/S1/2
Plantar response

Skin sensation

Big toe L4
Middle toes L5
Lateral border of foot S1
Heel S2

Palpation

Pressure on lumbar spine for pain, range and end feel

Lumbar capsular pattern

● Equal loss of side flexion, more loss of extension than flexion

Lumbar disc or nerve root pattern

● More loss of flexion than extension

Additional spinal tests if necessary

● These include repeated or combined spinal movements and resisted spinal muscle tests

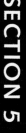

SECTION 5

SPINAL INJECTION TECHNIQUES

CAUDAL EPIDURAL

Acute or chronic low back pain or sciatica

Hx – Lifting heavy weights, prolonged sitting, insidious

OE – Central or bilateral pain in low back, with or without sciatica or root signs, and/or symptoms; painful flexion and usually side flexion away from pain

DD – Disc lesion, acute nerve entrapment; spinal tumour, ankylosing spondylitis

Equipment

Syringe	Needle	Adcortyl	Lidocaine	Total volume
5 ml	Green, 21 gauge 1.5–2 inches (40–50 mm)	40 mg	Nil	4 ml

Anatomy

The spinal cord ends at the level of L1 and the thecal sac ends at S2 in most individuals. The aim of this injection is to pass a disinflaming solution through the sacral hiatus and up the canal so that it bathes the posterior aspect of the intervertebral disc, anterior aspect of the dura mater and any affected nerve roots centrally. The sacral cornua are two prominences that can be palpated at the apex of an equilateral triangle drawn from the posterior superior spines on the ileum to the coccyx. There is a thick ligament at the entrance to the canal. The angle of the curve of the canal varies widely, and the placement of the needle reflects this.

Technique

- Patient lies prone over a small pillow
- Identify sacral cornua at base of an imaginary triangle with thumb
- Insert needle between cornua and pass it horizontally through ligament
- Pass needle a short distance up canal, adjusting angle to curve of sacrum
- Aspirate to ensure that needle has not penetrated thecal sac or a blood vessel
- Slowly inject solution into epidural space
- If using more volume, place a flat hand on sacrum to palpate for possible swelling caused by a suprasacral injection

Aftercare

Advise the patient to keep active within pain limits, and reassess about 10 days later. If the injection has only partially helped, it can be repeated as long as improvement continues. The causes of the back pain should then be addressed, such as weight, posture, work positions, lifting techniques, exercise routines and abdominal control.

Practice point

If clear fluid or blood is aspirated at any point, the procedure is abandoned and can be attempted a few days later. Occasionally, the canal is difficult to enter; this might be because of a bifid or very small canal or because the angle of the sacrum is very concave. In this case, a small amount of local anaesthetic can be injected into the ligament to make penetration more comfortable during reangulation of the needle.

If the affected level is higher than the common L5-S1 level or the patient is large, more volume may be required. We recommend using 40 mg of Adcortyl or adding up to 9 ml of normal saline to the Kenalog in these cases.

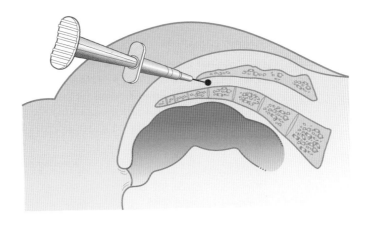

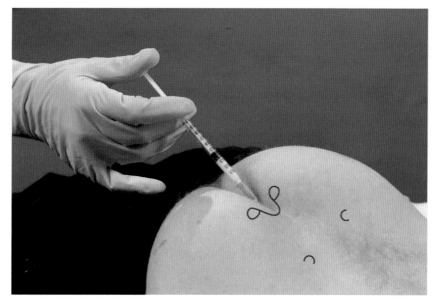

LUMBAR FACET JOINT

Chronic capsulitis

Hx – Gradual increasing low back pain and stiffness; traumatic incident

OE – Unilateral or bilateral low back pain, sometimes with dull vague aching down leg(s); CP: limited extension plus side flexions plus combined extension with side flexion toward the painful side

DD – Osteoarthritis, ankylosing spondylitis, spondylolysis, spondylolisthesis

Equipment

Syringe	Needle	Kenalog 40	Lidocaine	Total volume
1 ml	Spinal, 22 gauge 3–4 inches (75–90 mm)	40 mg	Nil	1 ml

Anatomy

The lower lumbar facet or zygapophyseal joints lie lateral to the spinous processes, approximately one finger width at L3, one-and-one-half at L4 and two fingers' width at L5. They cannot be palpated but are located by marking a vertical line along the centre of the spinous processes and horizontal lines *between* each process. The posterior capsule of the joint is found by inserting the needle the correct distance for that level laterally on the horizontal line.

Technique

- Patient lies prone on a small pillow to aid localization of spinous interspace
- Identify and mark one or more tender levels
- Insert needle at first selected level vertically
- Angle needle slightly cephalad and medially and pass slowly down to bone
- Aspirate to ensure that needle point is not intrathecal or in blood vessel
- Deposit solution into capsule
- Withdraw needle and repeat at opposite side and different levels if necessary

Aftercare

Avoid excessive movement while maintaining activity. Abdominal strengthening and mobilizing exercises should be performed regularly. Occasional mobilization and hamstring stretching will help maintain flexibility and lumbar support may be used during activities.

Practice point

It may be impossible to enter the joint, but controlled studies have shown that depositing the solution into and around the capsule can be therapeutically effective. These injections are often performed under imaging, but the additional cost of this should be considered.

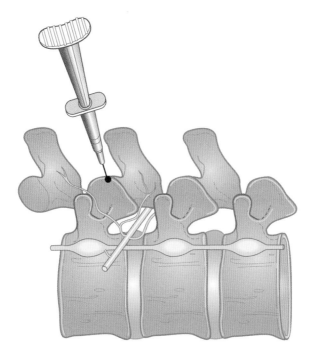

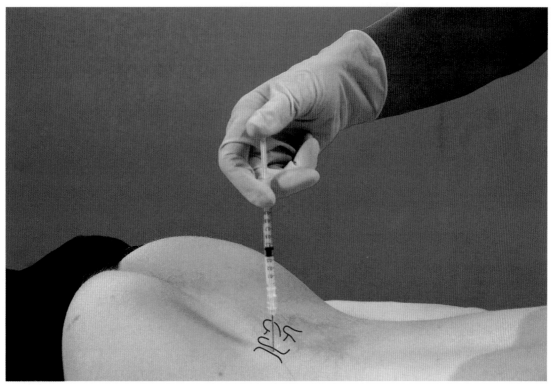

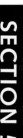

LUMBAR NERVE ROOT

Nerve root inflammation

Hx – Usually acute onset with possible paraesthesia

OE – Acute or chronic sciatica with or without root signs; painful flexion and usually side flexion away from pain plus nerve root tension signs

DD – Spinal stenosis, nerve root entrapment

Equipment

Syringe	Needle	Kenalog 40	Lidocaine	Total volume
1 ml	Spinal, 22 gauge 3–4 inches (75–90 mm)	40 mg	Nil	1 ml

Anatomy

The lumbar nerve roots emerge obliquely from the vertebral canals between the transverse processes at the level of the spinous process. Draw a vertical line along the centre of the spinous processes and horizontal lines *level* with each spinous process. A thumb's width laterally along the horizontal line marks the approximate entry site for the needle.

Technique

- Patient lies prone over a small pillow to aid localization of spinous processes
- Identify spinous process at painful level and mark a spot laterally along a horizontal line
- Insert needle and pass it perpendicularly to a depth of about 3 inches (7 cm)
- Aspirate to ensure that needle point is not intrathecal or in blood vessel
- Inject solution as a bolus around nerve root

Aftercare

The patient keeps mobile within pain limits and is reassessed a week or 10 days later. Repeat as necessary.

Practice point

This injection can be especially effective when the patient is in severe pain, and conservative manual therapy techniques are impossible to administer. It can also be given when caudal epidural has proved unsuccessful; the caudal technique is technically an easier procedure, but the solution might not reach the affected part of the nerve root. If the first level injected does not relieve the symptoms, a level above or below can be tried. This is well worth attempting before considering surgery.

The needle must be repositioned if it encounters bone at a distance of about 2 inches ($\approx$5 cm) because this means that it is touching the lamina or facet joint. Equally, repositioning is necessary if the patient complains of a sharp electric shock sensation because the needle will be in the nerve root. Two levels can be infiltrated at a time. A large patient may require a longer needle.

If clear fluid is aspirated, the needle is intrathecal and the procedure must be abandoned, although it can be attempted again a few days later.

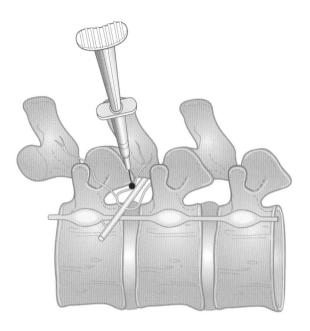

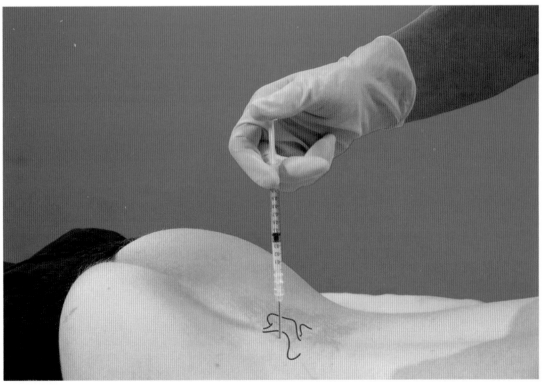

SACROILIAC JOINT

Acute or chronic sprain or capsulitis

Hx – Usually female, often prepartum or postpartum, or traumatic incident (e.g., fall onto the buttocks); pain after rest or long periods of sitting or standing; chronic ligamentous pain after successful manipulation

OE – Pain over buttock, groin or occasionally down the posterior thigh to the calf; painful stressing posterior ligaments in hip flexion, oblique and transverse adduction and anterior ligaments in hip flexion, abduction and/or external rotation, plus asymmetry in 'walk' test – see Sacroiliac examination p. 268

DD – Acute sacroiliitis, early ankylosing spondylitis, OA hip joint, referred from lumbar spine

Equipment

Syringe	Needle	Kenalog 40	Lidocaine	Total volume
2 ml	Spinal, 22 gauge 3–3.5 inches (75–90 mm)	20 mg	1.5 ml 2%	2 ml

Anatomy The SIJ surfaces are angled obliquely posteroanteriorly, with the angle being more acute in the female. The dimples at the top of the buttocks indicate the position of the posterior superior iliac spines. Injection of this joint can be difficult, but the easiest entry point is usually found in a dip just below and slightly medial to the posterior superior iliac spines.

Technique
● Patient lies prone over a small pillow
● Identify and mark posterior superior iliac spine on the affected side
● Insert needle a thumb's width medially and just below this bony landmark at level of second sacral spinous process
● Angle needle obliquely anterolaterally at an angle of about 45 degrees
● Pass needle between the sacrum and ilium until a ligamentous resistance is felt
● Inject solution as a bolus within joint if possible, or pepper posterior capsule

Aftercare Movement within the pain-free range is encouraged; a lunging motion with the foot up on a chair can help relieve pain, as can moderate walking. The patient should avoid hip abduction positions and should sit with the back supported. A temporary belt is worn if the joint is unstable, and sclerosing injections can be tried to increase ligamentous stability.

Practice point

This is not a very common injection; usually manipulation, mobilization and exercise techniques relieve most chronic sacroiliac joint symptoms.

The needle often comes up against bone when attempting this injection and then has to be manoeuvred around to allow for the variations in bony shape before entering the joint space. Deposit of a small amount of the solution aids in making the process less uncomfortable. It is unusual to have to repeat this injection, and the joint can often be successfully manipulated a week later if necessary.

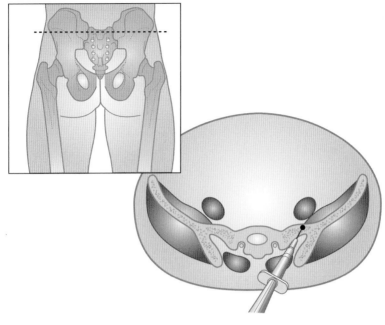

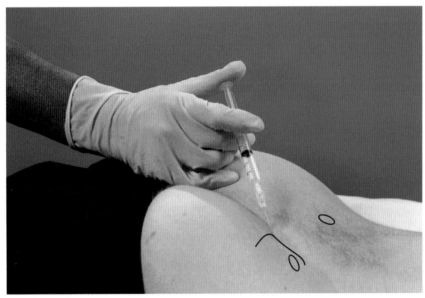

SACRO-COCCYGEAL JOINT

Coccydynia – strain of coccygeal ligaments, subluxation

Hx – Postnatal, prolonged sitting on hard surface or trauma, such as a fall onto the buttock

OE – Pain localized over sacrococcygeal joint on sitting or bearing down; tender on joint line, coccyx might be subluxed

DD – Fracture; occasionally psychological distress in female

Equipment

Syringe	Needle	Kenalog 40	Lidocaine	Total volume
1 ml	Blue, 23 gauge 1 inch (25 mm)	20 mg	0.5 ml 2%	1 ml

Anatomy

The ligaments at the sacrococcygeal joint line are usually tender and can be palpated both on the dorsal and ventral surfaces. The gloved finger palpates the angle of the coccyx rectally to check for subluxation of the bone.

Technique

- Patient lies prone over a small pillow
- Identify and mark tender site on dorsum of coccyx at joint line
- Insert needle down to touch bone
- Pepper solution around into tender ligaments

Aftercare

The patient should avoid sitting on hard surfaces, and use a ring cushion when seated. At follow-up about 10 days later, manipulation of the coccyx might be necessary to correct any subluxation; the anti-inflammatory effect of the steroid enables this to be performed with less discomfort. The clinician's gloved finger is inserted into the rectum, and a firm anteroposterior movement is applied with the other hand. Sometimes an audible click can be heard, and several days later the relief of pain is apparent.

Practice point

Pain in this area can be symptomatic of psychological or psychosexual distress, in which case the appropriate treatment and advice are required. With somatic pain, the protocol discussed appears to work either well or not at all. Surgery is not usually indicated or particularly successful.

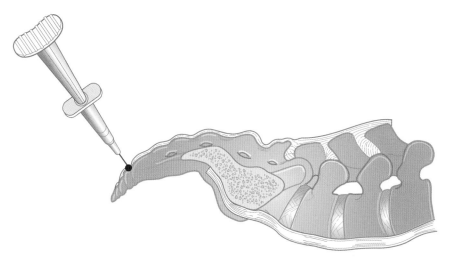

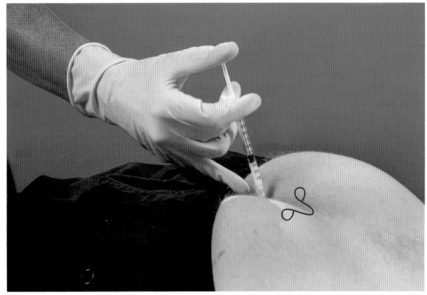

SUMMARY OF SUGGESTED SPINAL DOSAGES

Syringe	Needle	Corticosteroid	Lidocaine	Total volume (ml)
Caudal epidural				
5 ml	Green 21 gauge 1.5–2 inches	40 mg Adcortyl	Nil	4
Lumbar facet joint				
1 ml	Spinal 22 gauge 3–4 inches	40 mg Kenalog 40	Nil	1
Lumbar nerve root				
1 ml	Spinal 22 gauge 3–4 inches	40 mg Kenalog 40	Nil	1
Sacroiliac joint				
2 ml	Spinal 22 gauge 3–4 inches	40 mg Kenalog 40	1 ml 2%	2
Sacrococcygeal joint				
1 ml	Blue 23 gauge 1 inch blue	20 mg	0.5 ml 2%	1

REFERENCES

1. Parr AT, Diwan S, Abdi S. Lumbar interlaminar epidural injections in managing chronic low back and lower extremity pain: a systematic review. *Pain Physician*. 2009;12(1):163–188.
2. Deyo R, Mirza SK, Martin BI. Back pain prevalence and visit rates: estimates from U.S. national surveys, 2002. *Spine*. 2006;31(23):2724–2727.
3. Manchikanti L, Cash KA, McManus CD, et al. Preliminary results of randomized double-blind controlled trial of fluoroscopic lumbar interlaminar epidural injections in managing chronic lumbar discogenic pain without disc herniation or radiculitis. *Pain Physician*. 2010;13(4):E279–E292.
4. Riew K, Yin Y, Gilula L, et al. The effect of nerve-root injections on the need for operative treatment of lumbar radicular pain: a prospective, randomised, controlled, double-blind study. *J Bone Joint Surg Am*. 2000;82:1589–1593.
5. Staal JB, de Bie R, de Vet HC, et al. Injection therapy for subacute and chronic low-back pain. *Cochrane Database Syst Rev*. 2008;(3):CD001824.
6. Valat JP, Giraudeau B, Rozenberg S, et al. Epidural corticosteroid injections for sciatica: a randomised, double blind, controlled clinical trial. *Ann Rheum Dis*. 2003;62:639–643.
7. Arden NK, Price C, Reading I, et al. A multicentre randomized controlled trial of epidural corticosteroid injections for sciatica: the West study. *Rheumatology* (Oxford). 2005;44(11):1399–1406.
8. Buttermann GR. Treatment of lumbar disc herniation: epidural steroid injection compared with discectomy; a prospective, randomized study. *J Bone Joint Surg Am*. 2004;86:670–679.
9. van Tulder M, Koes B. Low back pain (chronic). *Clin Evid*. 2004;12:286–291.

10. Samanta A, Samanta J. Is epidural injection of steroids effective for low back pain? *BMJ*. 2004;328:1509–1510.

11. Cluff R, Mehio AK, Cohen SP, et al. The technical aspects of epidural steroid injections: a national survey. *Anesth Analg*. 2002;95:403–408.

12. Fanciullo GJ, Hanscom B, Seville J, et al. An observational study of the frequency and pattern of use of epidural steroid injection in 25,479 patients with spinal and radicular pain. *Reg Anesth Pain Med*. 2001;26(1):5–11.

13. Karppinen J, Malmivaara A, Kurunlahti M, et al. Periradicular infiltration for sciatica: a randomized controlled trial. *Spine*. 2001;26(9):1059–1067.

14. Barre L, Lutz GE, Southern D, et al. Fluoroscopically guided caudal epidural steroid injections for lumbar spinal stenosis: a retrospective evaluation of long term efficacy. *Pain Physician*. 2004;7(2):187–193.

15. Ghahreman A, Ferch R, Bogduk N. The efficacy of transforaminal injection of steroids for the treatment of lumbar radicular pain. *Pain Med*. 2010;11(8):1149–1168.

16. Huston CW, Slipman CW, Garvin C. Complications and side effects of cervical and lumbosacral selective nerve root injections. *Arch Phys Med Rehabil*. 2005;86(2):277–283.

17. Price CM, Rogers PD, Prosser AS, et al. Comparison of the caudal and lumbar approaches to the epidural space. *Ann Rheum Dis*. 2000;59(11):879–882.

18. Dashfield AK, Taylor MB, Cleaver JS, et al. Comparison of caudal steroid epidural with targeted steroid placement during spinal endoscopy for chronic sciatica; a prospective randomized, double-blind trial. *Br J Anaesth*. 2005;94(4):514–519.

19. Roberts ST, Willick SE, Rho ME, et al. Efficacy of lumbosacral transforaminal epidural steroid injections: a systematic review. *PM R*. 2009;1(7):657–668.

20. Kim DJ, Yun YH, Wang JM. Nerve-root injections for the relief of pain in patients with osteoporotic vertebral fractures. *J Bone Joint Surg Br*. 2003;85(2):250–253.

21. MacVicar J, King W, Landers MH, et al. The effectiveness of lumbar transforaminal injection of steroids: a comprehensive review with systematic analysis of the published data. *Pain Med*. 2013;14(1): 14–28.

22. Horlocker T, Bajwa ZH, Ashraf Z, et al. Risk assessment of hemorrhagic complications associated with non-steroidal anti-inflammatory medications in ambulatory pain clinic patients undergoing epidural steroid injection. *Anesth Analg*. 2002;95:1691–1697.

23. National Collaborating Centre for Primary Care (UK). Low back pain: early management of persistent non-specific low back pain. back.cochrane.org/sites/back.cochrane.org/files/uploads/PDF/4106 .PDF.

24. Botwin K, Brown LA, Fishman M, et al. Fluoroscopically guided caudal epidural steroid injections in degenerative lumbar spinal stenosis. *Pain Physician*. 2007;10(4):547–548.

25. Hansen H. Is fluoroscopy necessary for sacroiliac joint injections? *Pain Physician*. 2003;6:155–158.

SECTION 5

26. Manchikanti M, et al. Evaluation of effectiveness of lumbar interlaminar epidural injections in managing chronic pain of lumbar disc herniation of radiculitis: a randomized double-blind controlled trial. *Pain Physician.* 2010;13:343–355.
27. Ng LC, Sell P. Outcomes of a prospective cohort study on peri-radicular infiltration for radicular pain in patients with lumbar disc herniation and spinal stenosis. *Eur Spine J.* 2004;13(4):325–329.

Appendix 1 CLINICAL CASE HISTORIES – ANSWERS

The primary diagnosis is listed (confirmed by treatment result or by scanning), followed by two possible alternative diagnoses. Consider why these are less likely and how you would treat the primary diagnosis.

UPPER LIMB

1. Acute haemorrhagic subscapularis bursitis
   (acute capsulitis, fractured humerus)
2. Acromioclavicular joint strain
   (subacromial bursitis, fractured coracoid process)
3. Chronic glenohumeral capsulitis
   (subacromial bursitis, referred from C5)
4. Chronic subacromial bursitis
   (glenohumeral capsulitis, referred from C5)
5. C5-6 cervical nerve root entrapment
   (subacromial bursitis, glenohumeral capsulitis)
6. C4 osteosarcoma
   (subacromial bursitis, glenohumeral capsulitis)
7. Elbow extensor tendinitis – tennis elbow
   (wrist extensors, supinator tendinitis)
8. Elbow flexor tendinitis – golfer's elbow
   (wrist flexors, pronator tendinitis)
9. Loose body in elbow joint
   (tennis elbow, osteoarthritis (OA) of elbow joint)
10. Impingement of elbow capsule because of hyperextension
    (loose body, anconeus strain)
11. Fractured head of radius
    (acute capsulitis, infection)
12. Biceps tendon tendinitis
    (biceps belly, supinator tendonitis)
13. Wrist extensor tenosynovitis
    (thumb extensor tendinitis, tennis elbow)
14. Trapeziometacarpal capsulitis
    (metacarpophalangeal joint, gout)
15. Fractured scaphoid
    (Colles' fracture, fractured pisiform)
16. Thumb extensor tendinitis
    (wrist extensor tendinitis, trapeziometacarpal capsulitis)
17. Carpal tunnel syndrome
    (referred from cervical spine, thoracic outlet syndrome)
18. Triangular meniscus tear
    (ulnar collateral ligament strain, flexor tendinitis)

LOWER LIMB

19. Trochanteric bursitis
    (tensor fascia lata fasciitis, referred from lumbar spine)
20. Loose body in hip joint
    (OA hip, referred from lumbar spine)
21. Adductor tendon tear
    (fractured lesser trochanter, pubic symphysis)
22. Juvenile bilateral slipped epiphyses, with gross osteoarthritis
    (sacroiliac joint dysfunction, adductor strain)
23. Psoas bursitis
    (psoas tendinitis, lateral cutaneous nerve entrapment)
24. Avascular necrosis
    (OA hip, osteosarcoma)
25. Medial meniscus tear
    (medial ligament strain, sartorius strain)
26. Medial coronary ligament strain
    (medial meniscus tear, quadriceps insertion strain)
27. Superior tibiofibular joint strain
    (peroneal tendinitis, peroneal nerve entrapment)
28. Quadriceps insertion strain
    (quadriceps muscle strain, referred from L3)
29. Anterior cruciate ligament (ACL) tear
    (torn menisci, fractured patella)
30. Quadriceps belly tear, with adherent calcification
    (quadriceps muscle strain, OA knee joint)
31. Ankle joint capsulitis
    (lateral ligament strain, fractured fibula)
32. Anterior talofibular ligament strain, with bruising of sustentaculum tali
    (calcaneofibular, calcaneocuboid ligament strain)
33. First metatarsophalangeal joint capsulitis
    (hallux valgus, tibialis anterior strain)
34. Deltoid ligament strain
    (flexor digitorum, tibialis posterior strain)
35. Morton's metatarsalgia
    (dorsalis pedis nerve entrapment, referred from L4)
36. Achilles bursitis
    (Achilles tendinitis, plantaris strain)

Appendix 2 PREINJECTION CHECKLIST AND INFORMED CONSENT

Date of Discussion _____ Date of Procedure _____

Name of Patient _____ Name of Clinician _____

CHECKLIST (If "Yes," add details below)

	Yes	No
Systemically unwell (fever, rigors, sweats, malaise)		
Immunosuppressive illness		
Immunosuppressive drugs		
Coagulopathy		
Blood-thinning medication (warfarin, aspirin, novel oral anticoagulant)		
Diabetes		
Psychotic illness		
Prosthetic joint		
Joint replacement surgery pending		
Recent fracture		
Adverse reaction to local anaesthetics		
Infection at injection site		
Pregnant or breastfeeding		

INFORMED CONSENT
Other treatment options and anticipated benefits of injection
Possible injection side effects
Anaphylaxis
Joint, soft tissue infection
Tendon rupture, atrophy
Facial flushing
Temporary impairment of diabetic control
Skin depigmentation, atrophy
Menstrual disturbances
Temporary flare of symptoms
Bruising, bleeding
Other rare side effects (may be relevant to individual patients)

Appendix 3 ORTHOPAEDIC MEDICINE SEMINARS: SAMPLE OF PATIENT INFORMATION SHEET

What drug is used?
Usually two drugs are used:

- Corticosteroid – an anti-inflammatory medication that reduces pain and swelling.
- Local anaesthetic – temporarily numbs the part (for about an hour, as when the dentist injects your tooth). It also helps ensure that the diagnosis is correct, and the drug is placed in the correct area.

How does this differ from tablets?
This drug is administered directly to the cause of the pain so it does not go through your stomach first. The result is that pain is usually relieved more quickly and, because only a very small amount is given, there are fewer side effects.

How quickly does the drug work?
After the initial relief of pain, because of the effect of the local anaesthetic, it usually takes about 2 days for the corticosteroid to kick in, but this does vary. The anti-inflammatory effect of the drug usually lasts about 3 to 6 weeks.

Will I need another injection?
The aim is to relieve your symptoms with one injection, but if the first one only partially helped, or if the inflammation is very severe – as in frozen shoulder, for example – you may need a second one. Injections will not be repeated if they are not helping.

Will the injection hurt?
The clinician giving the injection will have been highly trained in this skill and, on our courses, will have been injected themselves. You may feel a small jab as the injection is given.

Will I be sore after the injection?
Sometimes there is a temporary increase of discomfort after the injection, but most patients report none. You may take your usual painkillers, if necessary.

What do I do after the injection?

- You will be asked to wait a short while to ensure you feel well enough to leave.
- You will also be advised on whether to rest the part afterwards (this is usual when the cause has been overuse) or you may be given an exercise routine to start when the pain has eased to prevent joint stiffness and muscle weakness.

- You should "listen to your body" and avoid any movement or position that increases your pain significantly. Some discomfort on movement can be expected to continue for a while if you have had the pain for a long time.

The injection should not be given if you:

- Are allergic to either drug
- Have an infection in any part of your body
- Are taking antibiotics
- Feel unwell
- Are due to have surgery in the next 3 months

You must tell the clinician if you:

- Have had any allergic reaction to drugs before
- Are taking warfarin or other blood thinners
- Are diabetic
- Have cancer anywhere
- Are taking oral steroids
- Have had a recent fracture
- Are pregnant or breastfeeding

Are there any possible side effects?
Apart from the occasional flushed face, which usually settles quickly, these are **very** rare. Possible mild side effects include the following:

- Sugar levels in the diabetic patient may increase for a short time, so you should check your sugar levels carefully for the first couple of weeks afterwards and report any significant rise to your doctor.
- Periods may become irregular for a short while.
- You may see some bruising around the area.

However, if your injection site becomes hot, red and swollen, and there is considerable increased pain, you must contact your doctor or go to the emergency department at your local hospital,

Allergic reaction to the drug
This is **extremely** rare and, provided you have told the clinician about any previous adverse reactions to drugs, and wait a while after the injection, there is no danger. However, if you start to have difficulty breathing, have swelling around or in your throat or develop a rash, you must go the hospital emergency department immediately.

Appendix 4 FREQUENTLY ASKED QUESTIONS

These are the most common questions asked by allied health professionals (AHPs) on our courses. We hope you find them helpful.

How do I manage with the no mixing of drugs rule for AHPs in the United Kingdom?

There are several ways in which an AHP can continue to mix drugs legally.

NOTE: This information is current (2018) but may be changed in the future.

The AHP should consult with their medical, pharmacological and/or management team to ensure they approve of whatever process is undertaken.

- Inject under a patient-specific directive (PSD).
- Use Lederspan (hexacetonide), 20 mg/ml, which is currently licensed to be mixed with local anaesthetic (LA) in the United Kingdom.
- Use Depo-Medrone (methylprednisolone) premixed with lidocaine by the manufacturer, but it is more difficult to control dosage.
- Inject LA first, change the syringe and inject corticosteroid through same needle, but there is a possible small increased risk of infection.
- Use two needles and two syringes but there is more discomfort for the patient and possibly a small increased risk of infection.
- Do not use LA at all; it is not absolutely necessary, but we recommend its use to make injections less painful especially when treating small tight joints with known difficulty of entry, such as the acromioclavicular joint, thumb or toe joints

What should I do if the top of a glass ampoule doesn't snap off?

Rather than crush the glass into your fingers and bleed everywhere, first check that the coloured dot (the weakest part found on the neck most of these ampoules) is facing you and that you are attempting to snap it off by pushing away from the dot.

If this doesn't work using moderate pressure, wrap protecting tissue around the top, or discard the ampoule and start again with a fresh one.

How do I detach a jammed-on needle from the syringe?

This happens to everyone at some point. The easiest way is to wrap a cotton wool ball or piece of tissue around the needle hub, grip it firmly and twist the syringe in the opposite direction to the way in which you attached it. You may find that it helps to wiggle the syringe while doing this, using a clean thumb nail to help pull it off.

It's best if you don't do this in front of the patient!

How do I prevent the syringe from blasting off the needle?

This also happens to everyone, usually when injecting tendons; it is somewhat embarrassing to have both patient and injector sprayed with white dots of corticosteroid, but it can be avoided.

First, expect there to be some resistance to introducing the solution and ensure the needle is very firmly attached to the syringe. Then, when you come across tough areas of tendon as you pepper around, very slightly reposition needle while gripping needle hub against syringe with your other hand. Attempt to deposit solution there. There is always a part which is less dense, but be aware that if there is no resistance at all you are probably subcutaneous; injecting corticosteroids here can cause fat atrophy and skin depigmentation.

How much do I have to cleanse the skin?

There is little sound evidence about this in the literature; opinions vary, from absolute aseptic conditions (in operating theatre, gowned, masked, gloved and with extensive iodine cleansing) to not bothering to wipe the skin at all.

We recommend the use of an appropriate cleanser using a spiralling movement from the injection point outwards. We do not usually wear gloves unless aspirating (and that is to protect the operator rather than the patient), but this rule varies, so check the policy in your place of work.

What is most important is that your hands are thoroughly cleansed, that the whole process is undertaken smoothly but quickly and that you follow strict nontouch techniques. Always assemble your drugs and equipment carefully and never rush an injection. (see Section 2).

What if the injection doesn't work?

Usually, correctly placed injections are remarkably successful, but in this case always review your diagnosis. First assume that the fault is yours, not the patient's possible failure to follow your aftercare instructions.

- It is possible that the patient had a double lesion, and you could have helped the first, but then exposed the second; this is quite common at the shoulder.
- You might have missed the target although, with the combined use of LA, this should have been obvious at the time.
- It could be that the lesion was not responsive to the drug.
- The patient might, having had complete relief from a painful tennis elbow, have decided to cook a meal for 40 people 3 days later, using heavy cast iron dishes. This has been known to happen!
- After carefully going back to the drawing board, re-examining and discussing the possibilities, you might be allowed to try again. If it fails a second time, you should arrange for a scan and/or get their blood work done and/or refer them to another expert.

How often can the injection be repeated?

The aim is to relieve all symptoms in one injection, but sometimes this does not happen. The questions to ask are as follows:

- Did the first injection help at all?
- Did the patient conform to his or her aftercare advice?
- Is he or she willing to try again? If so, and if you are sure of your diagnosis, it is certainly worth repeating the injection once, but not more if there is still no significant improvement of symptoms.

It can be quite usual to have to repeat the treatment in chronic conditions such as osteoarthritis of the hip or knee. These are, after all, worn-out joints, and the temporary relief of pain is welcomed. We recommend that the repeat injection in these cases be given at about 3-monthly intervals, but this depends on how painful the joint is. These patients may be on a waiting list for surgery, so it is important not to inject as they get near to this date. Some surgeons will not operate even many months after an injection, despite the fact that the drug has normally dissipated after about 6 weeks. Consultation with the surgeon to clarify their stance is essential; no-one wants the joint to become infected.

Acute shoulder capsulitis can also require more than one injection. Patients with severe symptoms should be warned at the first visit that they might need more than one injection. This should be regarded as a possible course of therapy, rather than a one-off treatment, and they should return straight away if the pain starts increasing, rather than wait too long. A reduced dose can be given on each occasion. The insulin-controlled diabetic patient should be warned to monitor their glucose level carefully and regularly.

Some clinicians cheerfully reinject patients with recurring symptoms – 10 or 12 times is not uncommon in difficult cases – but 2 or 3 is the most we would usually perform in any one attack, and only if the patient is getting some relief. Referral for imaging or other investigations should be carried out before continuing to reinject.

What should I do if the patient reports increased pain and swelling a few days after the injection?
Immediately review the patient in person, or ask him or her to go to the local hospital emergency department (see Patient Information, Appendix 3). Joint or soft tissue infections are luckily extremely rare in our experience, but you should always suspect that this could be more than just postinjection flare.

If it is an infection, you need to record the event (in the United Kingdom, this is done on a yellow card) and file this with the appropriate authorities.

Appendix 5 SURVEY OF 2051 CONSECUTIVE MUSCULOSKELETAL INJECTIONS ADMINISTERED IN AN OUTPATIENT SETTING

Total injections (%)	Peripheral injections (%)
Peripheral, 71.7	Upper limb, 72.5
Spinal, 28.2	Lower limb, 27.5

1472 peripheral injections	Number of injections	% of total
Shoulder	735	50
Elbow	261	17
Knee	176	12
Hip	125	9
Foot	103	7
Hand	72	5
Total	1472	100%

Top four peripheral diagnoses	Number of injections	% of area
Tennis elbow	214	81
Subacromial bursitis	546	74
Knee osteoarthritis	117	66
Shoulder capsulitis	141	19
Total	1018	69% of total

Each practice has its own bias towards certain conditions; in this case, nearly one-third of the injections recorded were for spinal lesions, including cervical, thoracic, lumbar (78%), sacroiliac and coccyx. The results show, however, a clear indication of the high percentage of injectable upper limb lesions, of which the shoulder area is invariably the most frequently treated. This information is supported by results from over 2000 clinicians who have attended our courses.

INDEX

Page numbers followed by "*f*" indicate figures, "*t*" indicate tables, and "*b*" indicate boxes.